AF774807

Conceptualizing Personality Disorder

This book offers an interdisciplinary perspective on personality disorder with chapters by philosophers, psychological scientists, and psychiatrists. Written to be accessible to all three disciplines, it updates traditional conceptualizations and offers new and novel perspectives on personality disorder with a special emphasis on borderline and narcissistic personalities. Featuring contributions from established senior researchers as well as early career scholars from across four continents, it offers a survey of contemporary research and clinical expertise that together plumb the foundational understandings of personality disorder.

KONRAD BANICKI is an assistant professor at the Institute of Applied Psychology, Jagiellonian University, Poland. He is a philosopher, psychologist, and cognitive-behavioral therapist as well as a convenor of the Understanding Personality Disorders network associated with St Catherine's College Oxford.

PETER ZACHAR is Professor of Psychology at Auburn University at Montgomery. He is the author of two previous books, *Psychological Concepts and Biological Psychiatry* (2000) and *A Metaphysics of Psychopathology* (2014) and has served as editor or co-editor of seven additional volumes.

Conceptualizing Personality Disorder

Perspectives from Philosophy, Psychological Science, and Psychiatry

Edited by

Konrad Banicki

Jagiellonian University

Peter Zachar

Auburn University at Montgomery

CAMBRIDGE
UNIVERSITY PRESS

CAMBRIDGE
UNIVERSITY PRESS

Shaftesbury Road, Cambridge CB2 8EA, United Kingdom

One Liberty Plaza, 20th Floor, New York, NY 10006, USA

477 Williamstown Road, Port Melbourne, VIC 3207, Australia

314–321, 3rd Floor, Plot 3, Splendor Forum, Jasola District Centre, New Delhi – 110025, India

103 Penang Road, #05–06/07, Visioncrest Commercial, Singapore 238467

Cambridge University Press is part of Cambridge University Press & Assessment, a department of the University of Cambridge.

We share the University's mission to contribute to society through the pursuit of education, learning and research at the highest international levels of excellence.

www.cambridge.org
Information on this title: www.cambridge.org/9781009445979

DOI: 10.1017/9781009445955

© Cambridge University Press & Assessment 2025

This publication is in copyright. Subject to statutory exception and to the provisions of relevant collective licensing agreements, no reproduction of any part may take place without the written permission of Cambridge University Press & Assessment.

When citing this work, please include a reference to the DOI 10.1017/9781009445955

First published 2025

A catalogue record for this publication is available from the British Library

A Cataloging-in-Publication data record for this book is available from the Library of Congress

ISBN 978-1-009-44597-9 Hardback

Cambridge University Press & Assessment has no responsibility for the persistence or accuracy of URLs for external or third-party internet websites referred to in this publication and does not guarantee that any content on such websites is, or will remain, accurate or appropriate.

Contents

Figures

Tables

Contributors

KONRAD BANICKI, Jagiellonian University, Poland

SIMON BOAG, University of Sydney, Australia

NINA S. DE BOER, Radboud University, The Netherlands

DENNY BORSBOOM, University of Amsterdam, The Netherlands

LÉON DE BRUIN, Radboud University, The Netherlands

MARTIN BRÜNE, Ruhr University, Germany

SIMONE CHELI, St. John's University, Italy; and Tages Charity, Italy

ANGÉLIQUE O. J. CRAMER, Amsterdam University Medical Center and University of Amsterdam, The Netherlands

COLIN G. DEYOUNG, University of Minnesota, Minneapolis, USA

ROY DINGS, Radboud University, The Netherlands

SUSI FERRARELLO, California State University – East Bay, Hayward, USA

THOMAS FUCHS, University of Heidelberg, Germany

GRANT GILLETT, University of Otago, New Zealand

GERRIT GLAS, Vrije University, The Netherlands

HUW GREEN, Addenbrooke's Hospital, Cambridge, UK

ADELA-MARIA ISVORANU, National University of Singapore, Singapore

STEFAN JEROTIC, University of Belgrade, Serbia; and University Clinical Centre of Serbia, Serbia

ANNEMARIE C. J. KÖHNE, University Medical Center Utrecht, The Netherlands; and GGZ Noord-Holland-Noord, The Netherlands

MILUTIN KOSTIC, University of Belgrade, Serbia; and Institute of Mental Health, Serbia

ROBERT F. KRUEGER, University of Minnesota, Minneapolis, USA

GARSON LEDER, Medical College of Wisconsin, Milwaukee, USA

KASPER LIPPERT-RASMUSSEN, Aarhus University, Denmark

MARCIN MOSKALEWICZ, Poznan University of Medical Sciences, Poland; Marie Curie-Skłodowska University, Poland; and IDEAS NCBR, Warsaw, Poland

SIENNA R. NIELSEN, University of Michigan, Ann Arbor, USA

ASTRID FLY OREDSSON, Independent, Denmark

NANCY NYQUIST POTTER, University of Louisville, Louisville, USA

JEANNE PROUST, University of California – Santa Cruz, Santa Cruz, USA

EISUKE SAKAKIBARA, The University of Tokyo, Japan

PHILIPP SCHMIDT-BODDY, University of Heidelberg, Germany

THOMAS SCHRAMME, University of Liverpool, Liverpool, UK

ANNA STERNA, Poznań University of Medical Sciences, Poland

ARMON J. TAMATEA, University of Waikato, New Zealand

MARK H. WAUGH, University of Tennessee, Knoxville, USA

LOUISE WILLIAMS, Empowerment Through Thought LLC, South Bend, USA

AIDAN G. C. WRIGHT, University of Michigan, Ann Arbor, USA

PETER ZACHAR, Auburn University at Montgomery, Montgomery, USA

TADEUSZ ZAWIDZKI, George Washington University, Washington DC, USA

Introduction

Personality Disorder and the Philosophy of Psychopathology

Peter Zachar and Konrad Banicki

Within the increasingly vast literature in the philosophy of psychopathology (a subset of the philosophy of psychiatry), little attention has been paid to personality disorder. This is somewhat surprising given that personality disorder has become one of the most conceptually contentious topics in clinical psychology and psychiatry (Kotov et al., 2017; Krueger et al., 2018). With this in mind, to encourage and support more interdisciplinary work on personality disorder, in 2019 Konrad Banicki established the Understanding Personality Disorders Network (as part of the Collaborating Centre for Values-based Practice in Health and Social Care: https://valuesbasedpractice.org/), invited members, and began a series of events and, with this book, publications.

The initial idea for the book was to potentially alter the scholarly landscape by encouraging more philosophers to tackle the complicated issue of personality disorder. A second important goal was to demonstrate to psychologists and psychiatrists the relevance of some philosophical theories and perspectives for conceptualizing personality disorder. Psychology and psychiatry books often address conceptual and historical issues for personality disorder, but less typically explicitly philosophical ones.

Our initial group of chapters were selected from responses we received after issuing a call for papers, and these were further augmented by asking additional colleagues to consider contributing a chapter. Some of the proposed chapters were about personality disorder in general and others were about one or more personality disorder types. As our ideas evolved, we also gravitated toward chapters that offer new and novel approaches to conceptualizing personality disorder.

As the writing commenced, we asked authors to be mindful of the ongoing transition to dimensional models. Dimensional models describe personality pathology using profiles of continuous traits on which every person in a population has a standing such as "neuroticism" and "impulsivity." One impetus for the transition to dimensional models was the discovery of unexpected comorbidity between different personality types such as borderline, histrionic, and narcissistic. This comorbidity calls into question the notion that these personality disorders are distinct categories. Many psychologists in particular consider well-known categories of personality to be scientifically invalid (Kotov et al., 2017).

One barrier to transitioning to dimensional models is that certain diagnostic categories have become a part of everyday psychology and cannot just be plucked out and eliminated from our language. An example of an entrenched everyday concept would be air. Although air is no longer considered an element in current scientific theory, it is still an understandable notion in the English language, especially in words like airplane and air conditioner. Depression is potentially like air in that sense. Even when someone claims we should not be talking about and studying depression, they often continue to refer to depression.

Although borderline personality disorder and narcissistic personality disorder are not as deeply entrenched in everyday psychology as depression, they have both everyday psychological and professional senses. Indeed, the *Diagnostic and statistical manual of mental disorders*, 5th edition (DSM-5)'s initial proposal to eliminate narcissistic personality disorder and the *International classification of diseases*, 11th revision (ICD-11)'s initial proposal to eliminate borderline personality disorder met with intense opposition (Campbell & Miller, 2011; Watts, 2019). These concepts are of historical importance for the concept of personality disorder; for many professionals they are part of their default conceptual schemata, and for dimensional models, borderline and narcissistic features are used to define the nature of personality disorder (Waugh, chapter 4). With these considerations in mind, if people were not writing about personality disorder in general, we asked that they focus on the borderline or the narcissistic patterns.

The book is divided into five sections. The first section includes three chapters with a historical focus. The first chapter examines how, after the concept of personality was popularized in the early twentieth century, personality disorder transitioned from being a feature of psychopathology in general to being an independent domain in psychopathology (Zachar). There is a chapter on Ribot's ground-breaking work on the importance of indecisiveness to personality and psychopathology. Ribot's ideas have been lost in history but can be seen as precursors to current interests in transdiagnostic concepts (Proust). A chapter rooted in Mischel's interactionist criticism of personality trait theory argues that maladaptive personality traits must be rooted in behavioral consistency across situations, which increases the risk of over-diagnosis. From this perspective, some dimensional personality disorder constructs such as negative emotionality and detachment may be too broad to be clinically informative (Sakakibara).

The second section includes a series of chapters describing contemporary approaches to traditional conceptual perspectives on personality disorder. There are chapters on psychodynamic (Waugh), systems theory (Cramer and

Borsboom), interpersonal (Wright and Nielsen), phenomenological (Sterna, Moskalewicz, Schmidt-Boddy, and Fuchs), pharmacological (Jerotic and Kostic), and evolutionary (Cheli and Brüne) approaches.

The third section includes chapters that address the call for novel conceptual approaches to personality disorder. These include a chapter on a cybernetic perspective, which argues that psychopathology understood as a persistent failure to move toward one's goals is inseparable from personality (DeYoung and Krueger). One chapter explores the ambiguity regarding whether a personality disorder reflects who someone is or rather reflects an imposed affliction – which may be particularly complex with personality disorder if one disidentifies with maladaptive traits (Dings, de Boer, de Buin, and Glas). A chapter calling into question the view that personality traits are causes of behavior casts doubt on scientific realism about the five-factor model and offers an alternative causal account grounded in motivation (Boag). A chapter advocating for a dual-aspect approach to personality disorder views personality pathology as in a dialectical relationship between disorders as residing in an individual versus disorders as constituted by external, social, and culture contexts (Green). A chapter rejecting an essentialist, common-cause model of comorbidity in the realm of personality disorder offers instead a relational, causally connected systems view from the perspective of network theory (Köhne and Isvoranu).

The next chapter in section three explores approaches that have recognizable spiritual or religious underpinnings. In particular, the ontological model of the Christian theologian Paul Tillich is discussed in terms of its dialectic character and the how dialectics can be applied to elucidate personality pathology. This framework is then compared with Marsha Linehan's dialectical behavior therapy rooted in Zen Buddhism and Thomas Lynch's radically open dialectical behavior therapy founded on Malâmati Sufism (Banicki). The last chapter in this section addresses the debate about whether cluster B personality disorders are actual disorders or are morally disvalued problems-in-living, showing that whether any action is one or the other depends on whether it results from a failure to self-regulate (Leder and Zawidzki).

The fourth section explores potential harmful consequences and misuses of personality disorder concepts. The first chapter in this section argues that the diagnosis of aversive and antagonistic personality disorder among indigenous people typically fails to take into account the importance of displacement in post-colonial worlds (Gillett and Tamatea). The second chapter in this section shows how injustifiably dismissing as inappropriate the anger associated with borderline personality disorder is a form of affective injustice that potentially undermines people's moral agency (Ordesson and Lippert-Ramussen).

The fifth section presents different approaches to conceptualizing borderline and narcissistic features. Feelings of emptiness can be excruciating and seem quite intractable, yet this criterion of borderline personality disorder is far less examined. The first chapter in this section argues that emptiness is not a distinct concept and, furthermore, is not specific to borderline personality disorder or, indeed, to people who are diagnosed with psychiatric disorders. Following Linehan's treatment model, the chapter argues that, albeit the concept of emptiness is distinct from its western concept, Buddhist meditation can, for some people struggling with feelings of emptiness, be a pathway toward healing (Potter).

The next chapter in section five examines empathy deficits in narcissistic personality disorder. Empathy – a complex phenomenon – is interpreted as a set of mechanisms that enable humans to understand others. Narcissistic personality disorder is construed as the result of persistent doubt about other people's perspectives and about one's own social standing. This is referred to as status blindness (Schramme). A chapter that combines both phenomenology and the perspective of philosophical counseling argues that narcissistic personality is a disorder of intentionality related to being disconnected from and out of resonance with one's interaffective community and thus with oneself (Ferrarello). The last chapter in this section offers a narrative account of pathological forms of narcissism. It argues that rather than seeking accurate self-understanding, narcissistic individuals curate a self-story that is constructed to ease their insecurities and then try to compel others to affirm that curated story (Williams).

References

Campbell, W. K., & Miller, J. D. (eds.). (2011). *The handbook of narcissism and narcissistic personality disorder*. The Guilford Press.

Kotov, R., Krueger, R. F., Watson, D., Achenbach, T. M., Althoff, R. R., Bagby, R. M., . . . Zimmerman, M. (2017). The hierarchical taxonomy of psychopathology (HiTOP): A dimensional alternative to traditional nosologies. *Journal of Abnormal Psychology, 126*(4), 454–477.

Krueger, R. F., Kotov, R., Watson, D., Forbes, M. K., Eaton, N. R., Ruggero, C. J., . . . Zimmermann, J. (2018). Progress in achieving quantitative classification of psychopathology. *World Psychiatry, 17*(3), 282–293. doi:10.1002/wps.20566

Watts, J. (2019). Problems with the ICD-11 classification of personality disorder. *The Lancet Psychiatry, 6*(6), 461–463. https://doi.org/10.1016/S2215-0366(19)30127-0

Part I

Historical Perspectives

1 How Personality Disorder Became an Independent Domain in Psychopathology

A History

Peter Zachar

1.1 From Psychopathology to Normal Personality

It would not be surprising for someone to claim that *certainly, people have personalities but asserting that a personality can be disordered is taking it too far.* To claim that the notion of personality pathology is medicalizing a normal psychological process, however, may be putting the cart before the horse. In a historical irony, the contemporary concept of personality was introduced in the nineteenth century to make sense of some puzzling psychiatric phenomena.

Lombardo and Foschi (2002, 2003) emphasize the origins of "personality" in abnormal psychology, pointing to Théodule Ribot, the founder of experimental psychology in France. Ribot claimed that clinical phenomena are akin to natural experiments that can be used to understand the components of normal psychology. The clinical phenomena that were most important at this time were dissociation and what was called the doubling of consciousness. An example of doubling would be the case of Félida – a woman who was usually sad, emotionally unstable, and beset with multiple physical ailments, but would switch to another state in which she was extroverted and happy – and there was no continuity of memory between those distinct states of personhood (Hacking, 1995). In *Diseases of the personality*, Ribot (1885) claimed that in normal psychology there is a coordination of intellectual, affective, and physical features that can break down in illness – and named the normal coordination of psychological features "personality."

Another contributor to the French tradition was the psychologist and physician Pierre Janet. For much of the nineteenth century, discussions of individuality, personhood, and continuity over time were framed using a metaphysical notion of the self. The metaphysical self is akin to an enduring essence that makes someone who they are and is known through introspection. Janet did not consider introspection a reliable way to study the self. Inspired by the work of the neurologist John Hughlings Jackson and Ribot, Janet argued that "the pathological method" (i.e., observations of individual clinical phenomena) pointed the way to developing an empirically based psychology rather than a metaphysical one (Berrios, 1996; Lombardo & Foschi, 2003).

Due to his extensive travels throughout Europe, William James was familiar with French ideas and promulgated them in the United States. For instance, Perry (1935) reports that James, referring to Janet, claimed that the study of psychopathology, especially dissociation, is worth more than all exact laboratory measurements put together. Indeed, James taught four classes on psychopathology in the 1890s, based in part on the idea that the best way to understand the normal is to study the abnormal (Richardson, 2006).

In *The principles of psychology*, James (1890) described hysterical phenomena, including a lack of feeling in one part of the body and blindness for part of the visual field. Rather than inferring that these phenomena represent a lack of conscious experience (tactile or visual), James said consciousness was split into parts that mutually ignore each other. According to James, even though the primary consciousness may have no awareness of feeling in the affected part of the body, the secondary consciousness does. He also used primary and secondary *self*, primary and secondary *personage*, and primary and secondary *personality* to describe these phenomena.

The psychiatrist Morton Prince also played a role in promulgating the concept of personality. Roback (1940) describes Prince as a Francophile who, like James, was familiar with the work of Janet and his advocacy for the clinical, case-study approach. Prince's 1906 book, *The dissociation of personality*, according to Henry Murray (1956), created a sensation wherever English was read.

Most assuredly, people recognized personality traits long before the twentieth century. Character types were present in the Greek tragedies and the characters of Theophrastus, in books such as the *Canterbury tales*, and the plays of Shakespeare. What seems to be different with the fin-de-siècle notion of personality is a shift in emphasis in which individuality takes center stage.

A relatively new feature of early twentieth-century American life was the growth of mass media. Various self-help books and self-improvement manuals associated with the mental hygiene movement promulgated the importance of personality in the 1910s. With advancements in photographic, radio, and film media, celebrity itself increasingly became associated with the larger-than-life "personality" (Grout, 2019).

This notion of personality became a trendy folk psychological concept (Barenbaum & Winter, 2003; Nicholson, 2003). In the new popular lexicon: everyone has a personality; it represents what they are like as an individual; and it is something they need to actively develop. For example, in *The Great Gatsby*:

Mrs. Wilson ... was now attired in an elaborate afternoon dress of cream-colored chiffon ... With the influence of the dress her personality had also undergone a change. The intense vitality that had been so remarkable in the garage was converted into an impressive hauteur. (Fitzgerald, 1925, pp. 30–31)

Or in *Arrowsmith*:

Knowledge is the greatest thing in the medical world but it's no good whatever unless you can sell it, and to do this you must first impress your personality on the people who have the dollars. (Lewis, 1925, p. 87)

In contrast, in 1896's *The red badge of courage*, we find:

He felt that something of which he was a part – a regiment, an army, a cause, or a country – was in crisis. He was welded into a common personality which was dominated by a single desire. For some moments he could not flee no more than a little finger can commit a revolution from a hand. (Crane, 1896, p. 56)

The incorporation of personality into the American cultural landscape raises the interesting issue of the relationship between folk psychological and scientific psychological concepts. Every new student brings their folk psychological understanding to their initial exposure to scientific psychology. Hopefully the exposure to scientific psychology alters some folk concepts, but newly emerging folk concepts can also be assimilated into psychology.

By the 1920s, the younger generation of Americans would think about themselves and others as having "personalities" and bring this perspective to psychology. Indeed, the time was ripe for a science of personality. As students in the history of psychology learn, in the late nineteenth and early twentieth century, psychology was a specialization within philosophy (i.e., experimental philosophy). When the United States entered World War I in 1917, psychologists believed that they could use their skills in intelligence testing to assign recruits to appropriate positions in the military and convinced the leaders of the military to fund such an effort. Greenwood (2015) reports that ultimately the military did not see the mass testing as useful, but after the war there occurred a perceptual shift in the public's opinion of psychology. It was newly seen as a scientific discipline that could produce practically useful knowledge.

This shift in perception resulted in large increases in economic support available for psychological research. To further increase the scope and utility of testing, psychologists began assessing nonintellectual traits. Given the great popularity of personality in the larger culture, personality traits were a natural choice. The psychologists also contrasted their preferred psychometric approach with the clinical–pathological approach of physicians such as Prince (Danziger, 1990).

Nicholson (1998) reports that in the 1920s when psychologists began offering personality courses, "personality" was seen as a value-neutral term that was more appropriate for an empirical science than the value-laden term of "character." In retrospect, this is at least a little strange, because personhood was also an unambiguously moral concept. Both Locke and Kant used "personality" as a synonym for "personhood." In any case, the measurement of personality (broadly construed) came to be seen as a distinguishing feature of psychology as a field. As stated by Roback (1933, pp. 214–215):

> That personality tests . . . would follow close upon the heels of the intelligence tests was after all to be expected, but could anyone have predicted . . . the avalanche which bids to sweep away from the foreground nearly all interest in American psychology, to the exclusion of personality measurement?

1.2 From Psychopathology to Personality Disorder

Doubtlessly, some readers have noticed that dissociation and split personality are not what is usually meant by personality disorder. The history just recounted describes the beginnings of a bifurcation between the clinical–pathological and the psychometric approaches to studying personality and psychopathology, but not the genesis of the contemporary concept of personality disorder.

In writing histories of personality disorder, many thinkers have looked back to Prichard's (1835/1963) concept of moral insanity, construing it as an early version of psychopathic–antisocial personality. Moral insanity played an important role in the history of personality disorder, but not in the way it is often discussed. Rather than psychopathic–antisocial personality disorder, moral insanity referred to insanity with an absence of delusions. Its symptoms included excitement or dejection, impulsivity and anger. According to Prichard, moral insanity was his preferred term for Pinel's *manie sans délire* (of 1801) and Esquirol's monomania (of 1810). The main idea behind each was that insanity can occur in people with intact intellects and adequate reality testing – thus expanding the scope of nineteenth-century psychiatry to include more than institutionalized patients.

Horwitz (2023) argues that the first "personality disorder" was Koch's concept of psychopathic inferiority, introduced in 1891. Psychopathic inferiority includes traits such as high-strung, capricious, rigid, and grandiose (Schneider, 1950/1958). It also has a significant blemish, because it was partly formulated in the context of degeneration theory. What was degeneration theory? Under the influence of the scientifically mistaken view that evolution aims at the development of more complex and advanced life-forms, in the latter part of the nineteenth century some thinkers inferred that the process could go the other way – a devolution to a more primitive, less-advanced form. This process, called degeneration, supposedly ran in families, with each subsequent generation being increasingly degraded, eventually culminating in the extinction of that family line. People with violent and aggressive personalities were readily considered to be degenerates.

Koch proposed three broad groups of psychopathic inferiorities, only one of which was tied to degeneration theory (Schneider, 1950/1958). Even so, in later years those who emphasized the biological and genetic determination of personality pathology seemed to prefer the term constitutional psychopathic inferiority.

It is important to note that the distinction between personality pathology and other forms of psychopathology was wobbly well into the twentieth century. Among the "types" identified by various thinkers were neurasthenic, hysteric, hypochondriacal, depressive, and manic personalities. A loose distinction between personality pathology and other forms of psychopathology is nicely illustrated by the Minnesota Multiphasic Personality Inventory (MMPI), which was developed in the early 1940s. Hysteria and psychopathic deviate were part of this personality inventory, but so was hypochondriasis, depression, schizophrenia, and mania (Hathaway & McKinley, 1940). To this day, moderately elevated MMPI-2 scores are given personality-trait interpretations. For example, a moderate score on hypochondriasis indicates being a complainer; on schizophrenia it indicates being alienated and withdrawn.

1.3 "Psychopathic" Personality

The concept of psychopathic personality is closely associated with Kurt Schneider (1950/1958), who in 1923 published a book titled *Psychopathic personalities*. Psychopathic was used broadly to mean "psychopathological." Those with psychopathic personalities were also called psychopaths. An English translation of the ninth edition of Schneider's book was published in 1958. In that edition he described 10 distinct types. Examples include the fanatic, depressive, and attention-seeking psychopaths.

Schneider was a German psychiatrist who publicly opposed Nazi eugenics and its advocacy for degeneration theory, stating that the concept of degeneration is worth mentioning for historical purposes only. He believed that pathological personality was rooted in one's innate dispositions and constitution, and claimed that dispositions are not morbid organic processes in the sense of physical disease or illness but just variations, nothing else.

He also made a distinction between personality pathology and neurosis. For personality pathology the concern is with what the person is like, for neurosis the concern is how experience has altered typical functioning. Unlike Kraepelin and Kretchmer, Schneider did not believe that psychopathic personalities were milder versions of serious mental illnesses such as schizophrenia. He accepted that there are recognizable premorbid personalities associated with schizophrenia and that psychosis is initially molded by the personality of the patient, but he rejected the notion of gradual transitions from one to another.

According to Schneider, when you call someone a fanatic psychopath rather than making a diagnostic claim about the essential features of the patient's personality, what one is doing is declaring that they are a person *of that sort*. Another way to put it is that one is saying *that is what they are like*. Fanatic psychopath is a general term for a group of people who are similar in clinically relevant ways but each individual is unique and cannot be reduced to a label. In this, Schneider anticipated the nonessentialist concepts used in prototype and exemplar models.

Rather than viewing psychopathic personalities as based on underlying dysfunctions, Schneider said that they were composed of variations in personal qualities that deviated from the average – either an excess or deficit relative to the norm. In Schneider's view, when people suffer or they make others suffer because of these personal qualities, the personality can be considered psychopathic. Rather than using a theory of normal personality as a systematic framework for understanding abnormal personality (e.g., extremely high and low extroversion are both abnormal), Schneider (1959) argued that abnormal personality is an unsystematic collection of traits that have been found to be clinically important:

> Descriptive labels . . . can only be given to a circumscribed set of personal qualities that have attained importance because they have been thought important (p. 29).

An example of a contrasting, systematic approach is Millon's (1986) theoretical model, which he claimed could be used to deduce what personality disorders should be in the classification system.

Another influential thinker who distinguished between psychopathic personality and other kinds of psychopathology was Hervey Cleckley (1950). In Cleckley's view, psychopathic personality is distinct from the normal irrationality of those who hold beliefs that are not supported by evidence and considered by many as unreasonable, such as giving away your possessions because you are convinced that the rapture is going to occur next week. Psychopathic personality, said Cleckley, is also distinct from psychoneurotic disorders, from the early manifestations of serious mental illness, and from florid psychosis. He further noted that many different personality types have been classified as psychopathic, but his interest was in a single clinical entity involving features such as superficial charm, lack of anxiety or remorse, and failure to learn from experience (all of which correspond to our current notion of psychopathic personality). Cleckley did not, however, demarcate personality disorder as an independent domain in psychopathology:

Personality disorder, a broader term, by-passes or side-steps many archaic assumptions, and into it as a concept fit both "nervous" and "mental" illness with minimum unnecessary confusion . . . All psychiatric illness, everyone will probably agree, can sensibly and accurately be called personality disorder. (p. 419)

In a similar vein, Horwitz (2023) suggests that the initial work on personality pathology in psychoanalysis did not segregate personality from other kinds of psychiatric problems. Freud's (1921/1960) structural theory (id, ego, superego) transformed his ideas about psychic conflict into a theory of personality. Later, character structure or character neurosis was seen as a version of neurosis that was resistant to change (Alexander, 1935/1949; Reich, 1949).

1.4 Personality Disorder in the Early DSMs[1]

In World War II, military physicians were confronted with large numbers of draftees who developed psychiatric problems in response to the stresses of the war. Most of these problems did not fit the psychiatric categories used for classifying institutionalized patients. Dealing with those who were not severely ill but at risk called attention to personality disturbances (Grob, 1991). In the classification developed to help military physicians deal with these new problems, called Medical 203, pathological personality types were conceptualized as manifesting in actions or behaviors, rather than symptoms of distress and anxiety (U.S. War Department, 1946).

The DSM-I, published in 1950, also conceptualized personality disorders as manifesting in behavioral reactions, not symptoms. It also simplified psychiatric classification by separating disorders of psychogenic origin into only three groups: psychosis, psychoneurotic disorders, and personality disorders.[2] However, alcohol and drug dependence, sexual deviations, enuresis, and gross stress reaction (an early version of post-traumatic stress disorder) were all classified under personality disorders. Furthermore, both psychotic and psychoneurotic disorders were described as representing how the personality struggles to adjust to stress.

In the DSM-II of 1968 sexual deviations, alcohol and drug dependence, and adjustment disorders were no longer listed as personality disorders. Some new personality disorders were added, including hysterical, asthenic, and explosive personalities. Although Medical 203 and the DSM-I noted that personality

[1] Although Schneider's views are usually described in histories of personality disorder, I have not found any evidence indicating that he had a direct influence on the DSM notion of personality disorder. Schneider's views are, however, recognizable in a glossary prepared by the World Health Organization and later added to the ICD-8 (Shepherd & Sartorius, 1974).

[2] Medical 203 placed personality disorder types in a category called character and behavior disorders.

disorders manifest in lifelong patterns of behavior, the DSM-II was more specific, stating that these patterns are often recognized by adolescence.

1.5 From the Borderlands to Borderline Personality

As noted, *manie sans délire*, monomania, and moral insanity expanded the scope of nineteenth-century psychiatry to encompass a broad range of conditions, some closer to normality than what we would now call psychosis. Psychiatrists referred to the transition zone between normal and abnormal as the borderlands of insanity (Clouston, 1892; Wynter, 1875).

In the middle part of the twentieth century, psychoanalysts began writing about patients who were not psychotic and looked like good therapy candidates, but rather than getting better with therapy they seemed to get worse. Among the names used to designate this group were the borderline group of neuroses (Stern, 1938) and pseudoneurotic schizophrenia (Hoch & Polatin, 1949). Pseudoneurotic meant appeared to be neurotic but was not.

At the beginning of the twentieth century, Kraepelin (1907) noted that personality pathology resides on the borderland between pronounced morbid states and personal eccentricities. The psychoanalyst's untreatable but not psychotic group of patients, however, were not conceptualized as being in the borderland between sanity and insanity but in the borderland between neurosis and psychosis (Knight, 1953). This borderland was placed in the realm of personality disorder. In the late 1960s and early 1970s the preferred concept became borderline personality. Some thinkers used borderline personality to denote the entire zone between neurosis and psychosis (Grinker Sr. et al., 1968; Kernberg, 1967) and others used it to denote a specific type of personality disorder in that zone (Gunderson & Singer, 1975; Masterson, 1971).

The borderline personality concept became clinically important because its proponents believed that rather than being untreatable, these conditions are treatable with a proper understanding of the nature of the psychopathology. For example, one way some clinicians think about people with borderline personality disorder is that they find it difficult to modulate negative emotions, which interferes with the establishment of a stable identity and cohesive sense of self. This can manifest in chaotic and unstable interpersonal relationship, particular kinds of maladaptive coping styles, and frequent crises. The focus of treatment is not on gaining insight into unconscious conflict but on becoming more integrated.

1.6 The DSM-III Makes Personality Pathology More Independent

The most important development in making personality disorders more independent in psychopathology was the publication of the DSM-III in 1980.

Although personality disorders were in a separate section in previous ICDs and DSMs and the DSM-II stated that personality disorders differ in quality from psychotic and neurotic symptoms, two developments in particular thrust personality disorder into a more independent foreground. First, personality disorders were segregated from disorders such as schizophrenia and depression. Schizophrenia and depression were placed on axis I and personality disorders on axis II. Placing personality disorders on axis II encouraged mental health professionals to evaluate every patient for the potential presence of a personality disorder even if they clearly had a primary diagnosis of an axis I disorder. Prior to this development, personality pathology would have been considered part of the background for most psychiatric problems (in psychodynamic models) or have often been overshadowed by a primary symptom disorder.

Second, some personality disorders that had been considered attenuated forms of axis I symptom disorders were reconceptualized as clinical syndromes and moved to axis I, which eliminated some of the overlap between personality pathology and the rest of psychopathology. For instance, what some thinkers called depressive personality disorder became dysthymia and cyclothymic personality disorder became cyclothymia. Arguably, the symptomatic features of asthenic personality disorder, anxiety neurosis, and neurasthenia were reshuffled to become generalized anxiety disorder and panic disorder.

In the period between the publication of the DSM-III in 1980 and the DSM-IV in 1994, personality disorders were increasingly recognized as important. One feature of this history that is well known is that the addition of borderline and narcissistic personality disorder in the DSM-III provided a large boost to psychodynamic clinicians during a period in which there was a paradigm shift from psychodynamic to biomedical psychiatry. Decker (2013) indicates that Robert Spitzer, the leader of the DSM-III revision, insisted on including a borderline personality diagnosis in the DSM-III and spent more time on what that disorder would look like than he did on all other personality disorders combined.

With some exceptions (such as the psychologist Theodore Millon) researchers were skeptical of personality disorders. For example, Decker (2013) reports that during the development of the DSM-III Aaron Beck told Spitzer that personality disorders were artificial, lacking in utility, and misleading fictions. The skeptics' wariness was especially directed at borderline personality disorder. This view is consistent with a popular perspective that personality disorder was a wastebasket category (Lewis, 1974).

This opposition of researchers to the borderline concept seems short lived. Between 1970 and 1979, APA PsycINFO and Medline list three articles with borderline personality disorder in the title. In the next decade that climbs to 485 articles and in the decade after that, 1,523 articles. In her influential book on cognitive-behavioral therapy for borderline personality disorder, Marsha Linehan (1993) reported that 11 percent of outpatients and 19 percent of inpatients meet criteria for borderline personality disorder. Even Beck himself published a book on cognitive therapy for personality disorders, including borderline personality disorder (Beck & Freeman, 1990).

1.7 Bringing It Full Circle – The Re-Assertion of Psychometrics

According to Allen Frances (A. Frances, personal communication, October 30, 2023), he was tasked with writing a portion of the introduction to DSM-III, including the section on the limits of diagnostic categories. According to that section, the DSM does not assume that there are sharp boundaries between normal and abnormal or between different disorders. Continuity between the normal and the abnormal is closely associated with dimensional models, which view the difference between the two to be quantitative rather than qualitative.

Frances told me that his thinking about the advantages of dimensions over categories was shaped by his reading of Robert Kendell's (1975) book *The role of diagnosis in psychiatry* and his own clinical experience. Kendell himself was influenced by a debate about hypertension in the late 1950s where one side argued that hypertension is a specific disease entity and the other (successfully) argued it represents a graded quantitative, not a categorical qualitative deviation from the norm – with no fixed separation between normal and abnormal (Oldham et al., 1960).

The view that personality disorders in particular are better suited for dimensional approaches became a running theme across future revisions and subtly set personality disorders apart from the rest of psychopathology in a different way. Interestingly, the resulting categorical versus dimensional debate has more than a passing resemblance to the bifurcation between the clinical–pathological and psychometric perspectives that emerged in the study of personality in the early twentieth century.

To contextualize this, let us examine a 1947 article by Karl Menninger (1947). Prior to World War II, psychiatry was a minor specialty within medicine, mostly concerned with the administration of mental hospitals, and clinical psychology was not an official specialization (Houts, 2000). Menninger oversaw the previously mentioned expansion of psychiatric services during the war, including the involvement of psychologists. Once the war ended, he clearly saw that this expansion was going to continue and believed that psychiatrists, psychologists, and clinical social workers should all be a part of it. According to Menninger, medical-psychiatric thinking should emphasize the study of personality for which psychology is a basic science. In his view, what psychologists could bring to this cooperative effort is training in psychometrics and objective measurement. In fact, even today, for many psychologists, training in psychometrics, measurement, and testing is a professional identity issue, one that sets them apart from psychiatry and other mental-health professionals.

Menninger was cautious, noting that psychologists are not accustomed enough to clinical settings to assert themselves and that psychiatrists would be inclined to enforce guild interests and keep psychologists out. Other than in a few places, such as the Menninger Clinic and the Austen Riggs Center, this seems to be what happened. For instance, focusing specifically on personality disorder, Aubrey Lewis (1974) claimed that it is surprising that psychiatrists have not paid attention to the concepts of the psychologists.

In a historically interesting chapter written just after the publication of the DSM-III, Klerman (1986) wrote that the development of ratings scales by thinkers such as Hamilton and Beck brought renewed attention to quantification and measurement in psychiatry. Furthermore, Klerman reports that in the 1960s psychologists interested in multivariate statistics, such as Hans Eysenck, criticized the use of diagnostic categories that implied sharp boundaries between the normal and the abnormal. For example, Eysenck (1986), typically contrarian, wrote a blistering derogation of the DSM-III, stating: “It is clearly necessary to throw out the whole approach, hook, line and sinker, before anything better can take its place” (p. 96). He suggested that what psychiatry needed was a Kuhnian revolution that would adopt an experimental and psychometric approach. Other thinkers who advocated for the use of multivariate statistics and dimensionality were less antagonistic and inclined to also acknowledge the benefits of categories and the limitations of multivariate statistics (Frances, 1982; Kendell, 1975; Lorr, 1986).

Just before and during the DSM-IV revision, more claims about the relevance of dimensional models for personality began to appear (Costa & McCrae, 1990; Frances & Widiger, 1986; Livesley, 1987). Frances, who led the DSM-IV revision, told me that he initially tried to get a consensus dimensional model for personality disorders in DSM-IV appendix, but there were too many competing models. The DSM-IV was importantly transitional because evidence in the form of measurement statistics was used to make incremental modifications to the diagnostic criteria, but the focus was not psychometric (Widiger et al., 1996).

After the DSM-IV was published, Jackson and Livesley (1995) suggested that the construct validation framework used in the development of psychological tests should be systematically applied to the development of diagnostic criterion sets. A similar argument had been made earlier by Skinner (1986) and Millon had put it into practice with the development of the *Millon Clinical Multiaxial Inventory* in the early 1980s (Millon, 1985). Later, Blashfield and Livesly (1991) noted that diagnostic criteria sets can be viewed as being like psychological tests. In an important respect, these works represented a call to arms for future research, which was answered by many people over the next few years.

In between the publication of the DSM-IV in 1994 and the beginning of the DSM-5 revision in 2008, psychologists actively asserted themselves in the way Menninger had earlier believed they could not. In part, this occurred in parallel with factor-analytic methods becoming a dominant statistic used in clinical psychology.

In the early 1970s doubt was cast upon the scientific validity of personality traits (Sakaibara, 2025). This trend was reversed with the introduction of the five-factor model of personality, which gained increasing prominence in the 1990s as factor-analytic personality traits were shown to have a high degree of temporal stability. The interest in factor-analytic (or dimensional) models of psychopathology was not limited to personality disorders, but they were a primary focus (Clark, 2005; Costa & Widiger, 2002; Harkness & McNulty, 1994; Livesley, 2003; Strack, 2006; Widiger et al., 2007).

At the beginning of the DSM-5 revision, the intention of those leading the revisions was to implement a dimensional model for personality disorders as a trial run for the rest of the manual in subsequent revisions (Zachar et al., 2019). This was partly predicated on the distinctiveness of personality pathology. To simplify this part of the history, the effort was not successful, and the DSM-IV personality disorder categories were reprinted in the DSM-5, while an Alternative Dimensional Model of Personality and Personality Disorder (AMPD) was published in the DSM-5 appendix.

There were many reasons for this outcome, one of which was that the standards used to evaluate proposals for making changes to the DSM-5 as developed by Kendler et al. (2009) were created to validate clinical syndromes rather than psychometrically derived dimensions. Indeed, although they were interested in dimensional models, many psychiatrists continued to think in terms of diagnostic categories. For example, even though those developing the ICD-11 successfully implemented a dimensional model for personality pathology, there was a strong outcry about the elimination of borderline personality disorder. As a compromise, the ICD working group had to retain borderline personality as a category (Tyrer et al., 2019).

1.8 Conclusion

As a new notion "personality" represented a shift in emphasis in which individuality takes center stage. Another way to say this is that personality previously referred to a kind of self-presentation, something external rooted in behavior, but around the turn of the century it was interiorized. Previously, people had the concepts of self, introspection, and looking inward. What changed was that the term "personality" became a framework for clustering together some disparate concepts, including behaviors, traits, thought patterns, interests, values, coping styles, dispositions, and personal history – all signifying expressions of one's "individuality." Indeed, another feature of the new notion of personality is that it pertained to the "whole person." If that is the case, then it is not surprising that in short order a good deal of what was called psychopathology was seen as being nested under personality.

If so, then how can we understand the idea expressed in this chapter that personality disorder came to be seen as an independent domain nested under the general concept of psychopathology? In part, the concept of personality disorder was introduced to describe certain kinds of psychiatric problems encountered in clinical work that were difficult to deal with. They seemed to be more entrenched than acquired afflictions like depression and anxiety, but not psychotic either.

I concur with Schneider that the personality disorder domain was constructed unsystematically. It has the structure of what I have called an imperfect community (Aftab, 2020; Zachar, 2014). The symptoms, types, and traits included in the domain are alike in many ways, but there is not one way in which they are all alike. According to this model, a cluster begins with seed disorders/symptoms and over time other disorders/symptoms are added because they resemble what is already there. In psychiatry, resemblance can include shared symptoms, but it can also include being manageable by the same skill set. If this model can be applied to personality disorders, I suspect that hysteria was one of the seeds, and likely compulsivity and paranoia as well.

The imperfect community model also offers another perspective on understanding comorbidity – as something written into the construction of the domain. New personality disorders would be added to the domain if they resembled something that was already there. Let me note that an imperfect community model would readily support making things more systematic, for example, using factor analysis to implement some mathematical rules for finding out which features in the domain best go together and which features fit less well.

The "open" nature of an imperfect community means that future developments may not be constrained by past developments. The DSM-III convention of segregating personality disorders from the rest of psychopathology was eliminated in the DSM-5 – potentially opening the door to again looking at resemblance relations between personality pathology and the rest of psychopathology.

Indeed, from a factor analytic perspective, DeYoung and Krueger (2025) specifically claim that most symptoms of psychiatric disorders, if persistent, can be considered maladaptive variants of normal personality traits. This involves a broad view of what counts as personality. For them, persistent traits such as attention problems can be considered personality. Thus, rather than making personality disorder distinct and independent from other psychiatric disorders, they would view other psychiatric disorders as personality disorders. From a casual symptom network perspective, Köhne and Isvoranu (2025) also argue that personality pathology and other kinds of psychopathology can be causally related systems rather than independent phenomena.

Separating personality pathology from the rest of psychopathology was a diagnostic convention, and arguably progressive in that it contributed to various empirical and theoretical advances about personality disorder. If re-nesting psychopathology under personality also supports empirical and theoretical advances in our understanding of psychopathology, adopting that convention could also be scientifically progressive.

Acknowledgements: Thanks to Jeannie Proust for double-checking what I wrote about Ribot and Janet and to Alan Horwitz for reading the first complete draft.

References

Aftab, A. (2020). Psychiatric disorders as an imperfect community: Interview with Peter Zachar, PhD. *Psychiatric Times*. www.psychiatrictimes.com/view/psychiatric-disorders-imperfect-community-peter-zachar-phd

Alexander, F. (1935/1949). *The psychoanalysis of the total personality: The application of Freud's theory of the ego to the neuroses* (B. Glueck & B. D. Lewin, trans.). The Coolidge Foundation.

Barenbaum, N. B., & Winter, D. G. (2003). Personality. In D. K. Freedheim (ed.), *Handbook of psychology: Volume 1 History of psychology* (pp. 177–203). John Wiley & Sons.

Beck, A. T., & Freeman, A. M. (1990). *Cognitive therapy of personality disorders* (2nd ed.). The Guilford Press.

Berrios, G. E. (1996). *The history of mental symptoms*. Cambridge University Press.

Blashfield, R. K., & Livesley, W. J. (1991). Metaphorical analysis of psychiatric classification as a psychological test. *Journal of Abnormal Psychology, 100*(3), 262–270. https://doi.org/10.1037/0021-843X.100.3.262

Clark, L. A. (2005). *Schedule for Nonadaptive and Adaptive Personality (SNAP): Manual for administration, scoring, and interpretation*. University of Minnesota Press.

Cleckley, H. (1950). *The mask of sanity: An attempt to clarify some issues about the so-called psychopathic personality* (2nd ed.). The C.V. Mosby Company.

Clouston, T. S. (1892). *Clinical lectures on mental diseases* (3rd ed.). J. & A. Churchill.

Costa, P. T., Jr., & McCrae, R. R. (1990). Personality disorders and the five-factor model of personality. *Journal of Personality Disorders*, *4*, 362–371.

Costa, P. T., Jr., & Widiger, T. A. (2002). Introduction: Personality disorders and the five-factor model of personality. In *Personality disorders and the five-factor model of personality* (2nd ed., pp. 3–14). American Psychological Association. https://doi.org/10.1037/10423-001

Crane, S. (1896). *The red badge of courage*. D. Appleton and Company.

Danziger, K. (1990). *Constructing the subject.* Cambridge University Press.
Decker, H. S. (2013). *The making of DSM-III®: A diagnostic manual's conquest of American psychiatry.* Oxford University Press.
DeYoung, C. G., & Krueger, R. F. (2025). What does personality have to do with mental disorder: A cybernetic perspective. In K. Banicki & P. Zachar (eds.), *Conceptualizing personality disorder: Perspectives from philosophy, psychological science, and psychiatry* (pp. 181–195). Cambridge University Press.
Eysenck, H. J. (1986). A critique of contemporary classification and diagnosis. In T. Millon & G. L. Klerman (eds.), *Contemporary directions in psychopathology: Toward the DSM-IV* (pp. 73–98). Guilford Press.
Fitzgerald, F. S. (1925). *The Great Gatsby.* Charles Scribner's Sons.
Frances, A. (1982). Categorical and dimensional systems of personality diagnosis: A comparison. *Comprehensive Psychiatry, 23*(6), 516–527.
Frances, A., & Widiger, T. A. (1986). Methodological issues in personality disorder diagnosis. In T. Millon & G. L. Klerman (eds.), *Contemporary directions in psychopathology: Toward the DSM-IV* (pp. 381–400). The Guilford Press.
Freud, S. (1921/1960). *The ego and the id* (J. Riviere, trans.). W. W. Norton & Company.
Greenwood, J. D. (2015). *A conceptual history of psychology* (2nd ed.). Cambridge University Press.
Grinker Sr., R. R., Werble, B., & Drye, R. C. (1968). *The borderline syndrome: A behavioral study of ego functions.* Basic Books.
Grob, G. N. (1991). Origins of DSM-I: A study in appearance and reality. *American Journal of Psychiatry, 148*(4), 421–431. https://doi.org/10.1176/ajp.148.4.421
Grout, H. (2019). Celebrity matters. *Aeon.* https://aeon.co/essays/the-history-of-celebrity-is-a-history-of-the-concept-of-self
Gunderson, J. G., & Singer, M. T. (1975). Defining borderline patients: An overview. *The American Journal of Psychiatry, 132*(1), 1–10. https://doi.org/10.1176/ajp.132.1.1
Hacking, I. (1995). *Rewriting the soul: Multiple personality and the sciences of memory.* Princeton University Press.
Harkness, A. R., & McNulty, J. L. (1994). The Personality Psychopathology Five (PSY-5): Issues from the pages of a diagnostic manual instead of a dictionary. In S. Strack & M. Lorr (eds.), *Differentiating normal and abnormal personality* (pp. 291–315). Springer Publishing Company.
Hathaway, S. R., & McKinley, J. C. (1940). A multiphasic personality schedule (Minnesota): I. Construction of the schedule. *Journal of Psychology, 10*(2), 249–254.
Hoch, P., & Polatin, P. (1949). Pseudoneurotic forms of schizophrenia. *Psychiatric Quarterly, 23*, 248–276.
Horwitz, A. V. (2023). *Personality disorders: A short history of narcissistic, borderline, antisocial, and other types.* Johns Hopkins University Press.
Houts, A. C. (2000). Fifty years of psychiatric nomenclature: Reflections on the 1943 War Department Technical Bulletin, Medical 203. *Journal of Clinical Psychology, 56* (7), 935–967.
Jackson, D. N., & Livesley, W. J. (1995). Possible contributions from personality assessment to the classification of personality disorder. In W. J. Livesley (ed.), *The DSM-IV personality disorders* (pp. 459–481). The Guilford Press.
James, W. (1890). *The principles of psychology.* Holt.

Kendell, R. E. (1975). *The role of diagnosis in psychiatry.* Blackwell Scientific Publications.

Kendler, K. S., Kupfer, D. J., Narrow, W., Phillips, K. A., & Fawcett, J. (2009). *Guidelines for making changes to DSM-5 revised 10/21/09*. Retrieved May 27 from https://web.archive.org/web/20100705210359/http://www.dsm5.org/ProgressReports/Documents/Guidelines-for-Making-Changes-to-DSM_1.pdf.

Kernberg, O. (1967). Borderline personality organization. *Journal of the American Psychoanalytic Association*, *15*(3), 641–685. https://doi.org/10.1177/000306516701500309

Klerman, G. L. (1986). Historical perspectives on psychopathology. In T. Millon & G. L. Klerman (eds.), *Contemporary directions in psychopathology: Toward the DSM-IV*, pp. 3–28. Guilford Press.

Knight, R. P. (1953). Borderline states. *Bulletin of the Menninger Clinic*, *17*, 1–12.

Köhne, A. C. J., & Isvoranu, A.-M. (2025). Network architectures of personality and its pathology. In K. Banicki & P. Zachar (eds.), *Conceptualizing personality disorder: Perspectives from philosophy, psychological science, and psychiatry* (pp. 244–260). Cambridge University Press.

Kraepelin, E. (1907). *Clinical psychiatry* (A. R. Diendorf, trans.). Macmillan.

Lewis, A. (1974). Psychopathic personality: A most elusive category. *Psychological Medicine*, *4*(2), 133–140. https://doi.org/10.1017/S0033291700041969

Lewis, S. (1925). *Arrowsmith*. Harcourt, Brace, & World, Inc.

Linehan, M. M. (1993). *Cognitive-behavioral treatment of borderline personality disorder*. The Guilford Press.

Livesley, W. J. (1987). A systematic approach to the delineation of personality disorders. *The American Journal of Psychiatry*, *144*(6), 772–777. https://doi.org/10.1176/ajp.144.6.772

Livesley, W. J. (2003). Diagnostic dilemmas in classifying personality disorder. In K. A. Phillips, M. B. First, & H. A. Pincus (eds.), *Advancing DSM: Dilemmas in psychiatric diagnosis*, pp. 153–189. American Psychiatric Association.

Lombardo, G. P., & Foschi, R. (2002). The European origins of 'personality psychology'. *European Psychologist*, *7*(2), 134–145. https://doi.org/10.1027//1016-9040.7.2.134

Lombardo, G. P., & Foschi, R. (2003). The concept of personality in 19th century French and 20th century American psychology. *History of Psychology*, *6*(2), 123–142.

Lorr, M. (1986). Classifying psychotics: Dimensional and categorical approaches. In T. Millon & G. L. Klerman (eds.), *Contemporary directions in psychopathology: Toward the DSM-IV*, pp. 331–346. Guilford Press.

Masterson, J. F. (1971). Treatment of the adolescent with borderline syndrome: A problem in separation-individuation. *Bulletin of the Menninger Clinic*, *35*(1), 5–18.

Menninger, K. A. (1947). Psychology and psychiatry. *American Psychologist*, *2*(4), 139–140. https://doi.org/10.1037/h0056668

Millon, T. (1985). The MCMI provides a good assessment of DSM-III disorders: The MCMI-II will prove even better. *Journal of Personality Assessment*, *49*(4), 379–391.

Millon, T. (1986). A theoretical derivation of pathological personalities. In T. Millon & G. L. Klerman (Eds.), *Contemporary directions in psychopathology: Toward the DSM-IV* (pp. 639–669). Guilford Press.

Murray, H. A. (1956). Morton Prince: Sketch of his life and work. *The Journal of Abnormal and Social Psychology*, *52*(3), 291–295. https://doi.org/10.1037/h0049369
Nicholson, I. A. M. (1998). Gordon Allport, character, and the "Culture of Personality." *History of Psychology*, *1*(1), 52–68. https://doi.org/10.1037/1093-4510.1.1.52.
Nicholson, I. A. M. (2003). *Inventing personality: Gordon Allport and the science of selfhood*. American Psychological Association.
Oldham, P. D., Pickering, G., Roberts, J. A., & Sowry, G. S. (1960). The nature of essential hypertension. *Lancet*, *1*(7134), 1085–1093. https://doi.org/10.1016/s0140-6736(60)90982-x
Perry, R. B. (1935). *The thought and character of William James: Volume II: Philosophy and psychology*. Little, Brown and Company.
Prichard, J. C. (1835/1963). Moral insanity (J. Swan, trans.). In R. Hunter & I. Macalpine (eds.), *Three hundred years of psychiatry (1535–1860)* (pp. 839–842). Oxford University Press.
Reich, W. (1949). *Character analysis* (3rd ed.). Farrar, Strauss and Giroux.
Ribot, T. (1885). *Les maladies de la personnalité*. Alcan.
Richardson, R. D. (2006). *William James: In the maelstrom of American modernism*. Houghton Mifflin Company.
Roback, A. A. (1933). Personality tests – whither? *Character & Personality; A Quarterly for Psychodiagnostic & Allied Studies*, *1*, 214–224. https://doi.org/10.1111/j.1467-6494.1933.tb02065.x
Roback, A. A. (1940). Morton Prince, 1854–1929: A memoir on the occasion of the tenth anniversary of his death. *American Journal of Orthopsychiatry*, *10*(1), 177–184. https://doi.org/10.1111/j.1939-0025.1940.tb05673.x
Sakaibara, E. (2025). What can the dimensional model of personality disorders learn from Mischel's classical challenge to the trait theory of personality? In K. Banicki & P. Zachar (eds.), *Conceptualizing personality disorder: Perspectives from philosophy, psychological science, and psychiatry* (pp. 40–55). Cambridge University Press.
Schneider, K. (1950/1958). *Psychopathic personalities* (M. W. Hamilton, trans.; 9th ed.). Cassell.
Schneider, K. (1959). *Clinical psychopathology* (M. W. Hamilton, trans.). Grune & Stratton.
Shepherd, M., & Sartorius, N. (1974). Personality disorder and the International Classification of Diseases. *Psychological Medicine*, *4*(2), 141–146. https://doi.org/10.1017/S0033291700041970
Skinner, H. A. (1986). A construct validation approach to psychiatric classification. In T. Millon & G. L. Klerman (eds.), *Contemporary directions in psychopathology: Toward the DSM-IV* (pp. 307–330). Guilford Press.
Stern, A. (1938). Psychoanalytic investigation of and therapy in the border line group of neuroses. *Psychoanalytical Quarterly*, *7*, 467–489.
Strack, S. (2006). *Differentiating normal and abnormal personality* (2nd ed.). Springer Publishing Co.
Tyrer, P., Mulder, R., Kim, Y. R., & Crawford, M. J. (2019). The development of the ICD-11 classification of personality disorders: An amalgam of science, pragmatism, and politics. *Annual Review of Clinical Psychology*, *15*, 481–502. https://doi.org/10.1146/annurev-clinpsy-050718-095736

U.S. War Department. (1946). Nomenclature of psychiatric disorders and reactions: War Department technical bulletin, medical 203. *Journal of Clinical Psychology, 2*, 289–296. https://doi.org/10.1002/1097-4679(194607)2:3<289::AID-JCLP2270020316>3.0.CO;2-O

Widiger, T. A., Frances, A., Pincus, H. A., Ross, R., First, M. B., & Wakefield Davis, W. (eds.). (1996). *DSM-IV sourcebook: Volume 2*. American Psychiatric Association.

Widiger, T. A., Simonsen, E., Sirovatka, P. J., & Reiger, D. A. (eds.). (2007). *Dimensional models of personality disorder*. American Psychiatric Press.

Wynter, A. (1875). *The borderlands of insanity*. G. P. Putnam's Sons.

Zachar, P. (2014). *A metaphysics of psychopathology*. MIT Press.

Zachar, P., Regier, D. A., & Kendler, K. S. (2019). The aspirations for a paradigm shift in DSM-5: An oral history. *Journal of Nervous & Mental Disease*, *202*(4), 346–352.

2 Ribot's Novel Approach to Character Pathology

From Normal Indecisiveness to the Madness of Doubt

Jeanne Proust

Théodule Ribot, considered as the father of experimental psychology in France and founder of the *Revue Philosophique de la France et de l'Etranger*, attained during his lifetime an undisputed and widely acknowledged authority that is not easily measured today. Known largely for his ambition to emancipate psychology from philosophy in order to constitute it as an independent science, his thought is often reduced, however, to a simple physiological – and deterministic – positivism, which fails to do justice to the imprint that metaphysics had left on his work and, more generally, to the complexity and originality of his "new" psychology. It is true that Ribot is critical of philosophy for having too often considered the physiological origins of our volitions as unworthy of study, and for being too exclusively devoted to the study of the highest, most sophisticated – and, to him, most fragile – forms of psychological activity. Philosophers have studied "the phenomena of the mind as logicians rather than psychologists, as reasoners rather than observers" (Ribot, 1870, p. 23). The abstract concepts of "memory," "will," or "attention," when violently amputated from their anchoring points within our physiology, give way to what Ribot considers vain metaphysical questions. Nonetheless, Ribot was particularly interested in the pathologies of our psychological functions; in this chapter, we will focus on indecisiveness, or irresolution (we will use both terms interchangeably), as one of the most puzzling impairments of our willpower.

Les maladies de la volonté (The diseases of the will), published for the first time in 1883, is Ribot's most republished book (printed 37 times since 1883). In this work, the founder of experimental psychology gathers and analyzes a considerable number of examples of pathologies, which he draws from different alienists and doctors of medicine.[1] The authenticity of the testimonies is not questioned, and the anecdotal nature of certain remarks undoubtedly leads the

[1] Some of which are Pinel (*Traité médico-philosophique sur l'aliénation mentale*, 1800), Briquet (*Traité clinique et thérapeutique de l'hystérie*, 1847), or Griesinger (*Traité des maladies mentales*, 1865).

reader to remain skeptical as to their scientific validity, but it is on the basis of these case studies that Ribot chooses to observe how the will gets "undone." He had previously formulated the "method of dissolution" and applied it to memory: inspired by the work of neurologist John Hughlins Jackson, "Ribot's law" (Ribot authors the law named after him) describes the order in which memories disappear, from the most recent to the oldest (*Les maladies de la mémoire*, 1881). This time, still faithful to this method, he observes how the disturbances of the will can enlighten us as to its nature and normal evolution. The method of *dissolution* is one of the most original aspects of Ribot's work. It focuses first on the physiological processes involved when a psychological function is altered or "dissolves": "in seeing how the ego is dissolved, we discover how it is made" (Ribot, 1885, p. 62). During the dissolution, everything that is unstable (the new states) is erased to let transpire the stable (the states anchored in the organism for a longer time): Ribot speaks of a "law of regression." Thus, the fact that conscious volitions appear later in the maturation of the individual makes them fragile, where reflexes and certain instincts remain unshakable. Ribot prefers the term *volitions* to *will*, abandoning the theory of the faculties – judged obsolete and inadequate to scientifically describe the human psychology – in favor of the observation of the psychophysiological tendencies: the neuronal, muscular, more or less complex nervous co-ordinations that determine the actions of the individual.

He starts by observing, in the first chapter of *The diseases of the will*, the situations in which there is an absence of action: the impulse to act is too weak, or is lacking completely. This is the case with *aboulia*, but also with irresolution, both of which we will explore in the next pages. The clinical typology proposed by Ribot doesn't fail to lay out the problem of the definition of the morbid state, but the continuity between pathological and normal phenomena makes certain cases harder to classify. Sudden impulses, irresolution, and laziness are not morbid within themselves. But they can be signs of a pathology when they permeate the character of the individual to the point of destroying any ability to combat the hypertrophied tendencies acting at their expense (in the case of impulses), or even to destroy any propensity to *want* at all (in the case of *aboulia*). It is the chronic aspect of this incapacity that constitutes the differentiating criterion – often implicit – that Ribot chooses to speak of as *disease*, even if he conceives the normal and the pathological as a difference in degree, rather than in kind. It is important to note here that the dimensional models of personality disorders today, with their emphasis on continuum, echo the spectrum-based symptomatology we already find in Ribot's work. The dimensional approach equally focuses on capturing the variability of personality traits along continuous dimensions, rather than categorizing individuals into distinct, often dichotomic diagnostic categories.

Likewise, Ribot's approach recognizes that individuals may exhibit varying degrees of certain traits associated with personality disorders.

For Ribot, the occurrence of punctual, ephemeral, isolated phenomena is not sufficient to qualify the individual concerned as sick: there is illness if there is a chronic condition, which has a lasting and profound effect on the character of the individual in the long run. The order of the chapters of *The diseases of the will* doesn't seem to be trivial in that regard, as it goes from the less-obvious pathological cases to extreme cases manifesting an annihilation of will. The theme of irresolution is addressed at the beginning of the book, which invites us to infer that Ribot does not consider it a disease, but a natural state that risks becoming pathological only if it chronically paralyzes the individual's ability to exert agency.

2.1 *Akrasia* and Intellectualism

The first two chapters of *The diseases of the will*, because they deal explicitly with the weakening of the will, do not fail to hint at the classic theme of *akrasia*. Ribot seeks to explain the defeat of self-control, but also the dispersion of inclinations, inconsistency, or *aboulia*, while avoiding resorting to the Socratic "intellectualism" (as he refers to it) that was – and still is – the starting point of the debate on the subject of *akrasia* in philosophy. He does not ignore, however, the influence of this intellectualism, which is why we will recall it here briefly.

Etymologically, the term *akrasia* meant, for Aristotle, absence of power or self-control, before being translated by the commonly accepted expression "weakness of the will." This choice of translation, common especially in the analytical tradition, is not devoid of a certain anachronism – as it is unclear whether Aristotle refers strictly to the concept of will – nor of a certain moralizing tone, which seems out of place when tackling this problem precisely from Ribot's experimental, "scientific" psychology standpoint.

The "intellectualist" tradition supposes that the intellect maintains a causal relationship with the will: the action of the agent echoes and translates in practice the content of their judgments. This intellectualist assumption is evidently startled by *akrasia* to the point of denying altogether the phenomenon. *Akrasia* gives rise to situations in which the reasons considered as the best by the agent are not the *causes* of their action – in fact, *cannot cause* their action. We are dealing with a conflict that renders the explanation of akratic actions challenging. The exact etiology of *akrasia* varies according to the authors who approach it: for some it includes irresistible impulses, conscious and unconscious; for others it refers exclusively to the inability to want what one thinks one wants to do – or to the inability to use one's best judgment. This last sense of the term, stricter, invites us to understand *akrasia* as a moral phenomenon of struggle between irrational forces (desire, passion) and the will – considered here as a rational faculty.

Medea's actions have traditionally served as an illustration of the inner contradiction that prevents the individual from acting in accordance with the moral evaluation that they are nevertheless capable of formulating rationally: *Video meliora proboque – deteriora sequor*: "I see the good, I approve of it, and I do evil" (Ovid, *Metamorphoses*: VII, 20). In Greek mythology, Medea is a powerful sorceress who assists Jason in obtaining the Golden Fleece. Jason betrays Medea by abandoning her to marry Glauce, the daughter of King Creon of Corinth, in order to secure his own political status. This act of betrayal deeply wounds Medea, who had sacrificed much for Jason, including betraying her own family and homeland to help him. After Jason betrays her, she seeks revenge by murdering their children, embodying the destructive consequences of unchecked passion. The murders of Glauce, Creon, and the infanticides committed by Medea can, however, be explained in the light of motives which we understand to have been decisive: the love she feels for Jason, and the revenge that her jealousy will impel her to orchestrate. There seem to be cases, however, where motives of this kind are missing, and where nothing seems to counteract the clear vision of the moral behavior which ought to be adopted.

We can take a look, for instance, at nineteenth-century Russian *Notes from underground*, sometimes considered one of the earliest existentialist novels. Dostoevsky explores the internal monologues of an unnamed narrator (the "Underground Man") on his life and offers a dark psychological exploration of his powerlessness and resentment towards societal norms and expectations. The Underground Man's descent into moral degradation and self-destructive behavior makes him wonder about his struggle for moral autonomy, and about the potential for human beings to freely embrace evil behavior. He does not clearly identify his reasons for committing actions that he knows are unjustifiable:

> Tell me this: why does it happen that at the very, yes, at the very moments when I am most capable of feeling every refinement of all that is "sublime and beautiful," as they used to say at one time, it would, as though of design, happen to me not only to feel but to do such ugly things, such that . . . Well, in short, actions that all, perhaps, commit; but which, as though purposely, occurred to me at the very time when I was most conscious that they ought not to be committed. The more conscious I was of goodness and of all that was "sublime and beautiful," the more deeply I sank into my mire and the readier I was to sink in it altogether. (Dostoevsky, 2009, p. 6)

The narrator of Dostoevsky's *Notes from underground* is thus indifferent to the reasons he perceives as right, which should, according to the intellectualist thesis, push him toward that good action – yet these reasons have no driving force. But in this passage, it almost seems that it is the very knowledge of the reasons to act right that motivates the individual to do wrong, to direct his action in the opposite direction from the one that these reasons clearly indicate. Here lies a perversity, a seemingly inexplicable call to transgression: it is no longer the weakness of the driving force of the good reasons (in relation to the bad ones, or independently of the latter) that is in question, but the force of a moral lucidity, which paradoxically provokes an action contrary to that prescribed by reason. It is therefore towards the problem of evil that the question of *akrasia* is directed, opened up by the possibility, contrary to the assertion of the Socratic adage, of voluntarily doing evil. Aristotle explains *akrasia* by invoking intemperance, also translated as incontinence, which makes the individual more sensitive to their appetites than to their intellect. But in this case the individual becomes sick, reckless, prone to anarchic passions. Aristotle is therefore not completely at variance with Platonic intellectualism, in the sense that he too believes that every lucid and healthy individual, that is to say, capable of deciding according to what dictates their reason, would not choose evil. But man seems to be capable of evil, "with no other motive for malice than malice itself," as Saint Augustine famously puts it.

The purpose of this chapter is not to undertake a comprehensive account of the history of the concept of *akrasia*. We will therefore reduce our scope to a few remarks on the approach of the moderns on the subject before going back to Ribot. It should be noted that Montaigne adopts an original position, which seems to free akratics of guilt by insisting on the opacity and natural contradiction of human motives. In the first chapter of Book II of his *Essays* (1580), titled "*On the Inconsistency of Our Actions*," Montaigne questions the freedom of a *naturally* unstable will, intermittent, inconstant in most humans; he quite uniquely *normalizes* the weakness of the will. But even so, we are nowhere near the a-moral physiological analysis suggested by Ribot. Descartes, meanwhile, does not hesitate to speak of "weak souls" in the *Discourse on the method* (1637), and subsequently, in *The passions of the soul* (1649). Descartes opposes irresolute character (denigrated) to the *generosity* of virtuous souls – a generosity which then adopts a very particular meaning. On the one hand, generous people use their will as they see fit; on the other hand, and most importantly, they have a firm and resolute character that enables them to make good use of this will. The will is healthy if it is constant. Indecisiveness is here again disapproved of. For Descartes, irresolution is a vice that one must fight against in order to not fall prey to the grip of passions. Spinoza, Locke, Leibniz, and Hobbes, by repudiating the *freedom of indifference* (which Descartes perceives as the lowest degree of freedom), continue to believe that the practical judgment of reason determines the will. If they give importance to the determining power of passions, they are still within the frame of the intellectualist logic that Ribot tries to detach himself from.

The moral dimension of *akrasia* is not of direct interest to Ribot. In fact, he does not once use the Greek term in his book *The diseases of the will*. Moreover, by employing the term "disease" in this title, Ribot directs his analysis toward a clinical typology that does not blame the "weak" more than it values the supposed merits of strong wills. Similarly, the choice of the term "*affaiblissements*" ("weakenings," also translated as "impairments" by Merwin Marie Snell), for the titles of the first three chapters, suggests not only a plurality of possible pathologies, but also a diachronic, evolutionary perspective, in opposition with the synchronic, more definitively stigmatizing one (perspective), implied by the term "weakness." Here again, we can draw a parallel between Ribot's nuanced approach and the ongoing transition to dimensional models of personality disorders: individuals cannot be easily assigned a fixed diagnosis that would make them belong to discrete, inflexible categories – either "normal" or "disordered." Ribot does insist on the fact that the disorders of the will often represent extreme manifestations of traits to be observed within common personality variations, and that they can overlap with other forms of psychopathologies.

Philosophers are being accused by Ribot of conveying too rigid and dichotomic perspectives, and of having confused the question of the nature of the will with that of the moral evaluation of our actions. He thus departs from philosophical considerations as to the origin of our intentions, and wishes to consider the will only from the perspective of experimental psychology. His methodological postulate rejects (or, shall we say, aims at rejecting) axiological and deontological insights. However, the paradoxical nature of the relationship between our will and our motives, the representations of our consciousness (specifically in the case of *akrasia*) does not leave him completely indifferent. He seems to abandon any causal, intellectualist theory of action, but he makes consciousness a necessary *attribute* of volition. He defends neither the existence of a causal link between state of consciousness and deliberate action, nor the idea of an absolute impermeability between the faculty of knowing, of judging and that of desiring and wanting – between our theoretical capacity to visualize goals to be attained, and the practical ability to implement the means to achieve these ends. By opting for an experimental, scientific approach, Ribot aims, not without difficulties, to eschew any risk of faulty dualism.

2.2 The Multiplicity of the Self

In *The diseases of the will*, Ribot draws attention first to the disappearance of the will insofar as it fails to translate into a muscular movement corresponding to the state of consciousness perceived by the individual. That is *aboulia*, which reduces the individual to observe their constantly aborted desires, the impotence of their acting tendencies despite the perfect conscience of the motives which should push them to act. The case of irresolution, or indecisiveness, seems more complex: here we face the confrontation of several impulses, and the incapacity of one of them to prevail over the others. As mentioned earlier, Ribot's physiological explanation first emphasizes that although irresolution can become pathological, it is primordially a normal phenomenon: the instability of the will is common, because the self is not a stable and unified entity. The self naturally has little cohesion, and rarely forms a unity without contradictions:

> Leaving apart characters that are perfectly consistent (in a rigorous sense of the word they do not exist), there are in every one of us tendencies of all sorts, all kinds of possible contradictions, and among these contradictions, all kinds of intermediate shades, and among those tendencies all possible combinations. This is because the ego is not solely a memory, a storehouse of recollections connected with the present, but an aggregate of instincts, tendencies, desires which are simply the activity of its innate and acquired constitution. (Ribot, 1885, p. 75)

The self is but a moving, unstable combination of various tendencies or chains of physiological processes of varied intensity. The images involved in these series of processes are more or less strong, regardless of their ability to produce consciousness. In fact, unconscious tendencies are often more powerful than conscious tendencies. The consensus of the body, which comes to light when one of the series ends up predominating over the others – thus allowing voluntary action – is not easily achieved. The multiplicity of organic tendencies is influenced by experiences that form new associations, reinforce certain tendencies, and attenuate others. The center of gravity of the self, that is to say, the prevailing tendency, moves and changes according to the way in which the combination of affective states, images, associations, nervous tensions within every tendency is built, and deconstructed.

The study of *akrasia* traditionally opposed, *grosso modo*, a rational tendency to an instinctual tendency. "Two souls live in my chest" (Goethe, Faust): this duality, although illustrating a certain dramatic force, is too reductive, as we mostly observe in reality (says Ribot) a multiplicity of tendencies succeeding one another usually too fast to allow the individual to act. Multiple inclinations and directions animate continually the individual subject to irresolution – which seems normal when considering the diversity of the perceptions involved, bringing into play different stimuli and images which only add to the complexity of the decision-making process. The social functions of the individual, their duties, the external events pull the self in different directions, thus wavering between various possibilities of expression.

> According to age, the various duties and events of life, and the excitations of the moment, certain complexes of ideas, at a given moment representing the ego, are more strongly developed than the others and take the first place. We become another

and are yet the same. My ego as a physician, as a scientist, my sensual ego, my moral ego, etc., that is, the complexes of ideas, inclinations, and directions of the will designated by these terms, may at a given moment enter into mutual combat and repel each other. The consequence of this state of things would be not only inconsistency and division of thought and will, but also a complete absence of energy for each of these isolated phases of the ego, if, in all these spheres there was not a more or less clear repetition for consciousness of some of these fundamental directions. (Ribot, 1885, pp. 77–78)

In addition to literature, physiology itself aimed to promote this idea of a duality between two coexisting selves. The theory, prevalent in Ribot's time, of an identity between the self and the brain thus contributed to the reductive vision of a self split in two – because the brain has two hemispheres, we would be double beings: the relative independence of the cerebral hemispheres would naturally cause internal disagreements, which the testimony of our consciousness seems so often to provide.

Some authors are inclined to go still further, holding that this cerebral dualism suffices to explain every discrepancy in the mind, from simple hesitation between two resolves, to the complete duplication of personality. If we will at the same time good and evil; if we have criminal impulses and a conscience that reproves them; if the insane at times recognizes their folly; if the delirious have moments of lucidity; if, in fine, persons believe themselves double, it is simply because the two hemispheres are in disaccord; the one is healthy, the other is morbid; one state has its seat to the right, its contrary to the left; it is a kind of psychological Manicheism. (Ribot, 1885, pp. 120–121)

The distortive aspect of this hypothesis is denounced from the outset by Ribot, who points out with humor the situations in which we hesitate between three (not merely two) possibilities: "Who has not hesitated between acting in two different ways or in neither, say between journeying northward or southward, or remaining at home? It happens repeatedly in our lives that we have to decide between three alternatives, of which each necessarily excludes the other two. Where shall we locate the third?" (Ribot, 1885, p. 121).

The cerebral specification of hesitation is here questioned by Ribot – who also rejects Gall's cranial topology, in vogue in the early nineteenth century. The hesitations that characterize irresolution do not spring from a *synchronic* conflict between two regions of the brain, but from a *diachronic* conflict between various tendencies which successively take the lead:

These contradictions in the personality, these partial scissions of the ego, such as are found in the lucid moments of insanity and of delirium, in the self-condemnation and reprobation of the dipsomaniac, while still drinking, are not oppositions in space (from one hemisphere to the other), but oppositions in time. They are – to use a favorite expression of Lewes – successive "attitudes" of the ego. (Ribot, 1885, pp. 119–120)

Again, it is not difficult to see how Ribot greatly contributes to a more holistic understanding of the complex phenomena at play within human behavior. By positing the interrelatedness of tendencies animating our will, and the hierarchical relationships between them through time, his work reflects a dimensional understanding of the rich and varied nature of our – mostly instable – will. Certain tendencies succeed in predominating, but this preponderance is short lived: they alternate too quickly, and thus do not acquire the force necessary to result in action. For Ribot, there is neither a naive unity of the self, nor a specious duality, but an intermittence of states of consciousness, a *diachronic multiplicity of the self*. This does not necessarily result in the dissolution of said self: just as "our body can successively and quickly assume two contrary attitudes without ceasing to be the same body" (Ribot, 1885, p. 120), we remain the same person, even in irresolution. However, the extreme cases of irresolution seem to lead to what Ribot refers to elsewhere as a dissolution of the personality. He stresses how much the self, to stabilize and be able to act, requires a strong character.

2.3 The Weakness of the Character: The "Changing Natures"

Despite his commitment to avoid moral evaluations of the will, Ribot insists on the driving force of an unambiguous and lasting idiosyncrasy: this is the prerogative of a strong character. Our character is the sum of tendencies, desires, tastes coordinated more or less coherently in our organism. It is this unidirectional coherence that is lacking in the unresolved. The strong character is a stable, predictable compound, with lasting aims: each decision of the self then emanates like a mature fruit, unhindered. When it wishes, this character expresses centrifugal tendencies, which are more easily oriented toward a final resolution, clearly identified, and rarely abandoned. The "weak" character, on the other hand, is incapable of feeling the predominance of a tendency over the others, and it ends up opting, passively, for what offers the least resistance: "In the irresolute who is poor in ideas, this can be seen more clearly. If they act it is always in the direction of the least action or of the feeblest resistance. Deliberation leads with difficulty to choice, and choice with more difficulty to an act" (Ribot, 1885 , p. 36).

The resolute individual draws their will from within their very unified character, which is the sum of coordinated tendencies inscribed in their organism – tantamount for Ribot to temperament or idiosyncrasy. The irresolute individuals, on the other hand, are too sensitive to the external environment, to the appeal of the various opinions, objects, and circumstances that are presented to them: they are scattered, so to speak, and distracted by extrinsic motives that come to impose on them alternately, creating an inner chaos from which no deliberate driving force can emerge:

> In fickle natures this definitive state is always provisional, that is to say, the willing ego is so unstable a compound that the most insignificant state of consciousness that may spring up modifies or wholly changes it. The compound formed at each instant has no force of resistance at the instant which follows. In that sum of conscious and unconscious states which from moment to moment represents the causes of volition, the part played by the individual character is a minimum, the share of the exterior circumstances a maximum. We fall back into that inferior form of volition studied above which consists in a "letting go." (Ribot, 1883, pp. 36–37)

We must clarify here that this hypersensitivity to external factors encountered in weak characters does not translate into a profound internalizing of motives, which, if they did acquire the force of *affect*, would then constitute an efficient drive. The hyper-receptivity to the external motives that Ribot mentions is in fact superficial, in that it gives rise only to states of consciousness, and not to affective states – only the latter are powerful enough to push the individual to act. Indeed, Ribot constantly stresses that the capacity to act comes from affective life, and not from states of consciousness. But the multiple and contradictory motives that blind the indecisive individual are nothing more than fickle, unanchored states of consciousness. In themselves, they have no efficacy: the emotional state that should accompany them is missing. This is where Ribot seems to disagree with the intellectualist tradition, which understands the weakness of the will as a sort of contamination by emotional impulses, affects, and passions, of rational deliberation. For Ribot, the will needs an emotional grounding to be effective: without affect, it is reduced to a mere superficial mental representation, devoid of effectiveness. This emotional deficit explains *aboulia* as well as irresolution: the various reasons that the individual perceives to act in one way or another do not "sink" into their character, leaving one's self intact, unaltered.

For the irresolute, thus, the impulses either succeed one another too quickly, or they are absent, and are replaced by states of consciousness amputated from their affective base. This is what makes the limit between *aboulia* and irresolution so tenuous, and one can understand why Ribot goes from one to the other sometimes without transition. In both cases, the nervous and muscular energy does not unfold. The irresolute individuals can be *aboulic*, that is to say, suffering from morbid apathy, perceiving various motives without being affected by them. Or they can be animated by a great diversity of physiological tendencies, truly anchored in themselves and affecting them, but none of which, for lack of time, manages to acquire this centrifugal, unidirectional force, necessary to lead to action.

A volition is not a mere decision, a velleity – it is already an act. Its conditions of possibilities are physiological, coordinated during the period of excitation, but it appears strictly speaking only when there is a transition from this period of excitation to the driving period, for which it constitutes the initial requirement.

After all it must never be forgotten that to will is to act, that volition is a transition to action. To reduce the will, as has sometimes been done, to a simple resolution, that is, to the theoretical affirmation that a thing is to be done, is to content oneself with an abstraction. Choice is but one stage in the process of volition. If it does not translate itself into action, immediately, or in due time, there is no longer anything to distinguish it from a logical operation of the mind. It resembles those written laws which are not enforced. (Ribot, 1883, p. 37)

Ribot seems here to equate resolution and choice, and thus to consider them as states of consciousness not necessarily involving action. But any state of consciousness associated with what we point out by the terms "choice" or "resolution" should naturally be translated into an action. Irresolution, or indecision, therefore constitutes a psychophysiological quirk on two levels: first, because the individual is unable to make a resolution (a "resolved" state of consciousness) prevail over others, and second because even if they succeed in doing so, this state of consciousness lacks the impetus necessary to carry out the action naturally called for. Effort is then impossible. What is the nature of this capacity for effort that is sorely absent in the undecided? And why do the irresolute individuals seem to exhaust themselves, if they are incapable of effort? Ribot points out that there are two types of effort: a muscular effort, but also, beforehand, a nervous effort that he calls "volitional effort." The muscular effort is often lacking in the unresolved, but the volitional effort is clearly felt. Drawing from the writings of William James (1880), Ribot describes this type of effort as a kind of inner thrust which, even if it does not translate into visible movements, tires the individual who feels it just as much. A predisposition is met with the resistance of other predispositions, conscious or not, which impede the action consciously decided upon. Ribot takes up James' example of "the man, who, after a long hesitation, decides to put arsenic into his wife's glass in order to poison her" (Ribot, 1883, p. 65). Volitional effort manifests in the resistance felt during hesitation, preceding the muscular act – which in this case is brief and easy. Whereas James saw the origin of volitional effort in a supra-sensitive domain, Ribot leaves it in the physiological realm. We know less about the organic, nervous processes at work in this type of effort, but there is certainly an expenditure of energy just as with muscular effort, perhaps even more. This explains the exhaustion of the irresolute: even if they barely act, even if there is little or no visible muscular effort, the volitional effort is at its height. This exhaustion is combined with the painful frustration of not being able to carry out a particular act, and can lead the irresolute, in time, to abandon all attempts to exert effort – then falling into *aboulia*.

2.4 The Madness of Doubt

Ribot identifies two types of inabilities to make decisions and to act, as we have previously mentioned: there is either paralyzing hypersensitivity, or there is weakening of sensory capacities, which corresponds to *aboulia*. In both cases, there is depletion of the nervous system, weakening of vital and motor functions. The first type of irresolution can lead to the second: by dint of being wobbled between different motives stimulating the nervous system with equal force, the latter, overworked, becomes unable to react. It becomes numb, so to speak, and can sink the individual into *aboulia*.

We now want to return to the case of hypersensitivity, this time applied to a particular type of irresolute with strong intellectual capacity. Ribot considers, as a possible cause for irresolution, the overabundance of motives available for an individual who would eventually lose themselves in trying to evaluate and compare them. The complexity of the calculations engendered by this wealth of ideas hampers the resolute action, creating a multiplicity of apparently conflicting tendencies.

> Among irresolute characters, some, a very small number are so on account of a wealth of ideas. The comparison of motives, reasoning, the calculation of consequences, constitute an extremely complex cerebral state wherein the tendencies to action counteract one another. But this opulence of ideas taken alone is not a sufficient cause of irresolution; it is only an adjuvant cause. The true cause here as everywhere is in the character. (Ribot, 1883, p. 36)

Ribot underlines again the weakness of the irresolute individual's character, which is combined here with the "*psychological rumination*" (Du Saulle, qtd. in Ribot, 1883, p. 60) characteristic of an excessively restless imagination. Here is an illustration:

> A very intelligent woman cannot go out in the street without asking herself: "Is someone going to fall out of a window at my feet? Will it be a man or a woman? Will the person be wounded or killed? If wounded, will it be in the head or the legs? Will there be blood on the sidewalk? If the person is killed how shall I know it? Ought I to call for help, or to run away, or to recite a prayer? Shall I be accused of being the cause of this occurrence? Will my innocence be recognized?" and so on. (Du Saulle, qtd. in Ribot, 1883, p. 59)

We are dealing here with the first type of "madness of doubt": it is a sort of morbid perplexity of the intellect that manifests in the patient by a "doubting-insanity or fumbling-mania (*Grübelsucht*)" (Ribot, 1883, p. 59). This perplexity paralyzes the individual or, at best, forces them to infinite precautions: we can recall here the common example of people who cannot help but check whether they have closed the door behind them. A flow of useless ideas results in a stream of useless actions and incessant questioning. This madness of doubt is reflected in a constant anxiety:

> Some do not pass beyond the region of every-day trivialities, as the man who will return twenty times to see whether he has really locked his door. Others exhaust themselves in abstruse and insoluble questions, never able to satisfy themselves or stop, like an ever-turning wheel. Others, the timid, lose themselves in endless scruples and puerilities. But whatever be the matter to which the mind applies itself, the psychological process remains the same. It is an interrogation without pause or limits, accompanied by distress, constriction of the head, epigastric oppression, vaso-motor troubles, etc. There is the ardent desire to find a fixed state for thought without the ability to do so. (Ribot, 1896, p. 366)

At its worst stage, this disease becomes a kind of *aboulia*, nourished by an absolute practical skepticism: it is the second type of "madness of doubt," stemming from the first, to which Ribot refers in his later work on *The psychology of feelings* (Ribot, 1896):

> Under its gravest form it is "the complete loss of all notion and fueling of reality." It is absolute skepticism, not theoretic and speculative, after the manner of the Pyrrhonians, but practical, bearing not only on ideas, abstract conceptions, memories, reasonings, but even on perceptions and actions; the exercise of the intellect is not accompanied by any belief, any state of mind which presupposes a reality. "I exist", says one of these patients, "but outside real life and in despite of myself . . . ; something which does not seem to be in my body impels me to act as I formerly did, but I cannot succeed in believing that my actions are real. I do everything mechanically and unconsciously. My individuality has completely disappeared; the way in which I see things makes me incapable of realizing them, of feeling that they exist . . . Even when I see and touch, the world appears to me like a phantom, a gigantic hallucination . . . I eat, but it is a shadow of food entering the shadow of a stomach, my pulse is only the shadow of a pulse . . . I am perfectly conscious of the absurdity of these ideas, but cannot overcome them." (Tuke, qtd. in Ribot, 1896, p. 367)

Once again, Ribot insists here that the states of consciousness linked to this disorder do not explain it in the least: the causes lie on the side of the muscular, nervous, and affective weakening. Doubt and endless questioning are rather *epiphenomena*, the effects of a morbid physiological state, deserted by the vital functions necessary for affirmation, certainty, and resolution. In *The psychology of feelings*, Ribot draws up a typology of characters where he mentions the contemplative characters, which are especially vulnerable to this type of morbidity: "their constituent elements may be enumerated in the following order: acute sensitivity, sharp and penetrating intellect, no activity" (1896, p. 385). Hamlet provides an example of this type of irresolution: he feels and thinks extensively, without being able to act.

It is worth noting that Ribot doesn't tackle anywhere in his work ways of strengthening a character or of reinforcing the will. The reason being that "the capacity for effort is, in the last analysis, a natural gift" (Ribot, 1883, p. 68), and irresolution, as we have seen, is an inability to link the volitional effort to the muscular effort. Habit can change behavior, of course, and physiological series of tendencies become stronger through repetition. But the innate element is essential: "Every organ develops by exercise; here, too, so repetition becomes easier. But if a first element, and with it a potential energy, is not given by nature, nothing succeeds" (Ribot, 1883, p. 69).

* * *

It is clear why Ribot finds the moral condemnation of a weakened will absurd; our character is naturally more or less susceptible to succumbing to morbid irresolution. The states of consciousness which appear in the individual whose ill intelligence ruminates in excess are, like all states of consciousness, the result of nervous, physiological processes out of our control, and too weak to positively influence the behavior. The moment of action, which never seems compelling enough, gets perpetually postponed.

Irresolution, in its most common form, consists of a succession of impulses that is too rapid for any one of them to be able to prevail over the others and translate into action. We are incapable of ranking the various physiological series that animate us, as they are equivocal, multidirectional, and often contradictory tendencies. However, Ribot also explains irresolution by the inefficiency of states of consciousness that lack, this time, the corresponding impulses: irresolution then resembles *aboulia*. The affective force, alone capable of generating an act, is absent, and the state of consciousness in itself remains sterile. When *aboulic*, we may believe we are decided, but we do not *feel* decided enough to actually want, and ultimately, to act.

By analyzing states of consciousness "amputated" from their organic roots, Ribot seems to be moving away from the pure physiologism that many think he is ascribed to. The epiphenomenalism of consciousness implies a certain renewed dualism, but the rupture between conscious mental states and physiological tendencies is only apparent: states of consciousness remain the manifestation of the latter; only, they are too weak or too quickly overlapping to generate movement. The question of the moral responsibility of the agent does not appear, and Ribot's experimental psychology seems consequently to depart from the intellectualist dualism of the traditional debate on *akrasia*. There is no longer wonder about the fact that the states of consciousness can no longer cause action, because these states of consciousness are devoid of all causal power – unless they are accompanied by an impulse capable of profoundly altering the physiology of the individual. The irresolute individuals suffer from the weakness of their overly spasmodic or apathetic character, to the point of losing their footing with the real if they fall into the extreme pathology of the madness of doubt. Ribot's effort to anchor our will in our physiology, and to illustrate a spectrum of various strengths of will fundamentally dependent on character, promotes an unprecedented biology-based approach of personality disorders. His work on the diseases of the will (1883) and, more broadly, of personality (Ribot, 1885) sheds a valuable light on the current development of a more descriptive, empirical account of quantitative rather than qualitative differences in personality disorders. Revisiting Ribot's contribution seems crucial today to adequately provide the historical context in which philosophy and psychology, both conjointly and competitively, have attempted to define the impairments of human character.

References

Aristotle. (2007). *Éthique à Nicomaque* (trans. J. Tricot). Vrin.
Descartes, R. (1964–1974). *Œuvres* (in C. Adam and P. Tannery, eds.). Vrin, C.N.R.S.
Dostoevsky, F. (2009). *Notes from underground* (trans. Constance Garnett). Hackett Publishing.
James, W. (1880). *The feeling of effort*. The Society.
James, W. (1888). What the will effects. *Scribner's Magazine*, 3(2), 240–250.
Montaigne, M. de. (2009). On the inconsistency of our actions. In E. Naya, D. Reguig-Naya, & A. Tarrête (Eds.), *Essais I, II, III*, Gallimard.
Plato, *Protagoras*, 345d–e and 357c–e.
Ribot, T. (1870). *La psychologie anglaise contemporaine (Ecole experimentale)*. Alcan.
Ribot, T. (1881). *Les maladies de la mémoire*. Baillière.
Ribot, T. (1883). *Les maladies de la volonté* (5th ed.). Alcan.
Ribot, T. (1885). *Les maladies de la personnalité* (2nd ed.). Alcan.
Ribot, T. (1896). *La psychologie des sentiments*. Alcan.

3 What Can the Dimensional Model of Personality Disorders Learn from Mischel's Classical Challenge to the Trait Theory of Personality?

Eisuke Sakakibara

3.1 Introduction

In addition to the alternative model of personality disorders (AMPD) in Section III of the fifth edition of the *Diagnostic and statistical manual of mental disorders* (DSM-5) and its Text Revision (DSM-5-TR), the 11th edition of International Classification of Diseases (ICD-11) adopted a dimensional model of personality disorders (American Psychiatric Association, 2013, 2022; World Health Organization, 2022). This was a milestone in psychiatry as findings established from trait-theoretic research on normal personality were applied to the clinical classification of personality disorders, replacing the categorical diagnostic system (Zachar et al., 2016).

However, since the 1960s, researchers led by Walter Mischel have raised fundamental issues with trait-theoretic studies of normal personality (Mischel, 1968, 1973; Mischel et al., 2007). Trait theory is an approach of personality psychology that attempts to capture a person's personality through a combination of personality traits, such as being meticulous, bossy, or sociable. Currently, as dimensional models of personality disorders are being adopted, it is worthwhile revisiting the significance of Mischel's concerns in the contemporary context, as the dimensional models employ a trait-theoretic conception of personality, and attempt to describe personality with a combination of domain-level and/or facet-level personality traits, which will be explained later. This chapter reviews the history of typology and trait theory in personality research and explains the characteristics of basic personality concepts. Subsequently, Mischel's criticisms are reviewed and some points to consider when using a dimensional diagnostic system for personality disorders are outlined.

3.2 Typology and Trait Theory of Personality Studies

Methodologies for characterizing personality have traditionally comprised typology and trait theory (Watanabe, 2010). These roughly correspond to categorical and dimensional diagnoses of personality disorders, respectively. Typology has been the norm in the field of medicine. Representative examples include the application of Galen's theory of the four humors to personality types (melancholic, choleric, sanguine, and phlegmatic) and Kretschmer's personality classification (cyclothymic, schizothymic, and ixothymic), which associates one's physique with personality. These typologies assumed a biological basis for classification.

Schneider's theory of psychopathic personality had profound influence on the understanding of personality disorders in the pre-DSM era (Schneider, 1950). Schneider's typology is independent of biological assumptions. However, it comprehensively discusses the kinds of beliefs, modes of experience, emotions, and behavioral patterns that are internally organized in those with extreme personality. Borderline personality disorder, which is of the utmost clinical importance in contemporary psychiatry, was originally a concept deeply embedded in psychoanalytic theories of personality organization and defense mechanisms (Kernberg, 1967).

By contrast, the trait theory is predominant in basic psychology. It was initiated by Allport and Allport (1921). Early studies collected trait-names from a dictionary (Allport & Odbert, 1936). The theory attempted to characterize an individual's personality by selecting a combination of trait-names, such as "shy" and "friendly," that describe an aspect of personality. This method is well suited for questionnaire-based research, and with the development of statistical methods and computers, it developed into the "psychology of individual differences" in the latter half of the twentieth century (Watanabe, 2010). A major achievement of trait-theoretic personality research is the Five-Factor Model (also known as Big Five personality traits), which was initiated by Goldberg (1980) and later refined and corroborated by independent researchers, such as Costa and McCrae (1992). The Five-Factor Model states that personality differences can be universally explained by five dimensions: neuroticism, extraversion, agreeableness, conscientiousness, and openness to experience. However, it had minor impact on clinical psychiatry before the advent of AMPD and ICD-11 personality disorder (ICD-11PD) because psychologists with training in psychometrics rather than medicine were at the center of these studies.

Since the DSM-III, the categorical model of personality disorder has been carried over to the DSM-5-TR without major modification – not because it has been validated, but rather because it lacks a sufficient body of research to warrant revision. Many disadvantages have been identified in the categorical diagnosis of personality disorders (Widiger & Trull, 2007). First, many patients do not meet the criteria for a specific personality disorder and are classified as having an "unspecified" or "other specified" personality disorder. Second, many people meet the diagnostic criteria for more than one personality disorder (i.e., greater than expected comorbidity). Third, considerable heterogeneity exists within a personality disorder category. These are not limited to personality disorders but are common to operational categorical diagnostic criteria for psychiatric disorders.

In response to these issues, the diagnostic criteria for AMPD in the DSM and ICD-11PD have adopted a dimensional model rather than a categorical model. AMPD and ICD-11PD have similar features (McCabe & Widiger, 2020). First, as shown in Table 3.1, pathological personality traits are dimensionally characterized by five factors, four of which are shared (negative affectivity, detachment, antagonism/dissociality, and disinhibition). The concept of personality functioning is introduced as a common and novel feature. In AMPD, a patient must have at least moderate impairment in either identity,

Table 3.1 *Correspondence between the five-factor model, AMPD domains, ICD-11PD domains, and AMPD facets*

Five-Factor Model	ICD-11PD domains	AMPD domains	AMPD facets
Neuroticism	Negative affectivity	Negative affectivity	*Anxiousness*, *Emotional lability*, Hostility, Perseveration, *Restricted affectivity*, *Separation insecurity*, Submissiveness
Extraversion	Detachment	Detachment	*Anhedonia*, *Depressivity*, Intimacy avoidance, Suspiciousness, Withdrawal
Agreeableness	Dissociality	Antagonism	Attention seeking, Callousness, Deceitfulness, Grandiosity, Manipulativeness
Conscientiousness	Disinhibition	Disinhibition	Distractibility, Impulsivity, Irresponsibility, Risk taking
	Anankastia		Rigid perfectionism
Openness to experience			
	(Schizotypal disorder)	Psychoticism	Eccentricity, Perceptual dysregulation, Unusual beliefs and experiences

Negative affectivity and anankastia are positively correlated with neuroticism and conscientiousness, respectively, whereas detachment, dissociality/antagonism, and disinhibition are negatively correlated with extraversion, agreeableness, and conscientiousness, respectively. Among AMPD facets, underlined ones are behavioral personality concepts, whereas italicized ones are emotional responses.

self-direction, empathy, or intimacy to be diagnosed with a personality disorder. ICD-11PD also divides personality disorders into mild, moderate, and severe personality disorders based on personality functioning, and has a category of personality difficulty as a subthreshold condition not included in mental disorders.

One difference between the two systems is that ICD-11PD does not further subdivide the five domains into smaller facets. Additionally, AMPD includes psychoticism as the fifth domain of pathological personality traits, whereas ICD-11PD includes anankastia as the fifth domain, because schizotypal disorders have traditionally been considered to be related to schizophrenia rather than a type of personality disorder in the ICD (Table 3.1). Anankastia, sometimes called obsessive-compulsive personality, refers to being overly focused on details, rules, and organization, aiming for perfection, and being rigid or inflexible about how things should be done. (Table 3.1). AMPD retains the diagnostic criteria for antisocial, avoidant, obsessive-compulsive, borderline, narcissistic, and schizotypal personality disorders because they were supported by research or clinicians objected to their removal (Zachar et al., 2016). By contrast, ICD-11PD only retains the borderline pattern qualifier.

The adoption of a dimensional model in the diagnostic criteria for personality disorders is a victory for scientific psychology over psychiatry. Dimensional diagnosis is a feasible solution to problems associated with categorical diagnoses, such as unspecified diagnoses, comorbid diagnoses, and heterogeneity within diagnostic categories. It solves these problems by providing more comprehensive and finer-grained characterization of pathological personalities with a combination of domain-level and facet-level traits. ICD-11PD, which has only five trait-domain specifiers and a borderline pattern qualifier, can distinguish 64 (i.e., 2^6) different personalities, among which only one is "unspecified." Furthermore, because the trait-domain specifiers were established using factor analysis, individual patients would be characterized by a small number of specifiers, because personality traits that are likely to co-occur are combined into one domain from the outset. Dimensional models will stimulate further research on personality disorders and deepen our understanding of the continuity between normal personality and personality disorders.

3.3 Behavioral Personality Concepts

Personality is a characteristic of human being as a person. We usually think of personality as an internal attribute of a person that manifests itself in their behavior and/or emotional responses. This chapter focuses on personality as it manifests itself in behavior. Personality manifested in behavior is typically described using what I call behavioral personality concepts. Behavioral personality concepts are characterized by their ability to apply to both the person and the behavior. For example, concepts such as "cautious," "bold," and "humorous" can be used in the form of "cautious behavior/cautious person," "bold behavior/bold person," and "humorous behavior/humorous person." However, a person who exhibits a behavior predicated by a certain behavioral personality concept does not necessarily have the corresponding personality. This is because, for example, for a person to be said to be a "frugal person," they must consistently engage in frugal behavior at different times and in different situations. For example, a person who is frugal regarding the clothes they wear but not frugal about electronics and eating out is not a frugal person.

The behavioral personality concept is the foundation of personality research. AMPD characterizes maladaptive personality traits into five domains that are further divided into 25 facets (Table 3.1). Of these, 17 facets can be classified as behavioral personality concepts (e.g., callous behavior/callous person, eccentric behavior/eccentric person). Six of the remaining eight facets represent characteristics of emotional reactions (e.g., anxiousness, emotional lability). Exceptions include perceptual dysregulation and unusual beliefs and experiences, which are derived from schizotypal personality disorder and are included in the domain of psychoticism.

The characterization of behavior using the behavioral personality concept involves labeling from a third-person perspective. Suppose that a man, S, takes a friend's book to his home without the owner's permission. S may believe that he simply borrowed the book from a close friend. However, from the third-person perspective, this behavior is perceived as "self-centered." From S's first-person perspective, S did not intend to act in a self-centered manner. In other words, the fact that he behaved in a self-centered manner was an unintended consequence of some actions that he performed intentionally. Moreover, S may reject the third party's later suggestion that his behavior was "self-centered."

When applying a behavioral personality concept, the characterization of behavior epistemically precedes that of personality. In other words, a person is regarded as brave because they act bravely, but their actions are not characterized as brave because they are a brave person. Conversely, once a behavioral personality concept is ascribed to a person, explanations of behavior using a behavioral personality concept is a type of explanation of events based on dispositions, wherein behavior is causally explained by an actor's personality (McKitrick, 2004). This explanation responds to the question, "why did S do B?" with the answer "because B is a P behavior and S is P," where "P" refers to a behavior personality concept. In practice, the statement "B is a P behavior" is usually not explicitly stated. Rather, the person who answers, "because S is self-centered," to the question is implicating that S's behavior is described as "self-centered.

The need to explain a person's behavior using behavioral personality concepts arises when the behavior is unexpected. According to attribution theory in social psychology, behaviors that occur with a high base rate in a given situation are explained by situational constraints or external stimuli, whereas behaviors that occur infrequently in a given situation tend to be attributed to factors within the person who performs them (Kelley & Michela, 1980). For example, everyone will run away if a fire breaks out and everyone will go to the bathroom if they experience the urge to do so, thus these kinds of behaviors are not considered to reflect personality. By contrast, a behavior is unexpected when it exceeds or fails to meet normative standards. A behavior exceeds expectations when a person performs an outstandingly good or supererogatory (i.e., more than what is obliged to do) action (e.g., "Because he is very courageous, he jumped into a mansion on fire to save those left behind"). Those behaviors are explained by one's virtue. However, in what follows, I will focus on cases where the behavior falls short of expectations, which is relevant to personality disorders.

3.4 Interaction between Situation and Personality

For the behavioral personality concept to be useful, it must be able to predict a person's behavior in various situations. For predictions to be possible, a person's behavior must be consistent. Behavioral consistency can be divided into two types: temporal stability and cross-situational consistency (Watanabe, 2010). Behavior is temporally stable when one behaves similarly in the same situation at different points in time. By contrast, a behavior is cross-situationally consistent when one behaves similarly across various situations.

However, since the 1960s, Mischel has cited various empirical evidence to deny the cross-situational consistency of personality-related behaviors, provoking the so-called "consistency debate" (Mischel, 1968, 1973; Mischel et al., 2007). For example, people's attitudes toward authoritative figures do not constitute a unitary tendency, but differ depending on the figures, such as fathers, superiors, and symbolic authorities, with little correlation between them. Moreover, observation of children lying and cheating in multiple settings, such as schools, homes, sports competitions, and parties, has shown that the degree to which their behavior was consistent with morality varies significantly between situations (Mischel, 1968).

These observations seem to contradict the general impression that personality is consistent. However, the paradox of personality is resolved if we recall that we typically have the opportunity to observe another's behavior only in some fixed situations when we interact with them in person (Mischel, 1968). For example, one may only see a colleague at the workplace and may not know how they behave among their family or friends outside of the workplace. When person

B meets person A in person, being in the same place as B is, in itself, a powerful situational determinant for A. Thus, even if person A usually exhibits behavior X when interacting with person B and behavior Y when interacting with person C, and the behaviors X and Y are not very similar, neither B nor C has the opportunity to witness the cross-situational behavioral inconsistency of A.

The personality traits defined by the Five-Factor Model are known to have high temporal stability. A meta-analysis revealed that the median aggregated dependability coefficients (test–retest reliability) for the five traits exceeded 0.8, when measurements were conducted twice within a two-month period (Gnambs, 2014). However, personality assessment with a self-rated questionnaire records a person's behavior (i.e., marking answers) in a situation in which the person sits at a desk and reads predetermined sentences. Thus, the high test–retest reliability of the questionnaire only implies temporal stability of behavior in a fixed situation, and it provides no information about the cross-situational consistency of behavior.

Mischel (1968) further suggested that humans experience cognitive dissonance when they observe phenomena contrary to their expectations. Therefore, a behavior that is not consistent with personality traits previously attributed to the person is likely to be ignored or explained away as atypical and is attributed to exceptional external conditions.

One crucial piece of evidence for Mischel's claim derives from a laborious study in which Mischel himself participated, systematically observing and counting the behavior of 84 children with social adjustment problems for an average of 167 hours per child at a six-week residential summer camp (Shoda et al., 1994). The camp included various activities such as woodworking and cabin meetings. The researchers categorized the interpersonal situations children encountered into five categories based on the valence (positive versus negative) of the interaction and type of person involved in the interaction (adults versus peers): peer-approach, peer-tease, adult-praise, adult-warn, and adult-punish. The children's behaviors were classified into five types: prosocial talk, whining, compliance, physical aggression, and verbal aggression. Each type of the children's behavior in each situation was then counted. Consequently, the frequency of the occurrence of 25 situation–behavior combinations was recorded.

The researchers found that, even within the same children, there were significant differences in the frequency of occurrence of each type of behavior depending on the situation. For example, one child exhibited verbal aggression consistently when warned by an adult but not when teased by peers. Furthermore, the behavior type that was more frequent in each situation differed between children. For example, in another child, teasing by peers was more likely to elicit verbal aggression than warning by adults. Thus, personality characterizations that presuppose cross-situational consistency of behavior, such as the frequency of verbal aggression averaged across different situations, do not provide a clear picture of children's individuality. Conversely, the study found that, within the same child, the behavioral profiles in the same situation at two different times were positively correlated, indicating that the inconsistency of behaviors across different situations was not due to random error, but arose from temporally stable personality structure.

The consistency debate was initially a radical challenge to the validity of trait-theoretic personality concepts. However, a consensus has been reached (Mischel et al., 2007). The first consensus is interactionism, which postulates that human behavior arises from the interplay between situational context and personal factors. The interactionism with regard to personality states that personality is not a factor that exerts a constant influence on behavior regardless of situation, but the impact of personality on behavior varies greatly depending on the situation. Mischel abandoned the presupposition of cross-situational consistency of behavior and argued that the coherence of *if ... then ...* profile characterizes an individual's personality (Mischel, 1973; Mischel et al., 2007). The if ... then ... profile is a stable pattern of behavior elicited in certain types of situations, such as if in situation A, then a person does X, whereas if in situation B, then the person does Y.

The second consensus is that cross-situational consistency of behavior exists, albeit very weakly (Mischel et al., 2007). Even in the studies that Mischel used to support his critique of the cross-situational consistency of behavior, the correlation of behavior in different situations, although low, was not zero. When behaviors in various situations are integrated, there are differences in the average behavioral tendencies among people. This finding is reinforced by the fact that personality traits are correlated with objective variables that are affected by a person's cumulative behavior. For example, there are weak but robust positive correlations between conscientiousness and life expectancy (Friedman et al., 1995) and a negative correlation between neuroticism and academic performance (Chamorro-Premuzic & Furnham, 2003).

Taken together, although trait-theoretic personality concepts are useful for capturing general trends in individual differences found in human populations, they are limited in their use for predicting individual behavior in specific situations. Mischel (1973) noted that to predict individual behavior, one must explore the person's competence, concepts, expectations, values, and plans instead of personality traits.

3.5 Personality Disorders and Cross-Situational Behavioral Consistency

Section 3.4 highlights a general lack of cross-sectional consistency in behavior. By contrast, the persistent and pervasive presence of problematic behaviors is required for the diagnosis of personality disorders, both in current categorical diagnoses and AMPD in the DSM-5-TR (American Psychiatric Association, 2022).

Criteria B and D of the current categorical diagnosis of general personality disorder are:

B: The enduring pattern is inflexible and pervasive across a broad range of personal and social situations.

D: The pattern is stable and of long duration, and its onset can be traced back at least to adolescence or early adulthood. (American Psychiatric Association, 2022, p.735)

Criteria C and D of the general criteria for personality disorder in AMPD are:

C. The impairments in personality functioning and the individual's personality trait expression are relatively inflexible and pervasive across a broad range of personal and social situations.

D. The impairments in personality functioning and the individual's personality trait expression are relatively stable across time, with onsets that can be traced back to at least adolescence or early adulthood. (American Psychiatric Association, 2022, p. 881)

In other words, both temporal stability and cross-situational consistency of maladaptive behavior are required to diagnose personality disorders in general. As discussed in Section 3.6, the ICD-11PD model adopts a more nuanced description.

Let us consider the implications of this from another perspective. Behavioral personality concepts include both positive and negative words for something like risk-aversive behavior (e.g., "timid" versus "prudent" and "bold" versus "reckless"). Appropriate behavior differs from situation to situation, with superficially similar levels of risk-averse behavior being positively rated as "prudent" in one situation, but negatively rated as "timid" in another. People with healthy personalities can select appropriate behaviors according to the standards/norms demanded by the situation; they behave prudently in one situation and boldly in another. Therefore, healthy personality is difficult to characterize using behavioral personality concepts, even if each behavior can be predicated by behavioral personality concepts.

By contrast, a person with a high degree of cross-situational behavioral consistency would have little room to change their behavior to match the situation, either because they are unable to discriminate between different situations or because they have little flexibility in their behavior. Therefore, behavioral consistency across different situations is itself a manifestation of pathology in personality (Mischel, 1973). Personality disorders are an exception to Mischel's argument against cross-situational consistency of behavior. Behavioral personality concepts are best applicable for characterizing personality disorders.

Maladaptive behaviors are pervasive in personality disorders. What, then, creates behavioral consistency? Positively valued behaviors may be consciously and intentionally created by individuals. For example, sincere people may have an intention or a policy to behave sincerely and may deliberately engage in behaviors that are evaluated as "sincere" by those around them.

Conversely, negatively evaluated behavior is not consciously created by individuals. This is because individuals do not intentionally attempt to be negatively evaluated by others. However, personality disorders are conditions wherein behaviors that are negatively evaluated by others are consistently observed over time and across situations. Therefore, the question remains: Why does it occur? Mischel (1973) noted that to predict a person's behavior, one should focus not on personality traits but on their competence, concepts they utilize, their expectations, their values, and their plans. As no one plans to have their behavior evaluated negatively by others, the last one is ruled out. The remaining alternatives are explanations based on beliefs, desires, and competence, if roughly categorized. This section, while reserving the question of what underlies maladaptive behavior associated with personality disorders, briefly discusses the clinical implications of considering the consistency of behavior to be based on aberrant beliefs, extreme desires, and incompetence rather than personality traits.

First, cognitive therapy adopts the idea that personality disorders are a matter of core beliefs or schemas held by a person (Beck et al., 2014). A schema is a cognitive framework that serves as a template for beliefs arising in individual situations. For example, a suspicious person may believe that everyone around them is a potential enemy. This concept is congruent with how personality disorders are treated in cognitive therapy; as beliefs are true or false, erroneous beliefs must be corrected based on collaborative empirical approaches.

Second, personality disorders may be viewed as problems involving extreme desires and values. Individual differences in desires and values are major factors that cause people to behave differently in the same situation. For example, a narcissistic person may strongly desire to be superior to others. If we believe that a type of personality disorder is caused by extreme desires and values, personality difference per se is tolerated because there is no right or wrong in desire or value itself, and clinical interventions should focus on modifying non-adaptive behaviors.

Finally, personality disorders may be considered to stem from lack of competence. According to one theory, the primary functional impairment in psychopaths is the inability to recognize others' sorrows and fears (Levy, 2007). One study found that personality disorders were diagnosable in about half of those with an autism spectrum disorder (Lugnegård et al., 2012). Common comorbidities with autism spectrum disorders are schizoid, obsessive-compulsive, and avoidant personality disorders. This finding suggests that part of the cases of personality disorders are caused by the incompetence associated with neurodevelopmental disorders. Taking such perspectives would motivate the opinion that individuals with personality disorders should be exempted or mitigated of their responsibilities with respect to problematic behavior committed by them.

If a personality disorder is considered to be a problem of competence, therapeutic interventions would focus on skills acquisition. For example, dialectical behavior therapy (DBT) for borderline personality disorder emphasizes skills training, including mindfulness skills, emotion regulation skills, and interpersonal effectiveness skills (Robins & Chapman, 2004). It reflects, at least in part, the fact that DBT views borderline personality disorder as caused by insufficient competence.

3.6 Cautions for Dimensional Diagnosis of Personality Disorders

In this section, I would like to offer some caveats to the dimensional models of personality disorders, based on what was discussed so far regarding the behavioral personality concept and the cross-situational consistency and inconsistency of behavior. Before moving on to specific points, I would like to clarify the relationship between dimensional models of personality disorders, behavioral personality concepts, and the issues raised by Mischel.

First, the domain concepts, such as detachment and disinhibition, which play a pivotal role in the dimensional models, are also personality traits in the sense that they are used in combination to characterize an individual's personality, but they are not behavioral personality concepts in themselves. Domains are the names given to the factor structure found to summarize basic trait concepts including behavioral personality concepts. Because domain concepts were established based on behavioral personality concepts, if there is a problem in applying behavioral personality concepts to healthy personality, the same issues should arise for domain concepts.

Second, although Mischel came to appreciate the significance of the Five-Factor Model to some extent in later years, his initial concerns stand in sharp contrast to the ideas that led to the development of the dimensional models of personality and personality disorders. On the one hand, it was studies based on self-rated questionnaires that advanced the development of the dimensional models. On the other hand, Mischel emphasized observation of behavior in real-life situations. The former is based on first-person conception of the self, whereas the latter is based on third-person observation of others. Mischel emphasized differentiation over integration, as evidenced by his belief that in order to understand and predict human personality, it is important to observe individual human behavior for each different situation. In contrast, what prompted the development of the dimensional models was to take data from a large number of participants and put them together to draw a big picture of personality.

Neither Mischel's view nor the view behind the dimensional models is superior to the other. However, given the fact that clinicians should work longitudinally with individuals with personality disorders, it seems that the dimensional models of personality disorders must be supplemented by Mischel's perspective in clinical settings.

The first caveat is that the diagnosis of a personality disorder requires the problematic behavior to be pervasive. The cross-situational consistency of behavior is not observable in people with normal personalities. Therefore, the pervasiveness requirement accompanied by personality disorders is an exception rather than a general rule for personality. Therefore, one should be very careful in ascertaining that the behavior in question is pervasive before assigning a personality disorder diagnosis.

The behavior that a patient exhibits in a consultation room is behavior that occurs in the fixed situation of "meeting the doctor in a clinic," and thus does not guarantee that similar behavior is observed outside the clinic. The same is true for a third party's report of a patient's behavior. This is because the behavior of the patient observed by a third party, if temporally stable, is the behavior that emerges in a fixed situation – fixed because that the third party is co-present with the patient, and similar behavior need not be observed in other situations.

ICD-11 lists the following essential features of mild personality disorder:

- There are problems in many interpersonal relationships or in performance of expected occupational and social roles, *but some relationships are maintained and/or some roles fulfilled.*
- Mild Personality Disorder may be associated with substantial distress or with impairment in personal, family, social, educational, occupational or other important areas of functioning that is either *limited to circumscribed areas (e.g., romantic relationships; employment)* or present in more areas but of milder severity. (World Health Organization, 2022, my italics)

In other words, disruptions in social functioning and problematic behaviors may occur in some situations, but not in others, among people with mild personality disorders.

This might be viewed as a lowering of the diagnostic threshold compared with the traditional personality disorder concept, which simply required that problematic behaviors be "pervasive across a broad range of personal and social situations" (American Psychiatric Association, 2022, p. 735). If this is so, the notion of mild personality disorder in the ICD-11 may invite criticism regarding it being a further medicalization of personality that was previously considered normal. However, another interpretation is available: Many people who were previously diagnosed with a personality disorder exhibited cross-situational variability in behavior and should not have been diagnosed with personality disorder under the conventional diagnostic criteria but can now be correctly diagnosed with mild personality disorder under the ICD-11 diagnostic requirements.

If the situation can be interpreted in this way, the concept of mild personality disorder would provide a significant contribution to illuminate an issue that has been neglected in the conventional diagnostic criteria for personality disorders. First, mild personality disorder bridges the gap between a healthy personality – wherein little cross-situational consistency of behavior is observed – and traditional personality disorder, wherein problematic behavior is pervasively observed – and provides a clearer sense of the continuum between the two. Second, mild personality disorders highlight the interactionism in personality. In mild personality disorders, in which problematic behavior occurs in one situation and not in another, it is important to probe why situational variations make such a difference to identify points of therapeutic intervention. For patients with mild personality disorders, social work that attempts to change the environment that triggers maladaptive behaviors may dramatically ameliorate their disorder.

A second caveat is that the clinical utility of the domain-level characterization of pathological personality traits may be limited. It is repeated problematic behaviors and persistent affective responses that bring patients with personality disorders to psychiatric attention. In other words, the facet-level characterization of AMPD is the level of description that more directly captures the *caseness* of personality disorders, namely the reason they visit a psychiatrist. By contrast, summarization according to the five domains may be useful for classifying personality disorders but seems to deviate from clinical reality. For example, it is easy to imagine what a "suspicious person" looks like, but it may not be easy to get a clear picture of what a person with "high detachment" looks like. Descriptions of personality disorders based on the five domains may not have incremental utility for clinicians. This is an important limitation of the ICD-11 model, which contained only domain level traits.

However, as noted in Section 3.3, it is also a characteristic of the behavioral personality concept that perception can diverge significantly between the first- and third-person perspectives. Characterizing personality using negative behavioral personality concepts is a third-person label for behavior. Therefore, characterizing personality disorders using facet-level concepts is easily accepted by those around the patient and healthcare providers. Conversely, facet-level characterizations may be unacceptable to the patient. No one would be happy to be labeled "a suspicious person." By contrast, of the five AMPD and ICD-11PD domains, all but psychoticism in AMPD correspond to four of the Big Five personality factors as shown in Table 3.1 (McCabe & Widiger, 2020). Therefore, domain-level characterization of personality may be more acceptable for individuals with personality disorders and may facilitate patients and those around them to share their perceptions of the problem. For example, patients would be more likely to embrace the description of having "a very high level of detachment than average." This is a major achievement of the dimensional models, which places personality disorders on a continuum with healthy personalities. The dimensional models normalize patients with personality disorders.

A third caveat is that the five domains of pathological personality traits are latent variables that are taken to explain individual differences in a population. In general, the causes of variance in behavior between individuals and the causes of a certain behavior in an individual are different, unless the condition of so-called "local homogeneity" is met (Borsboom, 2005). If this condition is not met, the factor-analytic dimensions of the AMPD and the ICD-11 cannot be used to explain the behavior of individual persons.

This distinction is especially important in clinical practice, because psychotherapeutic interventions for personality disorders require a theory that illuminates why a patient repeats problematic behavior and how it can be remedied. The dimension of detachment explains why individual differences in personality occur in a group (between person) but cannot be considered a (within person) cause of a certain person's suspicious behavior. In this regard, as Mischel (1973) points out, it is necessary to inquire into the cognitive processes, values, and competence that lead to their problematic behavior.

3.7 Conclusion

This chapter discusses the caveats of deploying a dimensional model of personality disorders following the challenges raised by Mischel against trait-theoretic personality research. Compared with conventional categorical diagnoses, the diagnosis of personality disorders based on a dimensional model has many advantages; however, it still shares the limitations of the trait-theoretic theory of personality. Therefore, in clinical practice, it is necessary to utilize a new diagnostic system with awareness of its limitations and advantages.

Acknowledgments: I would like to thank Yoshiyuki Watanabe at the Obihiro University of Agriculture and Veterinary Medicine for helpful suggestions and discussions on preliminary ideas for drafting this paper. I also thank Peter Zachar and Konrad Banicki for insightful comments to improve the initial draft.

References

Allport, F. H., & Allport, G. W. (1921). Personality traits: Their classification and measurement. *The Journal of Abnormal Psychology and Social Psychology*, 16(1), 6–40. https://doi.org/10.1037/h0069790

Allport, G.W., & Odbert, H.S. (1936). Trait-names: A psycho-lexical study. *Psychological Monographs*, 47(1), i–171. https://doi.org/10.1037/h0093360

American Psychiatric Association. (2013). *Diagnostic and statistical manual of mental disorders, 5th ed. (DSM-5)*. American Psychiatric Publishing.

American Psychiatric Association. (2022). *Diagnostic and statistical manual of mental disorders, 5th ed., text-revision (DSM-5-TR)*. American Psychiatric Publishing.

Beck, A. T., Freeman, A. & Davis, D. D. (2014). *Cognitive therapy of personality disorders*, 3rd ed. The Guilford Press.

Borsboom, D. (2005). *Measuring the mind: Conceptual issues in contemporary psychometrics*. Cambridge University Press.

Chamorro-Premuzic, T. & Furnham, A. (2003). Personality predicts academic performance: Evidence from two longitudinal university samples. *Journal of Research in Personality*, 37(4), 319–338. https://doi.org/10.1016/S0092-6566(02)00578-0

Costa, P. T. & McCrae, R. R. (1992). The five-factor model of personality and its relevance to personality disorders. *Journal of Personality Disorders*, 6(4), 343–359.

Friedman, H. S., Tucker, J. S., Schwartz, J. E., Tomlinson-Keasey, C., Martin, L. R., Wingard, D. L. & Criqui, M. H. (1995). Psychosocial and behavioral predictors of longevity. *American Psychologist*, 50(2), 69–78.

Gnambs, T. (2014). A meta-analysis of dependability coefficients (test–retest reliabilities) for measures of the Big Five. *Journal of Research in Personality*, 52, 20–28. https://doi.org/10.1016/j.jrp.2014.06.003

Goldberg, L. R. (1980). Some ruminations about the structure of individual differences: Developing a common lexicon for the major characteristics of human personality. Symposium Presentation at the Meeting of the Western Psychological Association, Honolulu, HI.

Kelley, H. H. & Michela, J. L. (1980). Attribution theory and research. *Annual Review of Psychology*, 31(1), 457–501. https://doi.org/10.1146/annurev.ps.31.020180.002325

Kernberg, O. (1967). Borderline personality organization. *Journal of the American Psychoanalytic Association*, 15(3), 641–685. https://doi.org/10.1177/000306516701500309

Levy, N. (2007). The responsibility of the psychopath revisited. *Philosophy, Psychiatry, & Psychology*, 14(2), 129–138. https://doi.org/10.1353/ppp.0.0003.

Lugnegård, T., Hallerbäck, M. U., & Gillberg, C. (2012). Personality disorders and autism spectrum disorders: What are the connections? *Comprehensive Psychiatry*, 53(4), 333–340. https://doi.org/10.1016/j.comppsych.2011.05.014

McCabe, G. A. & Widiger, T. A. (2020). A comprehensive comparison of the ICD-11 and DSM-5 Section III personality disorder models. *Psychological Assessment*, 32(1), 72–84. https://doi.org/10.1037/pas0000772

McKitrick, J. (2004). A defense of the causal efficacy of dispositions. *Sats: Nordic Journal of Philosophy*, 5(1), 110–130. https://doi.org/10.1515/SATS.2004.110

Mischel, W. (1968). *Personality and assessment*. Wiley.

Mischel, W. (1973). Toward a cognitive social learning reconceptualization of personality. *Psychological Review*, 80(4), 252–283. https://doi.org/10.1037/h0035002

Mischel, W., Shoda, Y., & Ayduk, O. (2007). *Introduction to personality: Toward an integrative science of the person*, 8th ed. John Wiley & Sons.

Robins, C. J. & Chapman, A. L. (2004). Dialectical behavior therapy: Current status, recent developments, and future directions. *Journal of Personality Disorder*, 18(1), 73–89. https://doi.org/10.1521/pedi.18.1.73.3277

Schneider, K. (1950). *Die Psychopathischen Persönlichkeiten*, 9th ed. Franz Deuticke.

Shoda, Y., Mischel, W., & Wright, J. C. (1994). Intra-individual stability in the organization and patterning of behavior: Incorporating psychological situations into the diographic analysis of personality. *Journal of Personality and Social Psychology*, 67(4), 674–687. https://doi.org/10.1037/0022-3514.67.4.674

Watanabe, Y. (2010). *What was personality? Psychology and folk concepts [Seikaku Towa Nandatta Noka?]*. Shin'yosha (in Japanese).

Widiger, T. A. & Trull, T. J. (2007). Plate tectonics in the classification of personality disorder: Shifting to a dimensional model. *American Psychologist*, 62(2), 71–83. https://doi.org/10.1037/0003-066X.62.2.71

World Health Organization. (2022). *ICD-11 for Mortality and Morbidity Statistics*. https://icd.who.int/browse11/l-m/en

Zachar, P., Krueger, R. F. & Kendler, K. S. (2016). Personality disorder in DSM-5: An oral history. *Psychological Medicine*, 46(1), 1–10. https://doi.org/10.1017/S0033291715001543

Part II

Contemporary Approaches to Traditional Conceptual Perspectives

4 The Psychodynamic Core of Personality Disorder

Contemporary Concepts and Methods

Mark H. Waugh

Two basic assumptions underpin contemporary psychodynamic approaches to personality disorder. First, personality disorder refers to the personality system. This is more than an objective description of personality problems. That is, the intrapsychic system of internal processes (dynamics) responsible for self-identity, traits, coping, and relationship patterns – as well as symptoms – is disordered in some way. Second, the person's functioning varies from adaptive to maladaptive and can be viewed on a latent dimension of level of personality functioning. Personality disorder exists in a middle range: more impaired than minor dysfunction and less so than psychotic-level functioning. This idea was first formally articulated by Otto Kernberg (1967).

The psychodynamic conception of personality disorder is consistent with the personological tradition in psychology beginning with Henry Murray (1938) and continued by the narrative psychologist Dan McAdams (1995) and personality theory systemist Theodore Millon (2016). Personology assumes personality must be viewed holistically. The many features and components of personality interrelate and integrate into a whole. This also implies an emphasis on idiographic study of the individual life history. Often multiple points of view and types of data are required to provide a full picture of the person. A personological point of view for personality disorder means malfunctioning inner personality processes are understood holistically and presuppose multiple points of view. This includes but is not restricted to observable behavior and symptoms such as in descriptive psychiatry. Furthermore, personality disorder is considered more than general psychosocial or psychiatric symptom impairment because it refers to internal personality processes giving rise to psychological problems, symptoms, and patterns of impairment. In other words, personality disorder is known by both objective indicators and by phenomenological experience. The latter realm involves subjective, narrative concepts such as self, personal identity, agency, motivation, and autobiographical narrative. The psychopathologist Karl Jaspers called the combined objective and subjective understanding of mental disorder methodological pluralism

(Jaspers, 1968). This inclusive approach is well-suited to personality disorder. Psychodynamic conceptions of personality disorder are inherently methodologically pluralistic in part because they focus on both objective and subjective phenomena.

At root, people are story-telling beings. The earliest oral traditions of human culture, including theatrical dramas and poetry, were stories about life and meaning. At the individual level, the stories of one's life are ways of making meaning of experience. Narrative understanding is a key function of the self, a central component of personality (McAdams, 2015). Modern neuroscience considers personal identity to be constituted by evolving and at times fluctuating narrative representations (stories) that arise from the functioning of the human frontal lobes. These stories enable the self to make sense of experience over time, providing feelings of coherence and unity and helping in understand others' behavior (Stuss, 1991; Flanagan, 1991).

Contemporary psychodynamic conceptions of personality and personality disorder draw on narrative psychology (Sarbin, 1986) and the "narrative turn" (Spence, 1982) in psychoanalytic theory. This narrative perspective departs from early psychoanalytic explanation that relied on models of mind that invoked (1) psychic energy and psychosexual stages of development (e.g., libidinal cathexes; oral, anal, oedipal stages), (2) a topographic view of the conscious, preconscious, and unconscious giving rise to the "iceberg" metaphor (i.e., much of mental life is beneath the surface), and (3) the structural model of intrapsychic conflict between ego, id, and superego forces. These early conceptions reflected the mechanistic and hydraulic metaphors consistent with the technology and science of their era.

Like science in general, psychodynamic theory employs metaphors to advance understanding (Brown, 2003). Modern psychodynamic thinking borrows metaphors from present-day scholarly discourse to include (1) computer and information processing (i.e., cognitive psychology; see Peterfreund, 1980), (2) adaptive systems and complexity theory (personality is a dynamic system producing emergent properties; see Stolorow, 1997), and (3) the formative role of shared social–emotional experience in early relationships (Benjamin, 1990). These metaphors blend within three major lines of contemporary psychodynamic thought: object relations, intersubjectivity, and attachment/mentalization theory. Object relations theory highlights the role of early interpersonal relationships that become internalized (represented) as relationship patterns or social–cognitive schemas (Greenberg, 1983; Kernberg, 1995). Intersubjectivity theory prioritizes the unique shared experience between people (usually two) as they co-narrate their experience (Stern et al., 1998). Attachment/mentalization theory focuses on the role of early emotional bonding experiences in configuring relationship styles (called *internal working models*) as well as capacities for understanding mental experiences of oneself and others (Bowlby, 1980; Fonagy et al., 2002). Central players in this narrative, relational turn in psychodynamic theory are internal experience, subjectivity, personal agency (including unconscious action), interpersonal schemas, reflective capacity (ability to understand internal experiences of self and others), and the co-construction of meaning in relationships.

Historical contexts of psychiatric nosology and personality disorder are helpful in situating developments within psychodynamic thinking reflected in contemporary personality disorder models. Modern psychiatric nosology was promulgated in the *Diagnostic and statistical manual of mental disorders Third Edition* (DSM-III; APA, 1980). The DSM-III prioritized objective description by operationalized criteria and reflected the influence of the neo-Kraepelinian paradigm (Klerman, 1986). This paradigm embraced the goal of improved inter-diagnostician reliability and advocated for an agnostic approach to etiology yet also advanced medicalization of psychiatry, tacitly favoring biological explanation and the influence of psychopharmacology (Shorter, 2013). Beginning with the DSM-III, the term neurosis (and to some extent its psychodynamic heritage) was removed from official nosology, and traditional categorical personality disorder syndromes were defined by operationalized criteria.

Over time, concerns with the modern DSM approach to personality disorder grew. These included overlap between diagnoses (co-morbidity), heterogeneity of symptoms within diagnoses, limitations of categorical classification relative to dimensional approaches, and preferred ways to model and assess personality disorder. Despite significant controversy over how to redress these concerns (Zachar et al., 2016), the traditional categorical personality disorder syndromes defined by operationalized criteria were retained in the DSM-5 (APA, 2013). However, a hybrid categorical–dimensional model called the Alternative DSM-5 Model was included as an emerging model and measure. More recently, the *International statistical classification of diseases and related health problems 11th edition* (ICD-11; World Health Organization, 2022) introduced a fully dimensional personality disorder model.

These two personality disorder schemes are very similar. They both define personality disorder by a dimension of impairment in self and interpersonal functioning. Although multiple conceptual traditions are represented in these personality disorder schemes, each are organized on a core axis that is largely psychodynamic in nature and reflecting modern points of view in psychodynamic thinking. This chapter identifies and explicates this psychodynamic core and its role in dimensional personality diagnosis. Importantly, because this psychodynamic core refers to subjective, first-person experience as well as narrative and intersubjective aspects of personality functioning, it complements the positivistic emphasis on objective behavioral description prevalent in modern psychiatric nosology.

4.1 Key Elements in the Contemporary Psychodynamic Approach

Contemporary psychodynamic thinking has evolved considerably from early orthodox psychoanalytic theory and now prioritizes narrative and relational psychology (Luyten et al., 2015). Modern psychodynamic theory is a holistic ecumenical systems approach woven from interrelated principles and points of view. These can be summarized broadly as reflecting (1) the dynamic unconscious and its corollary, psychological causation of experience, behavior, and symptoms; (2) the importance of early development; and (3) the influence of internalized cognitive–affective–interpersonal schemas in behavior. These are briefly discussed as separate topics although they are blended personality processes of the whole person.

4.1.1 The Dynamic Unconscious and Psychological Causation

Unconscious mental functioning is basic to psychodynamic theory. This is a rather unfashionable notion, however, despite extensive evidence from affective neuroscience as well as cognitive, experimental, and social psychology showing that unconscious mental processes operate in behavior (see Westen, 1998; Panksepp & Solms, 2012). The well-known novelist Cormac McCarthy (2017) described the unconscious as an animal's operating system. Because people are meaning-making beings, this requires perceiving, sorting, and synthesizing present and past patterns of information – and particularly so for experience that involves social relationships. The organism cannot act and adapt to the world if all information processing occurs consciously. The need for an unconscious operating system is greater when the organism is bestowed with human frontal lobes and subjectivity, engendering the proclivity to make sense of experience narratively by constructing stories (Stuss, 1991; Schafer, 1992).

Unconscious mental functioning arises from the need to automate processing of interactions with the environment, which is substantially interpersonal. Because people are social mammals requiring prolonged childhood dependency on caretakers, early interpersonal experience becomes a major crucible for who we are. From the object relations point of view, formative interpersonal experiences become internalized as socio-emotional–interactional templates ("object representations") that color much of personality functioning. These implicit templates provide quasi-automatic ways to respond to emotionally charged situations and are often thematically related to ways the individual navigated early developmental challenges. Much of the personality system pertinent to self-relationships (e.g., identity, self-esteem regulation) and interpersonal functioning (understanding of others' mental states, intimacy) is thought to be configured by such early environmental challenges. Because they provide ongoing but implicit response action tendencies for emotionally high-valent situations, they constitute what is called the *dynamic* unconscious, which can be distinguished from general non-conscious processing supporting automaticity in perceptual and cognitive functioning. Examples of non-conscious cognitive processes include mental shortcuts such as cognitive heuristics (Kahneman et al., 1982) and implicit biases to which we are prone (stereotypic thinking; Greenwald & Lai, 2020). In contrast, in the dynamic unconscious, cognitive–emotional–behavioral response patterns reflect the operation of "working models" or paradigmatic representations of formative relationships that influence current behavior. Because these internalized mental schemas unwittingly color and influence thought, feeling, and interpersonal relationships, they reflect psychological causation. In personality disorder, psychiatric symptoms and maladaptive personality patterns thus express the impact, influence across personality features, and representation of early experiences or relational traumas. This conception of the dynamic unconscious differs from early psychoanalytic views which considered symptoms to be displaced symbolizations of specific traumas (i.e., repressed focal trauma).

Scientific psychology and descriptive psychiatry tend to shy from these ideas, seemingly reluctant to venture from shadows of "black box" behaviorism and objective, often biological, explanations of psychopathology. In this regard, it is somewhat ironic that well-accepted treatment approaches in the cognitive behavior therapy tradition, such as Acceptance and Commitment Therapy (Hayes et al., 2011), among others, increasingly reference internal experience, relationship dynamics, and implicit processes – ideas which are the fabric of psychodynamic theory (for excellent exposition of these points, see Bornstein, 2005; McWilliams, 2020; Shedler, 2022). Despite the substantial evidence base for key psychodynamic ideas, they are generally neglected in educational and training settings (Levendosky et al., 2023).

4.1.2 The Developmental Point of View

Contemporary psychodynamic approaches prioritize the role of early experience in personality development and later functioning. The basic idea is that early development leaves traces in the personality that are expressed in relational themes in later life. This idea is supported by a large body of research on infant–caregiver interaction showing its influence on later personality functioning (Trevarthan & Aitken, 2001; Beebe & Lachmann, 2013). For example, early face-to-face non-verbal synchronization between two people creates a mutual intersubjectivity (Stolorow et al., 1994). This becomes the psychological space wherein mentalization (i.e., the capacity to be aware of and make use of others' mental states), social connectedness, and self-regulation of emotion develops (Winnicott, 1969; Schore, 2021). The profound impact of early experience is underscored also in the association between adverse childhood experiences and adult diagnosis of personality disorder (Afifi et al., 2011; see also Doyle & Cicchetti, 2017).

The importance of early development is captured in the idea that the past lives on in the present. This refers to the classical idea of *repetition compulsion* (see Freud, 1896/1962). We are inclined to "repeat" experiences associated with trauma. However, trauma is construed broadly. Trauma can range from child abuse and severe psychosocial stressors (Chu, 1991) to challenges impinging on the child's ability to develop secure and lasting emotional connections with caregivers as in attachment theory described by John Bowlby and Mary Ainsworth (Bowlby, 1979). Similarly, object relations theory posits that recurrent mismatches between a child's evolving emotional needs and the early relational environment can be a source of trauma (Winnicott, 1969; Van der Kolk, 1994). Furthermore, trauma experiences can be repeated (expressed) in ways other than intrusive memories, negative emotionality, and dissociative experiences (as typically found in post-traumatic stress disorders). Trauma can be manifested by re-enacting interpersonal themes and in the subjective experience associated with early influential events. For example, an adult who suffered repeated failures of caretaking and/or losses of security figures may become sensitized to fears of loss. This may be expressed in vigilance for threats of emotional abandonment and efforts to test the reliability of others' regard. The impetus for repeating themes associated with trauma is the drive to master unsalutary early formative experiences (Loevinger, 1966a). The legacy of such experiences is evidenced by the association of early abuse, deprivation, and disturbed attachment on the development of personality disorder (Lieb et al., 2004; Johnson et al., 1999; Fonagy & Luyten, 2009). In this vein, Evans and Simms (2023) empirically showed that the self and interpersonal dysfunction dimensions of the Alternative DSM-5 Model reflect the commonality of disturbed psychological mechanisms stemming from adverse childhood experiences. In psychotherapy, persons with personality disorder may require specialized techniques, supportive postures, and the therapist tolerating momentary ruptures in the relationship in order to develop trust because of the tendency to experience the helping relationship similarly to prior relationships (Clarkin et al., 2015; Fonagy et al., 2015). This is also seen when underlying pathogenic beliefs (e.g., "I am unworthy of love") are tested out in the therapeutic relationship (Gazzillo et al., 2019).

4.1.3 Internalized Interpersonal Schemas

Personality, of course, is composed of many interrelated elements and processes. These include narrative self-identity, value systems, and dispositional traits. In addition, contemporary psychodynamic thinking places strong emphasis on internalized schemas or scripts. These can be described as social–emotional–interactional templates that underly (and impel) certain behavioral patterns. As noted, they are acquired during development and generally are largely unconscious (they possess a degree of automaticity, given certain triggers). These social–cognitive templates or schemas are thought to originate from evolutionary processes involved in forming emotional bonds with caregivers (attachment theory; Bowlby, 1979) and basic biological motivational systems common to social mammals. These motivational systems include attachment, erotism, play, fight–flight, and separation–panic (Panksepp, 2004). Specifically, the attachment–separation–panic system is particularly important in object relational theory (Kernberg, 2016, 2022). This is because the child's interactions with primary caregiver(s) – constituting emotional bonding patterns – serve as a prototype for interpersonal relationships, hence the idea of schema or script. Importantly, these interpersonal schemas are infused with emotional valance and at times may be felt in mood states that reflect early prototypical relationship experiences (Bollas, 1987/2017). The personality and psychopathological correlates of attachment styles have been extensively investigated, and the *core conflictual relationship theme* (Luborsky & Crits-Christoph, 1998) approach to identifying internalized core relationship patterns of adaptation (schemas) from narrative data has seen empirical study. The notion of internalized schemas or scripts has also become an important part of some cognitive behavioral therapy traditions (see Young et al., 2006).

Fonagy et al. (2015) have put forth a transdiagnostic formulation of personality disorder built on the core concept of *epistemic (dis)trust*. This refers to the capacity to receive transformative knowledge about the social world, which is acquired developmentally via social cues within reciprocal interactions between the child and caregivers in secure relationships. This process is thought to engender adaptive capacities of social discernment and openness to learning from experience. If sufficient epistemic trust is not achieved (internalized), epistemic distrust colors much of adult interaction. Fonagy et al.'s (2015) conception integrates evolutionary theory and social communication science (Sperber et al., 2010), attachment theory (Bowlby, 1980), and general psychodynamic principles (McWilliams, 2011). The idea of epistemic trust has been used to explain aspects of psychopathology, inform approaches to psychotherapy, and describe wider contemporary cultural phenomena (Campbell & Allison, 2022).

4.1.4 Summing Up Contemporary Psychodynamic Ideas

It is helpful to consider the term "psychodynamic." McWilliams (2020) traces three meanings to the term: an approach to treatment, a knowledge base, and a personal and professional ethos. Treatment approach refers to the body of clinical lore and techniques of psychodynamic therapy (e.g., Caligor et al., 2018). The knowledge base consists of concepts and findings derived from psychodynamic investigation, such as the core themes discussed in this section. Ethos refers to the valuing of reflectiveness and the interior life. This ethos embraces existential realities such as death and isolation, personal limits, and does not subscribe to a world view of unbridled optimism.[1] This ethos is also a bit subversive, contending that people and society have a dark side, and offers a counter perspective to conforming social forces. McWilliams (2020) calls this ethos a *wisdom tradition*. Our discussion of the psychodynamic core of personality disorder focuses mainly on the knowledge base aspect, but implications related to treatment and this underlying ethos are close at hand.

4.2 Personality Disorder Is Psychodynamic

Psychodynamic ideas are inherent in personality disorders. For example, over 50 years ago the DSM-II (APA, 1968, p. 41) described personality disorder as "characterized by deeply ingrained maladaptive behaviors that are perceptibly different in quality from psychotic and neurotic symptoms . . . ." It is but a small step to see the influence of the dynamic unconscious and internalized schemas in this definition ("deeply ingrained maladaptive behaviors"). Furthermore, this early definition posited a spectrum of personality functioning between "psychotic and neurotic." This middle ground was anticipated in the early notion of pseudoneurotic schizophrenia (Hoch & Polatin, 1949) and the "as if personality" (Deutsch, 1942), but it was fully delineated by Otto Kernberg. Relatedly, in 1915 Karl Jaspers introduced a strong distinction between psychosis and non-psychotic psychopathology (see Burgy, 2008). Psychosis was viewed as an organic (biological) illness characterized by major disturbances in relationships with reality. In contrast, non-psychotic disorders were considered more psychological in nature and a function of personal history. Psychoanalytic theorizing of this era afforded a major role to personal history in the etiology of psychopathology, particularly with conditions called neuroses. Kernberg's (1967) important contribution was to theorize about a range of personality functioning more adaptive than psychosis, but less so than neurotic functioning. This he termed this *borderline personality organization.*

[1] Roy Schafer (1970) described four "visions of reality," based on grand tropes from literature, which capture the character of McWilliams' (2020) psychodynamic ethos. These visions may be paraphrased as: comic ("power of positive thinking"), romantic ("life is a great quest"), tragic ("the multitudinous poignancies of life"), and ironic ("detached, accepting view of all of the above"). For Schafer, the psychoanalytic world view draws on each vision but highlights the tragic and especially the ironic.

Borderline personality organization involves dysfunctional personality processes including problematic identity, immature psychological defenses, and poorly differentiated interpersonal schemas. For Kernberg (1967) all personality disorders possess the same general level of personality functioning (i.e., borderline organization). The different traditional personality disorder syndromes (avoidant, dependent, narcissistic, paranoid, etc.) vary in symptoms and style, but all reside and function at the borderline level of severity. It should be noted that Kernberg's (1967) transdiagnostic concept of borderline personality organization is broader and differs from the psychiatric diagnosis of borderline personality disorder, a specific category of personality disorder introduced in the DSM-III (APA, 1980).

Major contemporary conceptions of personality disorder such as those described by Kernberg (1967), Theodore Millon (2016), and Peter Fonagy and colleagues (2015) share psychodynamic principles. Millon (2016) characterized personality disorders as inflexible personality styles that develop as adaptive strategies to early environmental challenges. For Millon (2016), personality disorder is marked by recurring problematic interpersonal experiences engendered by interpersonal schemas originating from early development. As noted earlier, Fonagy et al. (2015) emphasize a general property of epistemic distrust in personality disorders. Epistemic distrust is viewed as an adaptation to adverse early environmental experience and is characterized by an overriding rigidity or inflexibility. This interferes with being able to receive and make use of social exchanges in ways different from the previously internalized pathogenic interpersonal schemas and beliefs. The *Psychodynamic diagnostic manual second edition* (PDM-2; Lingiardi & McWilliams, 2017) is a psychiatric nosology designed to redress perceived conceptual imbalances of the "neo-Kraepelinian" descriptive psychiatry influences in the modern DSMs. In the PDM-2, psychiatric diagnosis is formulated not just with respect to psychiatric symptoms but includes diagnosis of personality syndromes largely based on the Kernbergian notion of level of personality functioning.

Each of the above approaches to personality disorders are essentially psychodynamic. That is, they speak to a particular range of maladaptive functioning, emphasize the developmental origins of inflexible personality functioning, account for the tendency to repeat (re-enact) formative experiences in current relationships, and frame personality disorder in terms of both subjective experience and objective, outward behavior.

4.3 Dimensional Personality Disorder Diagnosis Is Psychodynamic

The field of personality disorder has been invigorated by dimensional models (Krueger, 2013). Similarly, modern personality study is strongly influenced by the dimensional five-factor model (Costa & McCrae, 1992) and the Big Five (Goldberg, 1993) psychometric trait models. A prominent dimensional model in psychopathology is the Hierarchical Taxonomy of Psychopathology (HiTOP; Kotov et al., 2017). This model maps psychiatric symptoms onto a factor-analytically derived hierarchical organization of underlying dimensions. Expanding dimensional characterization of disorders was an aspiration of the DSM-5 (Regier et al., 2013) and was reflected in the diagnoses of autism spectrum and substance use disorder. Before further discussion of personality disorder dimensions, however, we briefly examine the idea of dimension and its measurement.

4.3.1 Dimensions

Dimensional measurement refers to representing a construct along an underlying or latent continuous variable. This is distinguished from a categorical construct or dichotomous variable such as in traditional medical or psychiatric classification wherein an illness or disorder is either present or absent. Dimensional representation confers measurement advantages because a continuous variable contains more information than a dichotomous variable. This also permits the application of powerful statistical analyses (e.g., multivariate methods like factor analysis). However, construing personality and psychopathological constructs, syndromes, or disorders as dimensions is more than an advantageous quantification strategy supporting statistical analysis. The measurement model should be faithful to the nature of the underlying construct. This is a basic principle of construct or scientific validity (Loevinger, 1957). It should be noted that many commonly used statistical methods such as factor analysis (as well as the correlation coefficient) assume variables are measured on a continuous scale, display a normal distribution, and reflect a linear relationship (Fabrigar et al., 1999). Thus, if the studied variables refer to categorical or discrete phenomena but are analyzed by multivariate statistics, conceptual errors (assuming a continuous dimension) and methodological errors (of statistical assumptions) occur. Berrios and Markova (2013) argued that dimensions in psychopathology display only degrees of gradation or order. That is, they reflect relatively more or less of the construct, like an ordinal scale. This contrasts with the mathematical properties of equal intervals associated with, for example, standardized test measurement of intellectual level, and with ratio scale of measurement applicable to physical phenomena like height, weight, and time (Stevens, 1946). Furthermore, Hopwood et al. (2023) distinguished three uses of the term "dimension" in psychopathology. These are constructs with continuous measurement, homogenous constructs with continuous measurement, and distinct homogenous constructs within a multidimensional (factor-analytic) framework.

It should be noted that categorical phenomena can be analyzed with quantitative methods such as taxometrics (Meehl, 1992). Interestingly, taxometric study in psychopathology finds many disorders reflect a dimensional structure and this seems particularly the case for personality disorders. Exceptions to dimensionality are seen with schizotypal personality disorder, substance use disorders, suicide risk, pedophilia, and autism spectrum disorders; these appear to best fit a discrete or categorical classificatory scheme (Haslam et al., 2012, 2020).

Implications of these conceptual and technical concerns to personality disorders become complex. On the one hand, often these statistical procedures are robust to violations of their assumptions (see Knief & Forstmeier, 2021). On the other hand, the psychometric theory of factor analysis, the exemplar method of this approach, posits a realist ontology in which the underlying (latent) dimension causes or explains observable measurements in variables such as test scores or symptom counts (Borsboom et al., 2003; Borsboom, 2017). However, this realist assumption may be less appropriate in realm of personality and personality disorder where social, cultural, and narrative-constructivist explanation has strong purchase. These conceptual and methodological concerns continue to be debated, particularly in philosophically informed literature of psychopathology (e.g., Banicki, 2020; Kendler, 2016).

It is important to note that dimensional models have been advocated for some time. Extensions of the popular five-factor model (Costa & McCrae, 1992) and other factor-analytic models (Clark, 2007; Widiger & Trull, 2007) have enjoyed much recent interest. However, earlier influential dimensional approaches also exist (e.g., Cloninger et al., 1993), including a key model also featuring a defining dimension of personality impairment (see Livesley, 1998). Recently, the Alternative DSM-5 Model has achieved significant traction (Hopwood et al., 2018). This is particularly true in academic circles with some inroads occurring in applied practice (Bach & Tracy, 2022), although psychologists, with their background in psychometrics, may be more familiar and partial to this approach compared to other mental health professionals. Helpful introductions and reviews of the Alternative DSM-5 Model are available for the interested reader (see Waugh et al., 2017; Sharp & Wall, 2021).

4.3.2 Descriptions of the Dimensional Personality Disorder Models

In both the Alternative DSM-5 Model and the ICD-11, personality disorder diagnosis begins with a global rating of moderate or greater impairment in personality functioning referencing the spheres of self and interpersonal functioning. Although self and interpersonal functioning can be evaluated for component dimensions (see below), it is important to note that these models are designed to yield a global, holistic rating for level of personality functioning impairment. Once this is achieved, ratings of pathological traits may be applied to further characterize the personality disorder.

In the Alternative DSM-5 Model, impairment in self and interpersonal functioning (called Criterion A) is decomposed into the dimensions of Identity, Self-Direction, Empathy, and Intimacy. Each of these refers to a range of adaptation from severe impairment to healthy function. Identity refers to experiencing oneself as unique, with clear boundaries between oneself and others, and maintaining stable self-esteem and regulation of emotional experience. Maladaptive Identity functioning, for example, can be expressed in an unstable sense of oneself, confused interpersonal boundaries, and fragile or fluctuating self-esteem. Self-Direction refers to the capacity to pursue life goals, maintain internal standards, and engage effective self-reflection. Impairment in Self-Direction can be expressed in instability or lack of success in attaining personal goals (relative to ability and circumstance), an overly exacting or paucity of internal standards, and an undeveloped awareness of one's behavior and motivation. Empathy functioning pertains to the ability to understand others' experiences and mental states, tolerating differences with others, and appreciating the effect of one's behavior on others. Impairment may manifest in egocentricity, excessive attunement to others in the service of self-interests, and lack of awareness of one's impact on others. Intimacy functioning refers to the quality and extent of interpersonal connection and the capacity for closeness and reciprocal social relationships. Impairment variously can be seen in disinterest, few and/or superficial relationships as well as feeling needy and insecure in relationships, fearing emotional abandonment, and relating to others primarily in terms of self-needs.

The second step in applying the Alternative DSM-5 Model, called Criterion B, evaluates the person in terms of five pathological personality-trait domains (Negative Affectivity, Detachment, Antagonism, Disinhibition, and Psychoticism). Each of these broad domains also can be decomposed into narrower facets. For example, facets for Negative Affectivity include specific pathological personality traits of emotional lability, anxiousness, separation insecurity, submissiveness, hostility, perseveration, depressivity, and suspiciousness. Importantly, the five broad maladaptive personality trait domains approximately correspond to the pathological poles of the five normal personality traits in the five-factor and Big Five models of personality trait research. These are sometimes characterized by the acronym OCEAN, referring to traits of Openness to Experience (maladaptively expressed as Psychoticism), Conscientiousness (as Disinhibition), Extroversion (as Detachment), Agreeableness (as Antagonism), and Neuroticism (as Negative Affectivity).

The original goal for the Alternative DSM-5 Model was to eliminate all personality disorder traditional syndrome categories in favor of personality-trait dimensions. As a compromise with those psychiatrists and psychologists committed to categorical models, the Alternative DSM-5 Model includes diagnosis of five hybrid categorical–dimensional personality disorders (i.e., Antisocial, Avoidant, Borderline, Narcissistic, Obsessive-Compulsive personality disorder). These are based on the presence of component traits (after impairment in self and interpersonal functioning has been established), but not formal diagnostic criteria. To this end, these hybrid categorical–dimensional personality disorders reflect the continued influence of the descriptive psychiatry tradition. However, Alternative DSM-5 Model diagnosis often is accomplished in practice with the term *Personality Disorder-Trait Specified* rather than by syndrome name. This involves listing the prominent maladaptive traits, an approach supported by empirical findings (Clark et al., 2015). Research has shown that the traditional personality disorder syndrome categories can be reliably described by these pathological traits (e.g., for borderline personality disorder, see Mulay et al., 2019), so there is a degree of empirical isomorphism between the models. However, clinicians are familiar with traditional personality disorder syndromes (e.g., borderline personality disorder, paranoid personality disorder) and are not generally fluent in trait description of these syndromes. Thus, the clinical utility of the approach for day-to-day clinical practice is a work in progress (Bach & Tracy, 2022).

In the ICD-11, personality disorder diagnosis is determined by a threshold global rating for self and interpersonal functioning impairment with a metric like that of the Alternative DSM-5 Model for level of personality functioning. One difference between the two models, however, is the ICD-11 requires only the rating for severity of self and interpersonal functioning impairment to diagnose personality disorder. In the ICD-11, characterizing personality disorder functioning with pathological traits is optional. The five maladaptive trait domains in the ICD-11 are: Negative Affectivity, Detachment, Dissociality, Disinhibition, and Anankastia. Notably, the ICD-11 model includes the maladaptive trait domain of Anankastia, referring to pathological compulsivity, rather than the trait domain of Psychoticism found in the Alternative DSM-5 Model. The ICD-11 also offers an optional specifier for borderline pattern when signs and symptoms of the well-known traditional borderline personality disorder syndrome are present.

4.3.3 Conceptual Heritage

The metric for establishing presence of personality disorder in the Alternative DSM-5 Model, the Level of Personality Functioning Scale, derives largely from psychodynamic traditions (see Bender et al., 2011; Sharp & Wall, 2021) and is very similar to Kernberg's (1967) formulation of borderline personality organization referring to personality functioning between neurotic and psychotic functioning (Clarkin et al., 2020). Conceptually, the Alternative DSM-5

Model also draws on interpersonal theory (Pincus et al., 2020), developmental psychopathology (Sharp & Wall, 2021), and narrative psychology (Lind et al., 2022) traditions. In this regard, Mulay et al. (2018) showed that experts perceive a greater presence of psychodynamic, interpersonal, and narrative paradigms within the elements of the Level of Personality Functioning Scale (capturing Identity, Self-Direction, Empathy, and Intimacy impairment) relative to the maladaptive personality traits, which incorporate greater presence of psychometric trait and five factor model traditions.

The core axis or impairment dimension of the Alternative DSM-5 Model and the ICD-11 personality disorder models is conceptually pluralistic, encompassing many strands of psychodynamic theory. This includes ego psychology, self-psychology, and object relations theory (Yalch, 2020) as well as narrative psychological perspectives. For example, ego psychology is reflected in constructs related to regulation of impulses and integrity of reality testing. Level of personality functioning impairment also incorporates the idea of a hierarchy of more to less adaptive defense mechanisms (Vaillant, 1992), reflecting the seminal ego psychology formulation of mechanisms of defense described by Anna Freud (Freud, 1946/2018). Psychodynamic self-psychology (e.g., Kohut, 1966) is found in the emphasis on self-esteem regulation in the Identity domain and perspective taking in the Empathy component. Object relations theory is represented in the mutual, reciprocal interpersonal relationships of Intimacy, the ability to consider others' views and needs in Empathy, and personal identity functioning the Identity domain. Attachment (modes of emotional bonding) and mentalization theory (the capacity to perceive the mental states of self and others) are prominent in contemporary psychodynamic thinking and inherent in the Empathy and Intimacy components. Narrative psychology points of view are captured in the Identity dimension. Of note, narrative psychology studies have shown that problems in coherence and stability of the sense of self are associated with personality disorders (Lind et al., 2020), and derailment of normal self-identity processes in adolescence can lead to personality disorder.

The Alternative DSM-5 Model and the ICD-11 denote a global conception of level impairment in personality functioning. As such, they bear some resemblance to earlier lifespan personality development models. Both Erik Erikson's (1959) writings on identity development over the life cycle and Jane Loevinger's (1966b) stage theory of ego development viewed personality as a holistic, integrated expression of many strands of self and interpersonal functioning. This organismic system perspective persists in the Alternative DSM-5 Model and the ICD-11 approach. Sharp (2022) pointed out this holistic view of self and interpersonal dysfunction that references mental structures and processes means personality disorder diagnosis is a consequence of personality dysfunction, and not simply a descriptive statement of dysfunction.

McAdams and Pals (2006) described personality meta constructs that are useful in illustrating dynamic features of the Alternative DSM-5 Model and ICD-11 personality disorder model. These are dispositional traits, characteristic adaptations, and narrative identity. These meta constructs, respectively, convey the metaphors of *actor*, *agent*, and *author* (McAdams, 2015). *Dispositional traits* reflect the observable behaviors of an *actor*, the personal qualities by which others know us and the focus of trait psychology (McAdams, 1994). *Characteristic adaptations* are the intentions, aims, desires, motivations, and ways of coping and defending of an *agent*. These are involved in typical psychodynamic explanation. *Narrative identity* refers to personality processes *authoring* self-identity, deriving from stories about oneself over time.

The personality constructs within the self and interpersonal functioning domains of the Alternative DSM-5 Model and the ICD-11 approach chiefly represent the characteristic adaptation and narrative identity constructs, with some influence of psychobiological traits. For example, the Identity component refers to how a person experiences oneself, manages boundaries between self and others, and maintains self-esteem. In the language of McAdams and Pals (2006), these are agentic actions of a person, originating from internal personality processes supporting (authoring) personal identity. This dimension of Identity functioning subsumes self-agency and expresses internalized interpersonal schemas and prototypical responses to stress and conflict (i.e., characteristic adaptations; metaphor of *agent*).

4.4 Psychometrics and Structures: Conceptual and Empirical Issues

Conceptual and empirical distinctions between the Alternative DSM-5 Model impairment dimension (Criterion A) and the maladaptive personality traits (Criterion B) are not sharp. This is also the case for the ICD-11 personality disorder model, but the more recent ICD-11 system has not yet generated as much published research illustrating these issues. Overlap between the core impairment axis and the maladaptive trait dimensions occurs in part because they share similar psychodynamic personality processes or downstream effects of these processes (see Yalch, 2020). For example, the pathological trait of Psychoticism includes reality testing and one's sense of reality; these are basic constructs of ego psychology and are included in assessment of level of personality functioning. The pathological trait domain of Antagonism incorporates psychological grandiosity, a major construct in the psychodynamics of narcissism in self-psychology (Kohut, 1965; Ronningstam, 2022). Pathological grandiosity would also be reflected in impaired personality functioning of Criterion A.

One way to frame the connections between the self and interpersonal functioning domains and the maladaptive traits is to say that dysfunction in internal personality processes drives the expression of pathological traits. In this vein, Zimmermann et al. (2015) suggested that maladaptive trait expression occurs *because* of impaired capacities for self and interpersonal function. That is, the self and interpersonal functioning domains *explain* the "how" of the "what" of pathological traits. This is the fundamental point of Sharp's (2022) argument that the unique advance of these dimensional personality disorder models is they ascribe a central role to dysfunction within internal personality processes of self and interpersonal functioning, and that this gives rise to symptoms and maladaptive trait expression in personality disorder.

The psychometric trait tradition of academic psychology is captured in the pathological-trait domains of the Alternative Model DSM-5 and the ICD-11 approach. The paradigmatic method of this tradition is factor analysis and similar methods (Hopwood et al., 2019). Several measures of the pathological traits have been published, with the *Personality Inventory for the DSM-5* (PID-5; Krueger et al., 2012) being a popular self-report instrument. In this regard, it is important to note that most of the research on the Alternative DSM-5 Model has been on maladaptive traits typically using self-report instruments (for a revealing comparative tabulation, see Zimmermann et al., 2019). More recently, self-report scales for the self and interpersonal functioning impairment dimension have emerged (e.g., *the Level of Personality Functioning Scale-Self Report* [LPFS-SR]; Morey, 2017). These and similar instruments predating the Alternative DSM-5 Model have permitted study of the empirical convergence and divergence of the elements of these models as well as their respective contributions in predicting other criteria.

Correlational and factor analyses of joint elements of these dimensional personality disorder models have shown they contain substantial shared variance (Zimmermann et al., 2015; McCabe et al., 2021; Sleep & Lynam, 2022). Several studies compared the models to see which components better predict criteria such as traditional personality disorder symptom counts, other psychiatric symptoms, psychosocial impairment, personality traits and constructs, and clinician ratings. Sometimes results have shown that measures of maladaptive traits moderately outperform the self and interpersonal impairment dimension in predicting external criteria, but some studies have found the opposite outcome (see Morey et al., 2022a).

This has led to a veritable "box score" approach to evaluating the impairment versus trait components with competing claims as to which is more important. Some authors advocate parsing the Alternative DSM-5 Model to remove psychometric redundancy. Other authors claim that only one of its major components (either impairment in self and interpersonal functioning or the maladaptive traits) is sufficient. Another proposal has been to replace the maladaptive traits with normal personality traits, which are then used to complement the self and interpersonal functioning dimension (Morey et al., 2022b). In this regard, Clark and Ro (2014) showed that impairment in personality functioning can be empirically differentiated from both psychosocial impairment and personality traits. Similarly, Garcia et al. (2020) found that the impairment dimension of the Alternative DSM Model could be decomposed into separable variances of impairment personality functioning, psychosocial impairment, and pathological trait severity.

The scholarly debate on these matters is complex, involves conceptual and measurement nuance, and does not necessarily have to be an either–or proposition. In this regard, Zimmermann (2022) suggested a path forward could be to refine the underlying concepts and their nosological definitions. This might start, for example, by viewing the self and interpersonal functioning dimension as a set of personality *capacities*, which give rise to maladaptive trait expression in personality disorder. The task for nosology then becomes carefully defining diagnostic indicators of personality capacities and separable pathological traits.

Proponents of the psychometric-trait approach, however, emphasize results from factor-analytic studies. They argue that the appreciable covariation between measures of self and interpersonal impairment and of maladaptive traits reflects a large general factor dimension of personality disorder severity. In this regard, factor-analytic studies in the fields of personality, personality disorder, and psychopathology have found that each realm evidences a general factor, akin to the historic notion of "g," the general factor of intelligence (Spearman, 1946), in the study of intelligence. These are called general factor of personality (GFP), general factor personality disorder (*g*-PD), and general factor psychopathology (*p*-factor) (Oltmanns et al., 2018).

As noted earlier, interpretation of factor analysis is more than a technical matter. An assumption in factor analysis is that observed indicators are caused by an underlying latent factor dimension. This generates questions about causal relations and ontology. That is, one may ask are underlying personality disorder dimension(s) natural phenomena (an essentialist view), or are they better understood as social constructions and/or pragmatic representations, as many have suggested (see Zachar & Kendler, 2007)? One way to redress the hard causal implications of factor analysis is to view results as proxies with explanatory and heuristic value rather than as causal realities. A competing multivariate approach, network analysis, deals with causal relationships, and has been applied to psychopathology and to personality disorder. Network analysis systematically evaluates connecting links between symptom variables for their causal associations (Borsboom, 2017). For example, network analysis has been used to examine causal connections among the standard diagnostic operational criteria for borderline personality disorder (Richetin et al., 2017).

In this study, affective instability, identity dysfunction, and fears of abandonment demonstrated central network properties and exerted causal effects within the diagnostic criteria for borderline personality disorder. Furthermore, the authors interpreted results as supporting the self and interpersonal functioning dimension of the Alternative DSM-5 Model (particularly Identity), consistent with prominent conceptions of personality disorder within object relations and attachment/mentalization theory.

As noted earlier, much of empirical research on the Alternative DSM-5 Model has relied on self-report instruments. Thus, it is important to consider the implications of this method of measurement. Self-report assessment has advantages of relative ease of data gathering as well as being a form of direct questioning of an individual's introspection. However, advantages of self-report methods must be balanced against weaknesses. Self-report relies on the capacity, awareness, and willingness to report on personal experience. In this regard, it is known that people with internalizing personality styles and personality disorders (e.g., avoidant and dependent personality disorders) are more willing to self-report socially undesirable or negative personal and subjective qualities. However, for externalizing personality styles and personality disorders (e.g., antisocial and narcissistic personality disorders), outside observers provide more valid assessments (see Carlson et al., 2013). This phenomenon is referred to as self-observer asymmetry (Vazire, 2010). Strong arguments have been made that research in personality, personality disorder, and psychopathology relies too heavily on self-report methods (Bornstein, 2015). Similar concerns pertain to structured psychiatric interview methods. These interviews are often used as validators in psychopathology research, but they do not necessarily represent a so-called gold standard (see Noordgard et al., 2013). Notably, self-report occurs in both questionnaire and structured interview assessment, although structured interviews include a more explicit interactional component which provides some opportunity for clarifying questions. Because of their similarity, this means that validating a self-report inventory for personality disorder with a structured interview capitalizes on the shared method of assessment. Hence, this strategy may over-state relationships between the underlying constructs because the methods are similar.

Study of the Alternative DSM-5 Model and the ICD-11 approach would benefit from multi-method assessment. This refers to the practice of using different types of methods to assess and converge on constructs of interest, a longstanding desideratum in psychology (Campbell & Fiske, 1959; Cattell, 1966). Multi-method studies can use information from observer report, direct behavior samples, physiological data, family history, projective tests, life history, ecological monetary assessment, and clinician inference based on these data. Although some of these approaches have been used with these personality disorder models, the relative paucity of multi-method study has often been noted in the literature (e.g., Widiger et al., 2019).

Psychometric evaluation of the structure of the Alternative DSM-5 Model and the ICD-11 approach should be guided by construct validity concerns (i.e., fidelity to theory) as well as pragmatic needs and functions of a psychiatric nosology. To these ends, Jasperian methodological pluralism presents crucial advantages. Understanding personality disorder phenomena may require a range of concepts, theoretical paradigms, and perspectives. Furthermore, some personality disorder constructs may be best evaluated with certain methods. The self and interpersonal functioning components of the Alternative DSM-5 Model and the ICD-11 personality disorder approach may be preferentially suited to methods generally associated with their psychodynamic, narrative, and interpersonal theory heritage. Similarly, the maladaptive trait component may be well-served by the psychometric-trait and factor-analytic approaches.

4.5 Whither Dimensional Personality Disorder Diagnosis?

The two contemporary personality disorder nosologies of the Alternative DSM-5 Model and the ICD-11 represent a significant advance. First, they are dimensional models and thereby join the larger ambitions of the mental health sciences to make use of dimensional approaches. Second, these dimensional personality disorder models are connected to major clinical, theoretical, and empirical traditions in personality disorder. This is particularly evident in the self and interpersonal functioning impairment dimension. This dimension draws on multiple paradigms of personality assessment (see Hopwood et al., 2019), spanning interpersonal theory, narrative psychology, psychometric-trait approaches, and, perhaps most importantly, contemporary psychodynamic theory. This is particularly seen in the close relationship between Kernberg's (1967) seminal conception of level of personality functioning and the core axis of impairment in self and interpersonal functioning in both personality disorder models. As such, these dimensional personality disorder nosologies implicitly embody traditions and the advances in psychodynamic theory and empirical research. Speaking more broadly, one can say personality theory has been returned to personality disorder diagnosis.

Morey (1991) pointed out that, from a construct validity point of view, psychiatric diagnoses carry surplus meanings beyond operationalized diagnostic criteria. Andreasen (2007) argued advances in psychopathology require more than operationalized criteria definitions which carry risk of reification, and that humanism must be part of the picture. A strict focus on descriptive psychiatry and kindred psychometric trait conceptions of personality disorder are less accommodating of the subjective and intersubjective processes inherent in self and interpersonal functioning. Importantly, the Alternative DSM Model and the ICD-11 approaches are psychiatric nosologies. They are not comprehensive theories of personality, personality disorder, or psychopathology. Yet, they bring correctives to the reigning paradigm of operational psychiatric diagnosis introduced in the DSM-III in 1980 and admit personality theory into the diagnostic arena. These two contemporary dimensional personality disorder models invite Jasperian methodological pluralism, and they start with an idiographic, personological approach to diagnosis. This is where the underlying psychodynamic core of dimensional personality disorder returns "what it means to be human" to personality disorder diagnosis (Bender, 2019).

References

Afifi, T. O., Mather, A., Boman, J., Fleisher, W., Enns, M. W., MacMillan, H., & Sareen, J. (2011). Childhood adversity and personality disorders: Results from a nationally representative population-based study. *Journal of Psychiatric Research*, *45*(6), 814–822.

American Psychiatric Association. (1968). *Diagnostic and statistical manual of mental disorders* (2nd ed.). American Psychiatric Association.

American Psychiatric Association. (1980). *Diagnostic and statistical manual of mental disorders* (3rd ed.). American Psychiatric Association.

American Psychiatric Association. (2013). *Diagnostic and statistical manual of mental disorders* (5th ed.). American Psychiatric Association.

Andreasen, N. C. (2007). DSM and the death of phenomenology in America: An example of unintended consequences. *Schizophrenia Bulletin*, *33*(1), 108–112.

Bach, B., & Tracy, M. (2022). Clinical utility of the alternative model of personality disorders: A 10th year anniversary review. *Personality Disorders*, *13*(4), 369–379.

Banicki, K. (2020). Beyond the categorical–dimensional dichotomy: An exercise of conceptual geography in the domain of personality disorders. *Journal of Theoretical and Philosophical Psychology*, *40*(4), 219–239.

Beebe, B., & Lachmann, F. M. (2013). *Infant research and adult treatment: Co-constructing interactions*. Routledge.

Bender, D. S. (2019). The P-factor and what it means to be human: Commentary on criterion A of the AMPD in HiTOP. *Journal of Personality Assessment*, *101*(4), 356–359.

Bender, D. S., Morey, L. C., & Skodol, A. E. (2011). Toward a model for assessing level of personality functioning in DSM-5, part I: A review of theory and methods. *Journal of Personality Assessment*, *93*(4), 332–346.

Benjamin, J. (1990). An outline of intersubjectivity: The development of recognition. *Psychoanalytic Psychology*, *7*, 33–46.

Berrios, G. E., & Marková, I. S. (2013). Is the concept of "dimension" applicable to psychiatric objects? *World Psychiatry: Official Journal of the World Psychiatric Association*, 12(1), 76–78.

Bollas, C. (1987/2017). *The shadow of the object: Psychoanalysis of the unthought known*. Routledge.

Bornstein, R. F. (2005). Reconnecting psychoanalysis to mainstream psychology. Challenges and opportunities. *Psychoanalytic Psychology, 22*(3), 323–340.

Bornstein, R. F. (2015). Personality assessment in the diagnostic manuals: On mindfulness, multiple methods, and test score discontinuities. *Journal of Personality Assessment, 97*(5), 446–455.

Borsboom, D. (2017). Representation and explanation in psychometric modeling. In K. Kendler & J. Parnas (eds.), *Philosophical issues in psychiatry IV: Classification of psychiatric illness* (pp. 45–50). Oxford University Press.

Borsboom, D., Mellenbergh, G. J., & van Heerden, J. (2003). The theoretical status of latent variables. *Psychological Review, 110*(2), 203–219.

Bowlby, J. (1979). The Bowlby–Ainsworth attachment theory. *Behavioral and Brain Sciences, 2*(4), 637–638.

Bowlby, J. (1980). *Attachment and loss, Vol. 3: Loss: Sadness and depression*. Hogarth Press.

Brown, T. L. (2003). *Making truth: Metaphor in science*. University of Illinois Press.

Bürgy, M. (2008). The concept of psychosis: Historical and phenomenological aspects. *Schizophrenia Bulletin, 34*(6), 1200–1210.

Caligor, E., Kernberg, O. F., Clarkin, J. F., & Yeomans, F. E. (2018). *Psychodynamic therapy for personality pathology: Treating self and interpersonal functioning*. American Psychiatric Association.

Campbell, C., & Allison, E. (2022). Mentalizing the modern world. *Psychoanalytic Psychotherapy, 36*(3), 206–217.

Campbell, D. T., & Fiske, D. W. (1959). Convergent and discriminant validation by the multitrait–multimethod matrix. *Psychological Bulletin, 56*(2), 81–105.

Carlson, E. N., Vazire, S., & Oltmanns, T. F. (2013). Self-other knowledge asymmetries in personality pathology. *Journal of Personality, 81*(2), 155–170.

Cattell, R. B. (1966). The data box: Its ordering of total resources in terms of possible relational systems. In J. R. Nesselroade & R. B. Cattell (eds.), *Handbook of multivariate experimental psychology* (pp. 69–130). Springer.

Chu, J. A. (1991). The repetition compulsion revisited: Reliving dissociated trauma. *Psychotherapy: Theory, Research, Practice, Training, 28*(2), 327–332.

Clark, L. A. (2007). Assessment and diagnosis of personality disorder: Perennial issues and an emerging reconceptualization. *Annual Review of Psychology, 58*, 227–257.

Clark, L. A., & Ro, E. (2014). Three-pronged assessment and diagnosis of personality disorder and its consequences: Personality functioning, pathological traits, and psychosocial disability. *Personality Disorders: Theory, Research, and Treatment, 5*(1), 55–69.

Clark, L. A., Vanderbleek, E. N., Shapiro, J. L., Nuzum, H., Allen, X., Daly, E., . . . & Ro, E. (2015). The brave new world of personality disorder-trait specified: Effects of additional definitions on coverage, prevalence, and comorbidity. *Psychopathology Review, 2*(1), 52–82.

Clarkin, J. F., Cain, N., & Livesley, W. J. (2015). An integrated approach to treatment of patients with personality disorders. *Journal of Psychotherapy Integration, 25*(1), 3–12.

Clarkin, J. F., Caligor, E., & Sowislo, J. F. (2020). An object relations model perspective on the alternative model for personality disorders (DSM-5). *Psychopathology, 53*(3), 141–148.

Cloninger, C. R., Svrakic, D. M., & Przybeck, T. R. (1993). A psychobiological model of temperament and character. *Archives of General Psychiatry*, *50*(12), 975–990.
Costa Jr, P. T., & McCrae, R. R. (1992). The five-factor model of personality and its relevance to personality disorders. *Journal of Personality Disorders*, *6*(4), 343–359.
Deutsch, H. (1942). Some forms of emotional disturbance and their relationship to schizophrenia. *The Psychoanalytic Quarterly*, *11*, 301–321.
Doyle, C., & Cicchetti, D. (2017). From the cradle to the grave: The effect of adverse caregiving environments on attachment and relationships throughout the lifespan. *Clinical Psychology: Science and Practice*, *24*(2), 203–217.
Erikson, E. H. (1959). *Identity and the life cycle: Selected papers*. International Universities Press.
Evans, C. M., & Simms, L. J. (2023). Do self and interpersonal dysfunction cross-sectionally mediate the association between adverse childhood experiences and personality pathology? *Personality and Mental Health*, *17*(3), 259–271.
Fabrigar, L. R., Wegener, D. T., MacCallum, R. C., & Strahan, E. J. (1999). Evaluating the use of exploratory factor analysis in psychological research. *Psychological Methods*, *4*(3), 272–299.
Flanagan, O. (1991). *The science of the mind*. MIT Press.
Fonagy, P., Gergely, G., Jurist, E. L., & Target, M. (2002). *Affect regulation, mentalization, and the development of the self.* Other Press.
Fonagy, P., & Luyten, P. (2009). A developmental, mentalization-based approach to the understanding and treatment of borderline personality disorder. *Development and Psychopathology*, *21*(4), 1355–1381.
Fonagy, P., Luyten, P., & Allison, E. (2015). Epistemic petrification and the restoration of epistemic trust: A new conceptualization of borderline personality disorder and its psychosocial treatment. *Journal of Personality Disorders*, *29*(5), 575–609.
Freud, A. (1946/2018). *The ego and the mechanisms of defence*. Routledge.
Freud, S. (1896/1962). The aetiology of hysteria. In J. Strachey (ed.), *The standard edition of the complete psychological works of Sigmund Freud* (Vol. 3). Hogarth.
Garcia, D. J., Waugh, M. H., Skadberg, R. M., Crittenden, E. B., Finn, M. T. M., Schmidt, M. R., & Kurdziel-Adams, G. (2020). Deconstructing criterion a of the alternative model for personality disorders. *Personality Disorders*, *12*(4), 320–330.
Gazzillo, F., Genova, F., Fedeli, F., Curtis, J. T., Silberschatz, G., Bush, M., & Dazzi, N. (2019). Patients' unconscious testing activity in psychotherapy: A theoretical and empirical overview. *Psychoanalytic Psychology*, *36*(2), 173–183.
Goldberg, L. R. (1993). The structure of phenotypic personality traits. *American Psychologist*, 48, 26–34.
Greenberg, J. (1983). *Object relations in psychoanalytic theory.* Harvard University Press.
Greenwald, A. G., & Lai, C. K. (2020). Implicit social cognition. *Annual Review of Psychology*, *71*, 419–445.
Haslam, N., Holland, E., & Kuppens, P. (2012). Categories versus dimensions in personality and psychopathology: A quantitative review of taxometric research. *Psychological Medicine*, *42*(5), 903–920.
Haslam, N., McGrath, M. J., Viechtbauer, W., & Kuppens, P. (2020). Dimensions over categories: A meta-analysis of taxometric research. *Psychological Medicine*, *50*(9), 1418–1432.

Hayes, S. C., Strosahl, K. D., & Wilson, K. G. (2011). *Acceptance and commitment therapy: The process and practice of mindful change*. Guilford Press.
Hoch, P., & Polatin, P. (1949). Pseudoneurotic forms of schizophrenia. *Psychiatric Quarterly*, *23*, 248–276.
Hopwood, C. J., Kotov, R., Krueger, R. F., Watson, D., Widiger, T. A., Althoff, R. R., . . . & Zimmermann, J. (2018). The time has come for dimensional personality disorder diagnosis. *Personality and Mental Health*, *12*(1), 82–86.
Hopwood, C. J., Morey, L. C., & Markon, K. E. (2023). What is a psychopathology dimension? *Clinical Psychology Review*, *106*, 102356.
Hopwood, C. J., Mulay, A. L., & Waugh, M. H. (eds.). (2019). *The DSM-5 alternative model for personality disorders: Integrating multiple paradigms of personality assessment*. Routledge.
Jaspers, K. (1968). The phenomenological approach in psychopathology. *The British Journal of Psychiatry*, *114*(516), 1313–1323.
Johnson, J. G., Cohen, P., Brown, J., Smailes, E. M., & Bernstein, D. P. (1999). Childhood maltreatment increases risk for personality disorders during early adulthood. *Archives of General Psychiatry*, *56*(7), 600–606.
Kahneman, D., Slovic, P., & Tversky, A. (Eds.). (1982). *Judgment under uncertainty: Heuristics and biases*. Cambridge University Press.
Kendler, K. S. (2016). The nature of psychiatric disorders. *World Psychiatry*, *15* (1), 5–12.
Kernberg, O. (1967). Borderline personality organization. *Journal of the American Psychoanalytic Association*, *15*(3), 641–685.
Kernberg, O. F. (1995). *Object relations theory and clinical psychoanalysis*. Jason Aronson.
Kernberg, O. F. (2016). What is personality? *Journal of Personality Disorders*, *30*(2), 145–156.
Kernberg, O. F. (2022). Some implications of new developments in neurobiology for psychoanalytic object relations theory. *Neuropsychoanalysis*, *24*(1), 3–12.
Klerman, G. L. (1986). Historical perspectives on contemporary schools of psychopathology. In T. Millon & G. L. Klerman (eds.), *Contemporary directions in psychopathology: Toward the DSM-IV* (pp. 3–28). The Guilford Press.
Knief, U., & Forstmeier, W. (2021). Violating the normality assumption may be the lesser of two evils. *Behavior Research Methods*, *53*(6), 2576–2590.
Kohut, H. (1966). Forms and transformations of narcissism. *Journal of the American Psychoanalytic Association*, *14*(2), 243–272.
Kotov, R., Waszczuk, M. A., Krueger, R. F., Forbes, M. K., Watson, D., Clark, L. A., . . . & Zimmerman, M. (2017). The hierarchical taxonomy of psychopathology (HiTOP): A dimensional alternative to traditional nosologies. *Journal of Abnormal Psychology*, 126(4), 454–477.
Krueger, R. F. (2013). Personality disorders are the vanguard of the post-DSM-5.0 era. *Personality Disorders: Theory, Research, and Treatment*, *4*(4), 355–362.
Krueger, R. F., Derringer, J., Markon, K. E., Watson, D., & Skodol, A. E. (2012). Initial construction of a maladaptive personality trait model and inventory for DSM-5. *Psychological Medicine*, *42*, 1879–1890.

Levendosky, A. A., Turchan, J. E., Luo, X., & Good, E. (2023). A re-introduction of the psychodynamic approach to the standard clinical psychology curriculum. *Journal of Clinical Psychology*, *79*, 2439–2451.

Lieb, K., Zanarini, M. C., Schmahl, C., Linehan, M. M., & Bohus, M. (2004). Borderline personality disorder. *The Lancet*, *364*(9432), 453–461.

Lind, M., Adler, J. M., & Clark, L. A. (2020). Narrative identity and personality disorder: An empirical and conceptual review. *Current Psychiatry Reports*, *22*, 1–11.

Lind, M., Sharp, C., & Dunlop, W. L. (2022). Why, how, and when to integrate narrative identity within dimensional approaches to personality disorders. *Journal of Personality Disorders*, *36*(4), 377–398.

Lingiardi, V., & McWilliams, N. (eds.). (2017). *Psychodynamic diagnostic manual: PDM-2*. Guilford Press.

Livesley, W. J. (1998). Suggestions for a framework for an empirically based classification of personality disorder. *The Canadian Journal of Psychiatry*, *43*(2), 137–147.

Loevinger, J. (1957). Objective tests as instruments of psychological theory. *Psychological Reports*, *3*(3), 635–694.

Loevinger, J. (1966a). Three principles for a psychoanalytic psychology. *Journal of Abnormal Psychology*, *71*(6), 432–443.

Loevinger, J. (1966b). The meaning and measurement of ego development. *American Psychologist*, *21*(3), 195–206.

Luborsky, L., & Crits-Christoph, P. (1998). *Understanding transference: The core conflictual relationship theme method*. American Psychological Association.

Luyten, P., Mayes, L. C., Blatt, S. J., Target, M., & Fonagy, P. (2015). Theoretical and empirical foundations of contemporary psychodynamic approaches. In P. Luyten, L. C. Mayes, P. Fonagy, M. Target, & S. J. Blatt (eds.), *Handbook of psychodynamic approaches to psychopathology* (pp. 3–26). The Guilford Press.

McAdams, D. P. (1994). A psychology of the stranger. *Psychological Inquiry*, *5*(2), 145–148.

McAdams, D. P. (1995). What do we know when we know a person? *Journal of Personality*, *63*(3), 365–396.

McAdams, D. P. (2015). *The art and science of personality development*. Guilford Press.

McAdams, D. P., & Pals, J. L. (2006). A new Big Five: Fundamental principles for an integrative science of personality. *The American Psychologist*, *61*(3), 204–217.

McCabe, G. A., Oltmanns, J. R., & Widiger, T. A. (2021). Criterion A scales: Convergent, discriminant, and structural relationships. *Assessment*, *28*(3), 813–828.

McCarthy, C. (2017, April 17). The Kekule problem. *Nautilus*, *19*, 22–31.

McWilliams, N. (2011). *Psychoanalytic diagnosis: Understanding personality structure in the clinical process* (2nd ed.). Guilford Press.

McWilliams, N. (2020). The future of psychoanalysis: Preserving Jeremy Safran's integrative vision. *Psychoanalytic Psychology*, *37*(2), 98–107.

Meehl, P. E. (1992). Factors and taxa, traits and types, differences of degree and differences in kind. *Journal of Personality*, 60(1), 117–174.

Millon, T. (2016). What is a personality disorder? *Journal of Personality Disorders*, *30* (3), 289–306.

Morey, L. C. (1991). Classification of mental disorder as a collection of hypothetical constructs. *Journal of Abnormal Psychology*, *100*(3), 289–293.

Morey, L. C. (2017). Development and initial evaluation of a self-report form of the DSM-5 Level of Personality Functioning Scale. *Psychological Assessment*, *29*(10), 1302–1308.

Morey, L. C., Good, E. W., & Hopwood, C. J. (2022a). Global personality dysfunction and the relationship of pathological and normal trait domains in the DSM-5 alternative model for personality disorders. *Journal of Personality*, *90*(1), 34–46.

Morey, L. C., McCredie, M. N., Bender, D. S., & Skodol, A. E. (2022b). Criterion A: Level of personality functioning in the alternative DSM-5 model for personality disorders. *Personality Disorders: Theory, Research, and Treatment*, *13*(4), 305–315.

Mulay, A. L., Cain, N. M., Waugh, M. H., Hopwood, C. J., Adler, J. M., Garcia, D. J., . . . & Skadberg, R. (2018). Personality constructs and paradigms in the alternative DSM-5 model of personality disorder. *Journal of Personality Assessment*, *100*(6), 593–602.

Mulay, A. L., Waugh, M. H., Fillauer, J. P., Bender, D. S., Bram, A., Cain, N. M., . . . & Skodol, A. E. (2019). Borderline personality disorder diagnosis in a new key. *Borderline Personality Disorder and Emotion Dysregulation*, *6*(1), 1–16.

Murray, H. (1938). *Explorations in personality*. Oxford University Press.

Nordgaard, J., Sass, L. A., & Parnas, J. (2013). The psychiatric interview: Validity, structure, and subjectivity. *European Archives of Psychiatry and Clinical Neuroscience*, *263*, 353–364.

Oltmanns, J. R., Smith, G. T., Oltmanns, T. F., & Widiger, T. A. (2018). General factors of psychopathology, personality, and personality disorder: Across domain comparisons. *Clinical Psychological Science*, *6*(4), 581–589.

Panksepp, J. (2004). *Affective neuroscience: The foundations of human and animal emotions*. Oxford University Press.

Panksepp, J., & Solms, M. (2012). What is neuropsychoanalysis? Clinically relevant studies of the minded brain. *Trends in Cognitive Sciences*, *16*(1), 6–8.

Peterfreund, E. (1980). On information and systems models for psychoanalysis. *International Review of Psycho-Analysis*, *7*, 327–345.

Pincus, A. L., Cain, N. M., & Halberstadt, A. L. (2020). Importance of self and other in defining personality pathology. *Psychopathology*, 53(3–4), 133–140.

Regier, D. A., Kuhl, E. A., & Kupfer, D. J. (2013). The DSM-5: Classification and criteria changes. *World Psychiatry*, *12*(2), 92–98.

Richetin, J., Preti, E., Costantini, G., & De Panfilis, C. (2017). The centrality of affective instability and identity in Borderline Personality Disorder: Evidence from network analysis. *PLoS One*, 12(10), e0186695.

Ronningstam, E. (2022). Narcissistic personality disorder. In S. K. Huprich (ed.), *Personality disorders and pathology: Integrating clinical assessment and practice in the DSM-5 and ICD-11 era* (pp. 375–389). American Psychological Association.

Sarbin, T. R. (1986). *Narrative psychology: The storied nature of human conduct*. Praeger Publishers/Greenwood Publishing Group.

Schafer, R. (1970). The psychoanalytic vision of reality. *The International Journal of Psycho-analysis*, *51*, 279–297.

Schafer, R. (1992). *Retelling a life: Narration and dialogue in psychoanalysis*. Basic Books.

Schore, A. N. (2021). The interpersonal neurobiology of intersubjectivity. *Frontiers in Psychology*, *12*, 648616.

Sharp, C. (2022). Fulfilling the promise of the LPF: Comment on Morey et al. (2022). *Personality Disorders*, *13*(4), 316–320.

Sharp, C., & Wall, K. (2021). DSM-5 level of personality functioning: Refocusing personality disorder on what it means to be human. *Annual Review of Clinical Psychology*, *17*, 313–337.

Shedler, J. (2022). That was then, this is now: Psychoanalytic psychotherapy for the rest of us. *Contemporary Psychoanalysis*, *58*(2–3), 405–437.

Shorter, E. (2013). The history of DSM. In: J. Paris & J. Phillips (eds.), *Making the DSM-5* (pp. 3–19). Springer.

Sleep, C. E., & Lynam, D. R. (2022). The problems with Criterion A: A comment on Morey et al. (2022). *Personality Disorders: Theory, Research, and Treatment*, *13*(4), 325–327.

Spearman, C. (1946). Theory of general factor. *British Journal of Psychology*, *36*, 117–131.

Spence, D. P. (1982). *Narrative truth and historical truth: Meaning and interpretation in psychoanalysis*. Norton.

Sperber, D., Clément, F., Heintz, C., Mascaro, O., Mercier, H., Origgi, G., & Wilson, D. (2010). Epistemic vigilance. *Mind & Language*, *25*(4), 359–393.

Stern, D., Sander, L. W., Nahum, J. P., Harrison, A. M., Lyons-Ruth, K., Morgan, A. C., … & Process of Change Study Group (1998). Non-interpretive mechanisms in psychoanalytic therapy: The 'something more' than interpretation. *The International Journal of Psycho-Analysis*, *79*(5), 903–921.

Stevens, S. S. (1946). On the theory of scales of measurement. *Science*, *103*(2684), 677–680.

Stolorow, R. D. (1997). Dynamic, dyadic, intersubjective systems: An evolving paradigm for psychoanalysis. *Psychoanalytic Psychology*, *14*(3), 337–346.

Stolorow, R. D., Atwood, G. E., & Branchaft, B. (eds.). (1994). *The intersubjective perspective*. Rowman & Littlefield.

Stuss, D. T. (1991). Self, awareness, and the frontal lobes: A neuropsychological perspective. In *The self: Interdisciplinary approaches* (pp. 255–278). Springer New York.

Trevarthen, C., & Aitken, K. J. (2001). Infant intersubjectivity: Research, theory, and clinical applications. *The Journal of Child Psychology and Psychiatry and Allied Disciplines*, *42*(1), 3–48.

Vaillant, G. E. (1992). *Ego mechanisms of defense: A guide for clinicians and researchers*. American Psychiatric Association.

Van der Kolk, B. A. (1994). The body keeps the score: Memory and the evolving psychobiology of posttraumatic stress. *Harvard Review of Psychiatry*, *1*(5), 253–265.

Vazire, S. (2010). Who knows what about a person? The self-other knowledge asymmetry (SOKA) model. *Journal of Personality and Social Psychology*, *98*(2), 281–300.

Waugh, M. H., Hopwood, C. J., Krueger, R. F., Morey, L. C., Pincus, A. L., & Wright, A. G. C. (2017). Psychological assessment with the DSM-5 Alternative Model for personality disorders: Tradition and innovation. *Professional Psychology, Research and Practice*, *48*(2), 79–89.

Westen, D. (1998). The scientific legacy of Sigmund Freud: Toward a psychodynamically informed psychological science. *Psychological Bulletin*, *124* (3), 333–371.

Widiger, T. A., & Trull, T. J. (2007). Plate tectonics in the classification of personality disorder: Shifting to a dimensional model. *American Psychologist*, *62*(2), 71–83.

Widiger, T. A., Bach, B., Chmielewski, M., Clark, L. A., DeYoung, C., Hopwood, C. J., . . . & Thomas, K. M. (2019). Criterion A of the AMPD in HiTOP. *Journal of Personality Assessment*, 101(4), 345–355.

Winnicott, D. W. (1969). The use of an object. *The International Journal of Psychoanalysis*, *50*(4), 711–716.

World Health Organization. (2022). *ICD-11: International classification of diseases* (11th revision). https://icd.who.int/

Yalch, M. M. (2020). Psychodynamic underpinnings of the DSM-5 Alternative Model for personality disorder. *Psychoanalytic Psychology*, *37*(3), 219–231.

Young, J. E., Klosko, J. S., & Weishaar, M. E. (2006). *Schema therapy: A practitioner's guide*. Guilford Press.

Zachar, P., & Kendler, K. S. (2007). Psychiatric disorders: A conceptual taxonomy. *American Journal of Psychiatry*, *164*(4), 557–565.

Zachar, P., Krueger, R., & Kendler, K (2016). Personality disorder in DSM-5: An oral history. *Psychological Medicine*, *46*(1), 1–10.

Zimmermann, J. (2022). Beyond defending or abolishing Criterion A: Comment on Morey et al. (2022). *Personality Disorders: Theory, Research, and Treatment*, *13*(4), 321–324. https://doi.org/10.1037/per0000561

Zimmermann, J., Böhnke, J. R., Eschstruth, R., Mathews, A., Wenzel, K., & Leising, D. (2015). The latent structure of personality functioning: Investigating Criterion A from the Alternative Model for Personality Disorders in DSM-5. *Journal of Abnormal Psychology*, *124*(3), 532–548.

Zimmermann, J., Kerber, A., Rek, K., Hopwood, C. J., & Krueger, R. F. (2019). A brief but comprehensive review of research on the alternative DSM-5 model for personality disorders. *Current Psychiatry Reports*, *21*, 1–19.

5 Multiple Roads to Pathology

A Complex Systems Perspective on Personality Disorders

Angélique O. J. Cramer and Denny Borsboom

5.1 Introduction

The history of personality disorders is not without controversy and debate, if only because of (ongoing) disagreement concerning their fundamental nature. What are personality disorders (PDs) really (Berrios, 1993; Crocq, 2013)? Can PDs be successfully treated or is our only hope 'no cure but control' (e.g. Bateman et al., 2015; Katakis et al., 2023; Laws et al., 2000)? Generating answers to these fundamental questions is not merely an interesting academic pursuit. We owe it to people suffering from PDs in numerous ways, often from early adolescence onwards, who feature decreased physical and mental health and may not be able to finish an education or hold down a job (e.g. Hastrup et al., 2019; Moran et al., 2016; Skodol, 2016). The main aim of this chapter is to present a complex systems perspective as a potential contribution to answering the fundamental question: what are PDs?

To begin answering the question of what PDs are, one needs to start at the very core: is a PD something that is either present or absent in someone – that is, *categorical* in nature, akin to Down's syndrome; or is it something that one has to a certain extent – that is, *continuous* in nature, akin to height (e.g. Borsboom et al., 2016)? For quite a long time a categorical framework prevailed – not without early criticism (e.g. Frances, 1993; Widiger, 1993) – but ever since the inception of the latest edition of the *Diagnostic and statistical manual of mental disorders* (DSM-5; American Psychiatric Association, 2013) a continuous approach is embraced – the Alternative Model of Personality Disorders (AMPD) – in which PDs, among other criteria, are regarded to be some constellation of rather extreme manifestations of otherwise normal personality traits divided into five distinct domains, similar to the Big Five (e.g. Krueger et al., 2012; Krueger & Hobbs, 2020; Widiger & McCabe, 2020; Widiger & Mullins-Sweatt, 2009).

Although we view the move towards a more dimensional approach to PDs as more in line with reality, dimensional approaches such as AMPD still suffer from an underlying key assumption that we think is problematic. This concerns the relationship between a trait – say, negative affectivity – and the items – say, often feeling tense or jittery – used to measure someone's stance on the trait continuum. An important line of thought in personality theory (e.g. McCrae & Costa, 2008) holds that personality traits *cause* these (observable) item scores: for example, someone suffers from negative affectivity to a great extent and *this causes* the person to feel jittery or tense often. In this chapter, we start by outlining why this assumption might be flawed and argue for a relationship between (pathological) trait and its respective items that is exactly reversed (e.g. Cramer et al., 2012). Next, we will describe a dynamical systems model in which personality – relatively normal or a PD – is the ultimate outcome (i.e. equilibrium state) of dynamical couplings between thoughts, feelings, behaviours and environment. We will demonstrate some of the ways in which such a system might end up in a state of PD by means of a toy simulation model.

5.2 Personality Disorders: Not Common Causes But Potential Consequences

Both dimensional and earlier categorical approaches to PDs share the same underlying assumption, namely that, ultimately, a PD is the cause of its respective symptoms (i.e. the *common cause* assumption; Cramer et al., 2010; Cramer, van der Sluis, et al., 2012a). This assumption concretely means, for example, that narcissistic personality disorder is the very *reason* for, or the ultimate *cause* of, that person having an unreasonably high sense of self-importance and displaying a tendency to withdraw from situations in which failure might be imminent. If one would draw an arrow of time, the common cause assumption entails that the PD comes first and causes a set of observable symptoms that come at a later point in time. This assumption was borrowed from medical sciences, where it seems a sensible assumption for quite a few diseases: one only develops symptoms of lung cancer after a malignant tumour has started to grow in one's lungs (lung cancer → symptoms); analogously, one only develops the hallmark symptoms of Down's syndrome after abnormal cell division results in an extra partial or full chromosome 21 (Down's syndrome → symptoms).

We see two major reasons for doubting the veracity of the common cause assumption for mental health conditions. First, in contrast to lung cancer, in which case one can point to a computed tomography (CT) scan to show the actual presence of a malignant mass, we currently have no irrefutable evidence for the existence of a common cause anywhere in our brains, minds, immune systems and/or biology (Borsboom et al., 2019; Moncrieff et al., 2023). That is, a realist interpretation of mental health conditions as entities (e.g. a particular structural brain anomaly), particular content (e.g. memories of an unpleasant childhood) or certain properties (e.g. decreased availability of a particular neurotransmitter), separate from their observable symptoms, is simply unwarranted given the current body of evidence.

Second, in our view, common cause models do not provide the most compelling explanation for the one uncontested fact in clinical psychology and psychiatry, namely that symptoms tend to systematically covary with one another. Take two symptoms of narcissistic personality disorder: inability to recognize the needs and feelings of others and taking advantage of others. There is no need to invoke a hitherto undiscovered common cause to explain why these two symptoms covary with one another. A far more plausible explanation of this covariation is that these symptoms directly interact with one another: for example, if one is incapable of recognizing the needs and feelings of others, this makes it easier to use other people to one's own advantage (i.e. one symptom *facilitates* the development of another symptom). In PDs as in other disorders, myriad interactions between symptoms are likely, and these may in themselves be responsible for the reliable patterns of covariation between symptoms that we observe in the data.

So, suppose we accept that PDs are not common causes of their symptoms, and pursue the hypothesis that symptoms of PDs covary because they directly interact with one another: what is a PD then? From the *network perspective*, with its basic premise being that symptoms of mental disorders directly interact with one another (Borsboom, 2017; Cramer et al., 2010, 2016), the answer is that a PD is the potential *consequence*, not the cause, of these direct symptom–symptom interactions. So, for example, borderline personality disorder may arise from direct interactions between symptoms such as fear of abandonment, emotional outbursts and having intense yet unstable relationships (e.g. fear of abandonment → being angry at partner for perceived betrayal → unstable relationship; see von Klipstein et al., 2021).

However, although some of the symptoms of PDs constitute (perhaps in milder form) thoughts, behaviours or feelings that everybody has or displays from time to time – for example, being flirtatious (histrionic) or fearing abandonment (borderline) – many symptoms of PDs are in themselves quite problematic or extreme: for example, self-harm (borderline) or requiring constant and/or excessive admiration (narcissistic). This is quite different from common mental health conditions such as depression and anxiety, where relatively more symptoms seem to be comparatively normal (e.g. concentration problems in depression, experiencing heart palpitations in anxiety). In addition, common mental health conditions (i.e. depression, anxiety and addiction) develop on a faster timescale – with multiple episodes and recovery thereof across the lifespan – compared to personality, which develops on a slower timescale (Lunansky et al., 2020). As such, in our view, readily translating the network perspective on common mental disorders with a focus on symptom–symptom interactions into a version for PDs is perhaps insufficient. Therefore, in the next sections we will elaborate on a theoretical model whose elements are not primarily symptoms.

5.3 A Mutualism Model of Personality Disorders

In a seminal paper, Van Der Maas et al. (2006) proposed a so-called *mutualism model* to account for the positive covariation between various cognitive tasks and/or intelligence tests (e.g. arithmetic, vocabulary). The hitherto dominant explanation was to suppose that a common cause, general intelligence, was the main driver behind this positive covariation. This general intelligence, *g*, was hypothesized to be many things, ranging from 'mental energy' to working memory (e.g. Ackerman et al., 2005), but, analogous to the common cause hunt in clinical psychology and psychiatry, no one candidate turned out to be the sought-after material referent of 'general intelligence'.

The mutualism model accounts for the positive covariation between cognitive tasks by assuming that the cognitive processes needed to perform on such tasks interact with one another during development in a mutually beneficial or facilitating manner: for example, development of the cognitive process 'attention' facilitates the development of the cognitive process 'perception' – it is easier to perceive a trick question in an arithmetic test if one's attention is focused on the test at hand – and vice versa – the 'pop-out' phenomenon in which the rapid perception of, say, the letter M among a set of Ws focuses attention on the odd element M (Hochstein, 2012). Over time, these mutualistic relationships between cognitive processes during development culminate in an *equilibrium*, or stable state, in which someone possesses a certain level of intelligence (i.e. cognitive skills have *grown* towards a certain asymptotic maximum): highly optimized and strong beneficial relationships between cognitive processes will result in a stable state of a relatively high general intelligence, whereas less strong or less beneficial relationships will result in a stable state of a relatively lower general intelligence. So, analogous to the network perspective outlined in the previous paragraph, in a mutualism model general intelligence is a stable outcome of interactions between cognitive processes and not a common cause of these processes. Both the mutualism model and the network perspective operate from the assumption that a psychological construct (e.g. intelligence, or major depression) is a *complex dynamical system*: a system consisting of certain elements (e.g. symptoms of major depression) that interact with one another over time (e.g. insomnia → fatigue) culminating, over time, in the system being in a certain state (e.g. depressed state). In this chapter we propose an analogous model for personality disorders in which a PD is a potential – undesired – equilibrium state of a complex dynamical system.

We start with the building blocks of the development of personality that we explicated in earlier work (Cramer, van der Sluis, et al., 2012a; Cramer, van Der Sluis, et al., 2012b). These building blocks are *components* of personality that exert a unique pattern of causes and effects in relation to other personality components in a network structure (similar but not analogous to the concept of *nuances*, which are defined based on specific variance, e.g. see Condon et al., 2021; Mõttus et al., 2020). Typically, these components correspond to items used in personality measurement instruments – for example, the NEO-PI-3 (McCrae et al., 2005) – but this is not always the case. For example, the items 'social gatherings are usually boring to me' and 'I think most of the people I deal with are honest and trustworthy' are both personality components because they exert different effects on, for example, the component 'I like to have a lot of people around me'. In contrast, the items 'I am dominant and assertive' and 'I find it easy to take charge of a situation' are less likely to constitute two separate personality components as both items might exert similar effects on other components, for example 'I have often been a leader of groups I have belonged to'. These personality components (i.e. the squares in Figure 5.1) start interacting with one another from the early stages of development (i.e. the solid or dashed black lines between the squares in Figure 5.1) and can be categorized as belonging to one of four *domains*: thoughts, feelings, behaviours and environment.

For example, during early stages of development, a securely attached child believes that other people are essentially well-intentioned (thought), as a result of which the child loves to interact with familiar people and meet new ones (behaviour), tries to set up play dates (environment) and feels happy when there are other people around (feelings). These interactions between personality components, over time, form network structures, both within a particular domain – for example, one thought ('The world is a jungle and only the strongest survive') reinforcing or facilitating another thought ('I cannot be weak') – and across domains – for example, a thought ('I am worthy of love') facilitating a certain behaviour (engaging in some self-care practice).

As a result of these interactions over time between personality components at the *micro* level, certain couplings, broad tendencies to interact with one another in a certain way, between the four domains start to emerge at the *macro* level (see the middle of Figure 5.1, the thick black double-headed arrows (couplings) between the four domains thoughts, feelings, behaviours and environment): for example, certain thoughts ('The world is a dangerous place', 'Generally, people cannot be trusted') become coupled to certain feelings and (selection of certain, available) environments (e.g. feeling out of place and somewhat anxious in social situations, avoiding large crowds). If network structures gradually develop in this way, patterns that form at the micro level can lead to more general, macroscopic dispositions. Ultimately, when a person reaches young

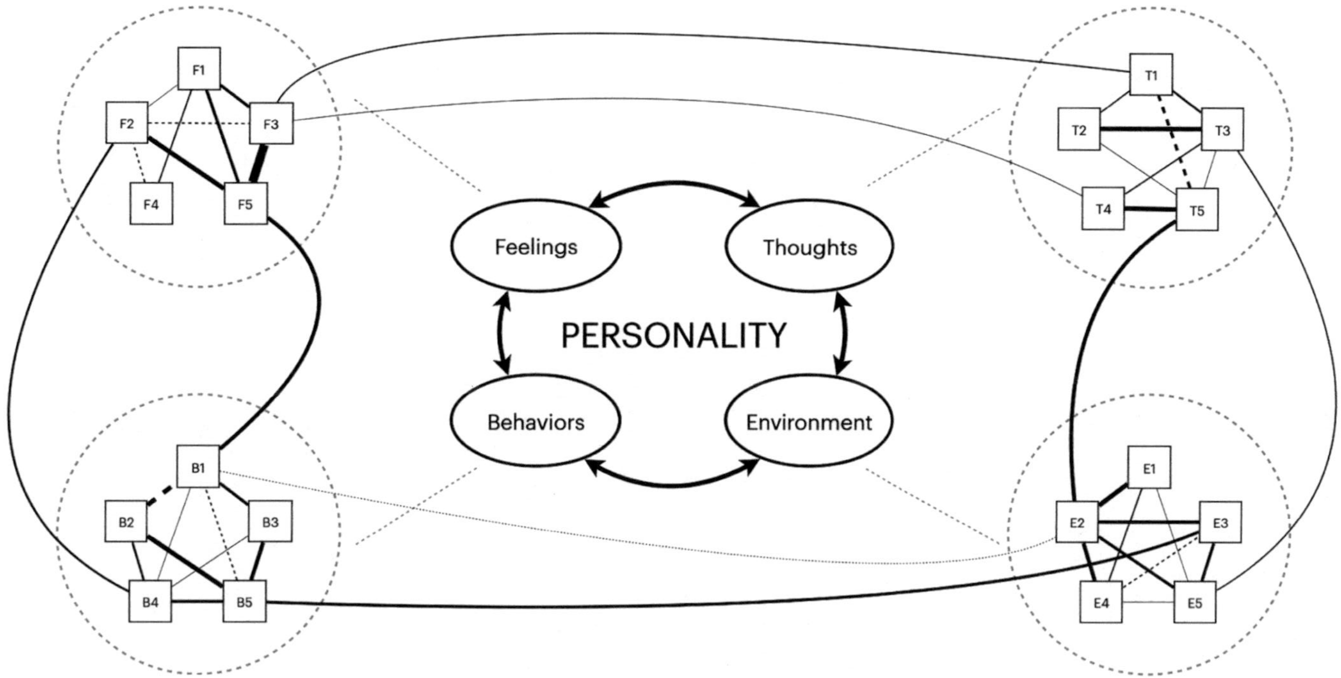

Figure 5.1 A dynamical systems perspective on (dysfunctional) personality. Personality components – visualized as squares – interact with one another – visualized as lines between these squares – in network structures: solid lines represent positive interactions while dashed lines represent negative interactions. The thicker the (dashed) line between two components, the stronger the interaction between them. Over time these interactions give rise to dynamical couplings (black double-headed arrows) between four domains (ovals): thoughts, feelings, behaviors and environment. These dynamical couplings eventually result in a certain personality.

adulthood, these couplings – like the grooves in a vinyl record – have become relatively stable, generic tendencies for a person to think, feel and behave in interaction with the environment: that is, a personality.

Importantly, in contrast to existing network and systems literature on common mental disorders in which the underlying assumption is that a mental disorder system has two states ('healthy' and 'disordered'; Borsboom, 2017; Cramer et al., 2016), our proposed personality system eventually settles in one state, some personality type, that lies somewhere on a spectrum with 'functional' at one extreme (i.e. not without its quirks but a relatively normal personality) and 'dysfunctional' at the other extreme (i.e. a PD). In that sense, we assume that personality, and disorders thereof, are potentially more akin to intelligence – with the exception of catastrophic events such as a traumatic brain injury, a person cannot transition from a highly intelligent state to a state of mental retardation but, instead, settles into a particular equilibrium state – than to common mental disorders where multiple recovery (i.e. transitioning from a disordered state into a healthy state) and relapse phases (i.e. transitioning from a healthy into a disordered state) are part and parcel of living with these disorders (Cuijpers et al., 2014; Fleury et al., 2016; Gueorguieva et al., 2017; Leichsenring et al., 2022). That is not to say that some sort of recovery is not possible when suffering from a PD: for example, some components might either change across the lifespan or be more modifiable in comparison with other components, such as impulsivity, the reduction of which might help in decreasing antisocial tendencies. In another example, alleviation of suffering from the most frequently diagnosed PD, borderline personality disorder, is certainly attainable via interventions that, for example, aim at decreasing risk taking behaviours and aggressive outbursts (Bateman et al., 2015; Grenyer et al., 2022). However, core symptomatology of PDs – for example, identity problems and impairment of interpersonal functioning (Bateman et al., 2015) – seem much harder to treat as is evidenced, for example, by the sobering observation that almost half of all borderline PD patients do not respond to psychotherapy treatment, the treatment option with the largest evidence base, at all (Leichsenring et al., 2024). In that sense, our outlook on the stability of and wiggle room for lasting changes in personality, and disorders thereof, is as optimistic as one can afford to be when it comes to 'treating' intelligence: it is certainly possible, with extensive training, to make a person of slightly below-average intelligence perform better than expected on various cognitive tasks, but that person can never become the new Einstein. That does not mean that we should not try to help people suffering from PDs to attain the best possible version of their lives, given their problems. It does mean that we should be cautious, just as we would be when it comes to intelligence, in framing what an optimal result would look like.

5.4 Potential Drivers of the Dynamical Couplings of Thoughts, Feelings, Behaviour and Environment

As we proposed in the previous paragraph, a personality type is thought to emerge as a result of dynamic couplings between the domains thoughts, feelings, behaviours and environment. In order to shed some light on how PDs might develop from this systems perspective, it is useful to investigate how these couplings between domains might arise: what are their potential drivers (see also Kendler, 2025)?

One potential driver is *resource competition* (De Ron et al., 2023). Thinking a thought, feeling a feeling or initiating behaviour all require certain resources, many of which are not available in infinite amounts. Take for instance the finite resource of *time*: time spent on thinking a certain thought cannot be spent on thinking another thought. Or: contemplating one's own thoughts and feelings on the couch leaves less time for initiating certain behaviours. As such, time as a finite resource is one of the drivers of why certain (patterns of) thoughts, feelings, behaviors and environments prevail over others: there simply is not enough time to think and feel other things, and to behave differently or be somewhere else during a given day.

Time might also play a (modest) role in maintaining PDs (and other mental health conditions). For example, PDs – perhaps most notably borderline PD – tend to be associated with the inability of holding down a job (Caruana et al., 2018; Chanen et al., 2020; Juurlink et al., 2020). Not having a job means that someone has more time on their hands, which might facilitate having more time to 'spend' on the core dysfunctions of the PD itself (e.g. entering and exiting fragile, doomed relationships). As such, time might trigger an undesired feedback loop in which a PD results in 'epiphenomena' (Bateman et al., 2015) such as not being able to hold down a job, which, in turn, might result in more time to maintain the disorder.

Another finite resource that might play a role in the development of (dysfunctional) personality systems is conscious *attention*. Analogous to time, paying attention to something means simultaneously not paying attention to other things. Competition for attention among various personality components might facilitate harmful couplings: for example, paying attention to one's own negative train of thought (e.g. 'I am worthless, the world is an awful place') might result in that person not paying attention to a cute little dance their child is performing in the living room. Over time, a potentially harmful coupling might, for example, ensue between the thought 'The world is an awful place' and a sad, empty and/or angry feeling. Paying conscious attention to the child's cute little dance in the living room might have 'protected' that person from developing sad or angry feelings.

Another driver of (harmful) dynamical couplings might be our innate desire for *self-consistency*. That is, in many cases we feel the need to, for example, align what we feel with what we think, or to behave in accordance with our feelings. For example, if one thinks that other people are less worthy than you, it would feel strange – inconsistent – to volunteer for distributing hot meals to homeless people twice a week (i.e. dissonance discomfort; Harmon-Jones & Mills, 2019). Or: if one regularly feels really angry at one's spouse because of misperceiving a harmless joke as an insult, it would be inconsistent to have only rosy thoughts about that spouse. And: if one feels awkward around other people, it would not make sense to select a work environment with only an open-office plan. As a result of this drive to be consistent, over time, dynamical couplings between the four domains might emerge that could be harmful or dysfunctional: for example, thinking that other people are less worthy than you (thoughts), having angry outbursts when other people do not recognize your superiority (feelings), manipulating a colleague into giving you public credit for work you did not actually do (behaviour) and frequently changing jobs after only the slightest perceived insult (environment).

5.5 Multiple Roads to Developing Personality Disorders from a Dynamical Systems Perspective

The ultimate question now is: how can one develop a PD if we assume personality to be the ultimate outcome of dynamical couplings between thoughts, feelings, behaviours and environment? We do not think there is a singular blueprint that outlines how certain dynamical interactions between personality components over time will ultimately, or necessarily, result in a PD; similar to the observation that although two people can have roughly the same IQ score, this does not imply they had similar developmental trajectories towards that level of intelligence, nor does it imply that their intelligence level is qualitatively comparable (e.g. two people with the same IQ score but one excels at math while the other excels at verbal skills).

Here, we highlight three possible ways in which a personality system can generate a PD as its ultimate outcome: (1) stronger *positive interactions* between certain components relative to other interactions, (2) stronger *negative interactions* between certain components relative to other interactions, and (3) *resource competition* where all personality components are in need of the same resource. We stress that these three possibilities are by no means an attempt at providing an exhaustive account of all the ways in which a personality system might end up in a dysfunctional – PD – state. Rather, we aim at providing a first pass at some potentially novel ways of thinking about the pathogenesis of PDs by means of an illustrative simulation, the particulars of which are derived from the work of De Ron et al. (2023) on the multiple trajectories to cognitive (mal) development via mutualistic, dynamical couplings between cognitive processes (see Appendix for the R script of the simulation).

The foundation of the simulation is a mutualistic model in which 10 personality components grow over time and interact with one another. For example, a component such as the belief that other people are essentially good-hearted and well-intentioned needs to grow from a rough 'idea' to a core belief, over time, based on interaction with other people – first one's own parents and later predominantly peers – that serve as evidence either corroborating or undermining that 'idea'. As explicated earlier, in a mutualistic dynamical systems model, we assume that these components interact with one another over time. In that sense, these interactions impose a limitation on how 'big', or dominant, a personality component can become in someone's personality architecture: the stronger two components interact with one another, the larger the impact of one component will be on the growth of the other.

The top left plot in Figure 5.2 highlights the development of a relatively normal personality system in which all components interact with one another with the same – relatively weak – strength. The end result of these interactions is that all components (represented by a line) over time grow to relatively similar levels; that is, in a relatively normal personality system, there are no components that are either under- or over-developed relative to other components. The top right plot in Figure 5.2 highlights what happens when two components interact far more strongly with one another than with the other components in a personality system (stronger *positive interactions*), for instance when there is an inappropriately strong drive for consistency of the components. These two components – the two black lines $x1$ and $x2$, with the highest levels in the plot – show, compared to the other personality components, excessive growth, that is, their levels are much higher compared to the other personality components. Substantive examples of such excessive growth of a personality component might include the grandiose sense of self-worth associated with narcissism (i.e. inflated version of the normal experience of self-worth), the feeling of being absolutely terrified to be abandoned associated with dependent PD (i.e. inflated version of an otherwise normal feeling not wanting to lose the most important people in one's life) and the overly sexually charged interactions with others associated with histrionic PD (i.e. inflated version of normal, slightly flirtatious behaviour if the other person is truly appealing).

The bottom left plot in Figure 5.2 highlights the consequences for personality development if two components, $x1$ and $x2$, interact (strongly) negatively with one another in an otherwise positively coupled system (stronger *negative interactions*). The end result is that one of these components ($x2$ in our example) tends to be pushed towards zero density, that is, is not developed. A substantive example might be under-developed (or total lack of) feelings of empathy towards others, pushed to low levels during development as a result of a strong dampening effect of early beliefs about one's own superiority, possibly fuelled by certain parenting styles (narcissistic PD).

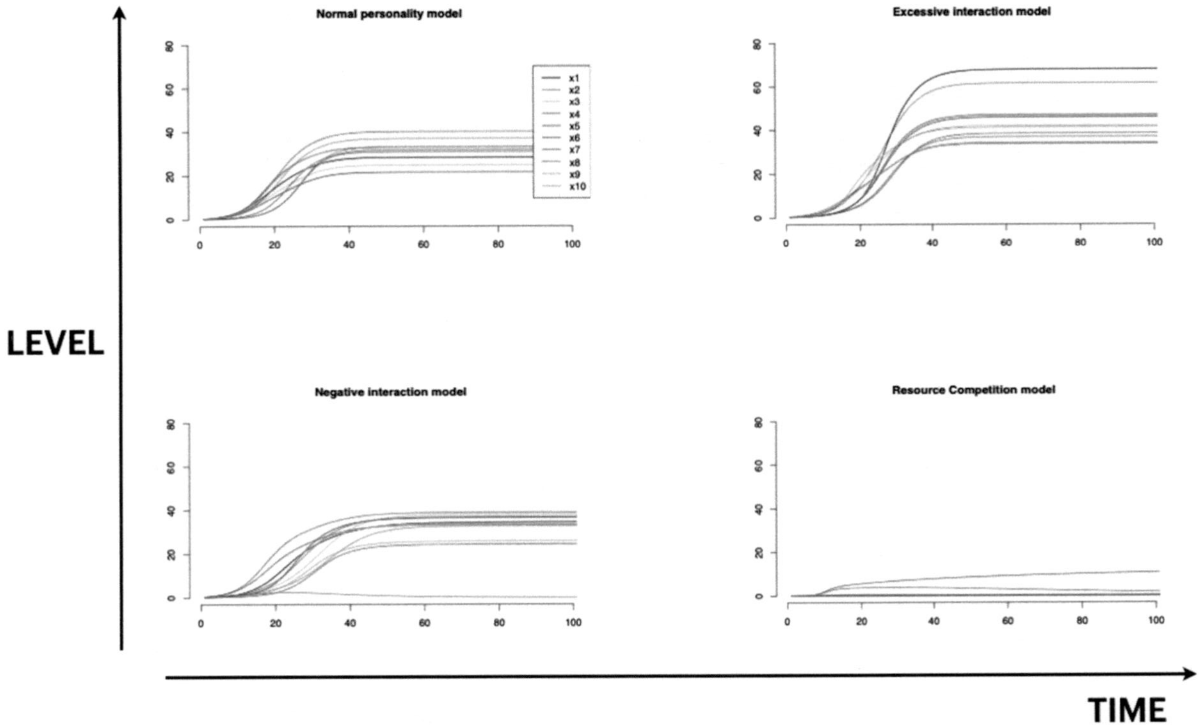

Figure 5.2 Four potential personality outcomes in a dynamical model. The x-axis represents time and the y-axis represents level of growth of personality components. The lines represent 10 fictitious personality components that grow to a certain level over time. The top left plot contains the legend for these lines. Top left: the development of a relatively normal personality where all components are relatively weakly coupled. Top right: the development of a personality where two components interact very strongly (positively) with one another resulting in those two components having grown excessively. Bottom left: the development of a personality where two components strongly interact with one another in a negative manner resulting in one component being strongly underdeveloped. Bottom right: the development of a personality where resource competition results in a winner-takes-all scenario where one component dominates all others.

Finally, the bottom right plot in Figure 5.2 highlights what could happen if all personality components are similarly coupled (positively) to one another but in order to grow, they rely on the same 'fuel' or resource (e.g. time or attention). The end result is a winner-takes-it-all scenario in which one component (*x5* in our example) dominates all others that are either under-developed or not developed at all. Here, one can think of a person for whom one particular behaviour takes up all time resources; an example would be a person whose behavioural repertoire is dominated by excessive attention-seeking at the expense of other modes of behaviour (histrionic PD).

5.6 Implications for Future Research

In this chapter we have outlined the contours of a theory in which a PD is a potential outcome of a system in which broad domains – thoughts, feelings, behaviours and environment – become coupled to one another throughout development as a result of dynamic interactions between smaller building blocks (personality components) of personality. This theoretical perspective on personality and its dysfunctions might have a number of implications for the way we think about ('abnormal') personality and do research.

First, a PD is not a common cause of its observable (dysfunctional) thoughts, feelings and behaviours. Importantly, this viewpoint implies that it would be rather fruitless to search for dysfunctional gene variants, brain structures, parenting failures or any other dysfunction that might explain away the positive covariation between symptoms of a certain PD. That is not to say that such physiological or psychological factors are not worthwhile to investigate yet, not as a common cause but as one of many possible factors that are implicated in shaping the architecture of someone's personality system (e.g. certain gene variants that have an impact on the speed of growth of certain personality components).

Second, from our systems perspective on PDs, two (related) research areas (extending previous work on personality change by, for example, Mõttus et al., 2017, 2020; Roberts et al., 2008; Roberts & Mroczek, 2008) would be (1) *growth* of personality components, their individual differences and factors – besides interaction strength – influencing that growth; and (2) *interactions* between personality components, their individual differences and factors influencing their strength. In particular, it would be paramount to develop a more sophisticated understanding of the relationship between growth and interaction patterns on the one hand and the various PDs on the other hand. In addition, in terms of intervention design, it could be worthwhile to investigate which interactions between personality components are more amenable to change compared to others. Given that much of personality development takes place during childhood, we would expect quite a few of these interactions (e.g.

feeling fearful that an important person might leave and responding to this by picking an unreasonable fight with that same person) to be rather old and thus inflexible and possibly hard to change.

Third, we have outlined a systems perspective with one equilibrium state: a certain personality, whether it be dysfunctional or not. Importantly, as we have stressed earlier, this one-state model implies that we view a PD as being somewhat more akin to intelligence – both are not amenable to huge change when subjected to an intervention – than to common mental health conditions. This hypothesis has potentially sizeable implications for our outlook on the prospects of treatment: lasting, sustainable recovery of a PD (i.e. core symptomatology) might be a moonshot at best instead of a highly probable outcome of treatment. It is therefore crucial to test the veracity of this hypothesis. One avenue could be to investigate the so-called stability landscapes of PD system architectures with an important caveat being that this method is currently not available for architectures based on intra-individual data (Cui et al., 2023). Another crucial question that is currently unanswered is whether there are differences between PDs in terms of the stability of their equilibrium state. When inspecting PD symptomatology some of the wording already hints towards certain possibilities: for example, symptoms of borderline PD include a pattern of unstable relationships, quick changes in how you see yourself and wide mood swings; all indicative of instability. Within a complex systems framework, an unstable PD equilibrium would be reason for (cautious) optimism in terms of treatment prospects as instability might leave enough wiggle room for (lasting) change.

Fourth, and final, with a toy simulation model, we have carved out some of the potential ways in which a personality system could result in a PD. It was beyond the scope of the present chapter to thoroughly investigate all potential roads to personality pathology, but such an endeavour is an important priority when a system's research agenda would be pursued. Importantly, the mere existence of multiple roads to developing a PD implies that (1) PD A might not have a similar pathogenesis compared to PD B, and (2) even within one PD, two people might have different trajectories towards the same end result (e.g. excessive interactions versus resource competition for example). This idea is congruent with the observation that, within the realm of PDs, there seem to be few robust empirical phenomena that hold across all PDs – besides the stability of personality from adulthood onwards and comorbidity with other (common) mental health conditions.

On a final note, we wish to stress that we have barely scratched the surface of what is theoretically and empirically possible when thinking about a PD as the ultimate, potential outcome of interactions within a dynamical system. This chapter is therefore not meant to be a comprehensive resource. Rather, we have aimed at providing some of the theoretical boundaries within which more sophisticated and articulated system models of (dysfunctional) personality might come to fruition. That said, given the absence of evidence for, for example, common causes of PDs and empirical evidence congruent with a systems perspective in other research areas (e.g. depression), we do see enough smoke coming from a systems' perspective to start looking for the fire.

Appendix

See below for the R code that we used – slightly adapted from De Ron et al. (2023) – to simulate four different scenarios under the assumption of a dynamical systems model in which personality is the outcome of mutualistic interactions between 10 personality components:

1. *Normal development* (ND), in which all components interact with one another with the same, relatively weak, strength
2. *Excessive interaction* (EI), in which two components interact strongly, positively, with one another
3. *Negative interaction* (NI), in which two components interact strongly, negatively, with one another
4. *Resource competition* (RC), in which all components are fuelled by the same resource but not by each other (i.e. no mutualistic, dynamical interactions between personality components)

In the basic model for the first three scenarios (ND, EI and NI), personality components x_i are hypothesized to grow over time. This growth is influenced by three factors: (1) the rate of growth of each component a_i; (2) the asymptote of the growth function of each component i, carrying capacity K_i; and (3) the strength of the interactions between the personality components, denoted in matrix M. The growth function is then written as the following equation:

$$\frac{dx_i}{dt} = a_i x_i \left(1 - \frac{x_i}{K_i}\right) + a_i \sum_{j=1}^{X} \frac{M_{ij} x_i x_j}{K_i}$$

The values of both K_i and a_i remained the same throughout the simulation of the first three scenarios. These three scenarios only differed with respect to matrix M, the strength of the interactions between the 10 personality components.

For the simulation of resource competition (RC) we used the following growth equations (see De Ron et al., 2023):

$$\frac{dx_i}{dt} = x_i\left(\left(\sum_{j=1}^{R}\mu_{ij}r_j\right) - d_i\right)$$

$$\frac{dr_j}{dt} = r(r_{\max} - r_j) - r_j\left(\sum_{i=1}^{X} b_{ij}x_i\right)$$

The first equation describes the growth of each personality component i, which is determined by its current 'size' x_i and the sum over all available resources r_j. How much each personality component benefits from the availability of resource j is represented by μ_{ij}. Without any resources available, a component will 'die out' (i.e., be pushed towards zero) with speed d_i. The second equation describes the growth of each resource r_j, which is determined by the steepness of the growth r and its asymptotic limit r_{max}. In addition, the depletion rate – the second part of the second equation – is determined by the sum of all personality components multiplied by their consumption rate b_{ij}: the larger a personality component becomes, the more resources it consumes and, thus, the more that resource becomes depleted.

```
# Packages
install.packages("remotes")
remotes::install_github("hansschepers/grindr")
library(Grind)

# Load packages:
library(deSolve)
library(rootSolve)
library(FME)

X = 10
col_set <- rainbow(X)

#####################
#NORMAL DEVELOPMENT#
#####################

# This is a basic mutualism model with slow development combined
with relatively weak interactions between personality components

# Define the model:
model <- function(t, state, parms){
  with(as.list(c(state, parms)),{
    x <- state[1:X]
    dx <- a*x*(1-x/K) + a*(x * M %*% x)/K
    return(list(dx))
  })
}
```

```
# Choose parameter values:
M <- matrix(0.05, X, X); diag(M) <- 0
a <- rnorm(X, 0.2, 0.05)
K <- rnorm(X, 20, 5)

# Set the parameter and initial values:
p <- c(a = a, K = K, M = M)
s <- c(x = runif(X, 0.1, 0.5))

result <-run(timeplot = TRUE,table = TRUE, tmax =100,legend = TRUE)
matplot(result[,2:(X+1)], type = "l",
    ylab = "", bty = "n", lty = "solid", col = col_set, main =
"Normal personality model", ylim = c(0,80))
legend("right", legend = dimnames(result)[[2]][2:(X+1)], lty =
c(1,1), col = col_set)

#######################
#EXCESSIVE INTERACTION#
#######################

# Deviation from the basic model: two personality components are
too strongly connected resulting in excessive growth of both

# Define the model:
model <- function(t, state, parms){
  with(as.list(c(state, parms)),{
    x <- state[1:X]
    dx <- a*x*(1-x/K) + a*(x * M %*% x)/K
    return(list(dx))
  })
}

# Choose parameter values:
M <- matrix(0.05, X, X); diag(M) <- 0
a <- rnorm(X, 0.2, 0.05)
K <- rnorm(X, 20, 5)
M[1,2]=M[2,1]=0.4 #excessive interaction

# Set the parameter and initial values:
p <- c(a = a, K = K, M = M)
s <- c(x = runif(X, 0.1, 0.5))

# Run the model:
result <- run(timeplot = TRUE, table = TRUE, tmax = 100, legend =
FALSE)
matplot(result[,2:(X+1)], type = "l",
```

```
    ylab = "", bty = "n", lty = "solid", col = col_set, main =
"Excessive interaction model", ylim = c(0,80))

########################
#NEGATIVE INTERACTION#
########################

# Deviation from the basic model: two personality components are
negatively connected resulting in one of the two being pushed to
(almost) zero

# Define the model:
model <- function(t, state, parms){
 with(as.list(c(state, parms)),{
  x <- state[1:X]
  dx <- a*x*(1-x/K) + a*(x * M %*% x)/K
 return(list(dx))
 })
}

# Choose parameter values:
M <- matrix(0.05, X, X); diag(M) <- 0
a <- rnorm(X, 0.2, 0.05)
K <- rnorm(X, 20, 5)
M[1,2]=M[2,1]=-1 #negative interaction

# Set the parameter and initial values:
p <- c(a = a, K = K, M = M)
s <- c(x = runif(X, 0.1, 0.5))

# Run the model:
result <- run(timeplot = TRUE, table = TRUE, tmax = 100, legend =
      FALSE)
 matplot(result[,2:(X+1)], type = "l",
     ylab = "", bty = "n", lty = "solid", col = col_set, main =
"Negative interaction model", ylim = c(0,80))

########################
#RESOURCE COMPETITION#
########################

# All personality components feed on one resource r with the result
that one component dominates all others

# Define the model:
model <- function(t, state, parms){
```

```
  with(as.list(c(state,parms)),{
   x <- state[1:X]
   r <- state[(X+1):(X+R)]
   dx <- x * (apply(t(mu) * r, 2, sum) - d)
   dr <- rj * (rmax-r) - r * apply(b * x, 2, sum)
   return(list(c(dx, dr)))
  })
}

# Determine the number of resources the 10 personality components
share:

R <- 1

# Set parameter values:
set.seed(1)
mu <- matrix(runif(X*R, 0.1, 0.3), X, R)
d <- runif(X, 0.05, 0.2)
rj <- 0.1
rmax <- runif(R, 1, 5)
b <- matrix(runif(X*R, .05, .2), X, R)

# Set initial values:
x <- runif(X, 0, 0.02)
r <- runif(R, 1, 2)

# Run model:
p <- c(mu = mu, d = d, rj = rj, rmax = rmax, b = b)
s <- c(x = x, r = r)
result <- run(timeplot = TRUE, table = TRUE,
         tmax = 100, legend = FALSE)

# Plot trajectory:

matplot(result[,2:(X+1)], type = "l",
    ylab = "", bty = "n", lty = "solid", col = col_set, main =
"Resource Competition model", ylim = c(0,80))
```

References

Ackerman, P. L., Beier, M. E., & Boyle, M. O. (2005). Working memory and intelligence: The same or different constructs? *Psychological Bulletin*, *131*(1), 30–60. https://doi.org/10.1037/0033-2909.131.1.30

American Psychiatric Association. (2013). *Diagnostic and statistical manual of mental disorders* (5th ed.). American Psychiatric Association.

Bateman, A. W., Gunderson, J., & Mulder, R. (2015). Treatment of personality disorder. *The Lancet*, *385*(9969), 735–743. https://doi.org/10.1016/S0140-6736(14)61394-5

Berrios, G. E. (1993). European views on personality disorders: A conceptual history. *Comprehensive Psychiatry*, *34*(1), 14–30. https://doi.org/10.1016/0010-440X(93)90031-X

Borsboom, D. (2017). A network theory of mental disorders. *World Psychiatry*, *16*(1), 5–13. https://doi.org/10.1002/wps.20375

Borsboom, D., Cramer, A. O. J., & Kalis, A. (2019). Brain disorders? Not really: Why network structures block reductionism in psychopathology research. *Behavioral and Brain Sciences*, *42*, e2. https://doi.org/10.1017/S0140525X17002266

Borsboom, D., Rhemtulla, M., Cramer, A. O. J., Maas, H. L. J. van der, Scheffer, M., & Dolan, C. V. (2016). Kinds versus continua: A review of psychometric approaches to uncover the structure of psychiatric constructs. *Psychological Medicine*, *46*(8), 1567–1579. https://doi.org/10.1017/S0033291715001944

Caruana, E., Cotton, S. M., Farhall, J., Parrish, E. M., Chanen, A., Davey, C. G., Killackey, E., & Allott, K. (2018). A comparison of vocational engagement among young people with psychosis, depression and borderline personality pathology. *Community Mental Health Journal*, *54*(6), 831–841. https://doi.org/10.1007/s10597-017-0197-5

Chanen, A. M., Nicol, K., Betts, J. K., & Thompson, K. N. (2020). Diagnosis and treatment of borderline personality disorder in young people. *Current Psychiatry Reports*, *22*(5), 25. https://doi.org/10.1007/s11920-020-01144-5

Condon, D. M., Wood, D., Mõttus, R., Booth, T., Costantini, G., Greiff, S., Johnson, W., Lukaszewski, A., Murray, A., Revelle, W., Wright, A. G. C., Ziegler, M., & Zimmermann, J. (2021). Bottom up construction of a personality taxonomy. *European Journal of Psychological Assessment*, *36*, 923–934. https://econtent.hogrefe.com/doi/10.1027/1015-5759/a000626

Cramer, A. O. J., Borkulo, C. D. van, Giltay, E. J., Maas, H. L. J. van der, Kendler, K. S., Scheffer, M., & Borsboom, D. (2016). Major depression as a complex dynamic system. *PLoS One*, *11*(12), e0167490. https://doi.org/10.1371/journal.pone.0167490

Cramer, A. O. J., van der Sluis, S., Noordhof, A., Wichers, M., Geschwind, N., Aggen, S. H., Kendler, K. S., & Borsboom, D. (2012a). Dimensions of normal personality as networks in search of equilibrium: You can't like parties if you don't like people. *European Journal of Personality*, *26*(4), 414–431. https://doi.org/10.1002/per.1866

Cramer, A. O. J., Van Der Sluis, S., Noordhof, A., Wichers, M., Geschwind, N., Aggen, S. H., Kendler, K. S., & Borsboom, D. (2012b). Measurable like temperature or mereological like flocking? On the nature of personality traits. *European Journal of Personality*, *26*(4), 451–459. https://doi.org/10.1002/per.1879

Cramer, A. O. J., Waldorp, L. J., Maas, H. L. J. van der, & Borsboom, D. (2010). Comorbidity: A network perspective. *Behavioral and Brain Sciences*, *33*(2–3), 137–150. https://doi.org/10.1017/S0140525X09991567

Crocq, M.-A. (2013). Milestones in the history of personality disorders. *Dialogues in Clinical Neuroscience*, *15*(2), 147–153. https://doi.org/10.31887/DCNS.2013.15.2/macrocq

Cui, J., Lunansky, G., Lichtwarck-Aschoff, A., Mendoza, N. B., & Hasselman, F. (2023). Quantifying the stability landscapes of psychological networks [Preprint]. *PsyArXiv*. https://doi.org/10.31234/osf.io/nd8zc

Cuijpers, P., Karyotaki, E., Weitz, E., Andersson, G., Hollon, S. D., & van Straten, A. (2014). The effects of psychotherapies for major depression in adults on remission, recovery and improvement: A meta-analysis. *Journal of Affective Disorders*, *159*, 118–126. https://doi.org/10.1016/j.jad.2014.02.026

De Ron, J., Deserno, M., Robinaugh, D., Borsboom, D., & Van Der Maas, H. L. J. (2023). Towards a general modeling framework of resource competition in cognitive development. *Child Development*, *94*(6), 1432–1453. https://doi.org/10.1111/cdev.13973

Fleury, M.-J., Djouini, A., Huỳnh, C., Tremblay, J., Ferland, F., Ménard, J.-M., & Belleville, G. (2016). Remission from substance use disorders: A systematic review and meta-analysis. *Drug and Alcohol Dependence*, *168*, 293–306. https://doi.org/10.1016/j.drugalcdep.2016.08.625

Frances, A. (1993). Dimensional diagnosis of personality – Not whether, but when and which. *Psychological Inquiry*. https://doi.org/10.1207/s15327965pli0402_7

Grenyer, B. F. S., Townsend, M. L., Lewis, K., & Day, N. (2022). To love and work: A longitudinal study of everyday life factors in recovery from borderline personality disorder. *Personality and Mental Health*, *16*(2), 138–154. https://doi.org/10.1002/pmh.1547

Gueorguieva, R., Chekroud, A. M., & Krystal, J. H. (2017). Trajectories of relapse in randomised, placebo-controlled trials of treatment discontinuation in major depressive disorder: An individual patient-level data meta-analysis. *The Lancet Psychiatry*, *4*(3), 230–237. https://doi.org/10.1016/S2215-0366(17)30038-X

Harmon-Jones, E., & Mills, J. (2019). An introduction to cognitive dissonance theory and an overview of current perspectives on the theory. In E. Harmon-Jones (ed.), *Cognitive dissonance: Reexamining a pivotal theory in psychology*, 2nd ed. (pp. 3–24). American Psychological Association.

Hastrup, L. H., Kongerslev, M. T., & Simonsen, E. (2019). Low vocational outcome among people diagnosed with borderline personality disorder during first admission to mental health services in Denmark: A nationwide 9-year register-based study. *Journal of Personality Disorders*, *33*(3), 326–340. https://doi.org/10.1521/pedi_2018_32_344

Hochstein, S. (2012). Reciprocal effects of attention and perception. In J. Wolfe, & L. Robertson (eds), *From perception to consciousness: Searching with Anne Treisman* (pp. 278–287). Oxford University Press.

Juurlink, T. T., Lamers, F., van Marle, H. J. F., Michon, H., van Busschbach, J. T., Beekman, A. T. F., & Anema, J. R. (2020). Employment in personality disorders and the effectiveness of individual placement and support: Outcomes from a secondary data analysis. *Journal of Occupational Rehabilitation*, *30*(2), 255–262. https://doi.org/10.1007/s10926-019-09868-9

Katakis, P., Schlief, M., Barnett, P., Rains, L. S., Rowe, S., Pilling, S., & Johnson, S. (2023). Effectiveness of outpatient and community treatments for people with a diagnosis of 'personality disorder': Systematic review and meta-analysis. *BMC Psychiatry*, *23*(1), 57. https://doi.org/10.1186/s12888-022-04483-0

Kendler, K. S. Parnas, J. and Zachar, P. (Eds.). (2025). Causal concepts in psychiatry. Cambridge University Press.

Krueger, R. F., Derringer, J., Markon, K. E., Watson, D., & Skodol, A. E. (2012). Initial construction of a maladaptive personality trait model and inventory for DSM-5. *Psychological Medicine*, *42*(9), 1879–1890. https://doi.org/10.1017/S0033291711002674

Krueger, R. F., & Hobbs, K. A. (2020). An overview of the DSM-5 Alternative Model of personality disorders. *Psychopathology*, *53*(3–4), 126–132. https://doi.org/10.1159/000508538

Laws, D. R., Hudson, S. M., & Ward, T. (2000). *Remaking relapse prevention with sex offenders: A sourcebook*. SAGE.

Leichsenring, F., Fonagy, P., Heim, N., Kernberg, O. F., Leweke, F., Luyten, P., Salzer, S., Spitzer, C., & Steinert, C. (2024). Borderline personality disorder: A comprehensive review of diagnosis and clinical presentation, etiology, treatment, and current controversies. *World Psychiatry*, *23*(1), 4–25. https://doi.org/10.1002/wps.21156

Leichsenring, F., Steinert, C., Rabung, S., & Ioannidis, J. P. A. (2022). The efficacy of psychotherapies and pharmacotherapies for mental disorders in adults: An umbrella review and meta-analytic evaluation of recent meta-analyses. *World Psychiatry*, *21*(1), 133–145. https://doi.org/10.1002/wps.20941

Lunansky, G., van Borkulo, C., & Borsboom, D. (2020). Personality, resilience, and psychopathology: A model for the interaction between slow and fast network processes in the context of mental health. *European Journal of Personality*, *34*(6), 969–987. https://doi.org/10.1002/per.2263

McCrae, R. R., Costa, Jr., Paul T., & Martin, T. A. (2005). The NEO-PI-3: A more readable revised NEO personality inventory. *Journal of Personality Assessment*, *84*(3), 261–270. https://doi.org/10.1207/s15327752jpa8403_05

McCrae, R. R., & Costa, P. T. (2008). Empirical and theoretical status of the five-factor model of personality traits. In G. J. Boyle, G. Matthews, & D. H. Saklofske (eds), *The SAGE handbook of personality theory and assessment: Volume 1 – Personality theories and models* (pp. 273–294). SAGE Publications Inc.

Moncrieff, J., Cooper, R. E., Stockmann, T., Amendola, S., Hengartner, M. P., & Horowitz, M. A. (2023). The serotonin theory of depression: A systematic umbrella review of the evidence. *Molecular Psychiatry*, *28*(8), Article 8. https://doi.org/10.1038/s41380-022-01661-0

Moran, P., Romaniuk, H., Coffey, C., Chanen, A., Degenhardt, L., Borschmann, R., & Patton, G. C. (2016). The influence of personality disorder on the future mental health and social adjustment of young adults: A population-based, longitudinal cohort study. *The Lancet Psychiatry*, *3*(7), 636–645. https://doi.org/10.1016/S2215-0366(16)30029-3

Mõttus, R., Kandler, C., Bleidorn, W., Riemann, R., & McCrae, R. R. (2017). Personality traits below facets: The consensual validity, longitudinal stability, heritability, and utility of personality nuances. *Journal of Personality and Social Psychology*, *112*(3), 474–490. https://doi.org/10.1037/pspp0000100

Mõttus, R., Wood, D., Condon, D. M., Back, M. D., Baumert, A., Costantini, G., Epskamp, S., Greiff, S., Johnson, W., Lukaszewski, A., Murray, A., Revelle, W., Wright, A. G. C., Yarkoni, T., Ziegler, M., & Zimmermann, J. (2020). Descriptive, predictive and explanatory personality research: Different goals, different approaches, but a shared need to move beyond the big few traits. *European Journal of Personality*, *34*(6), 1175–1201. https://doi.org/10.1002/per.2311

Roberts, B. W., & Mroczek, D. (2008). Personality trait change in adulthood. *Current Directions in Psychological Science*, *17*(1), 31–35. https://doi.org/10.1111/j.1467-8721.2008.00543.x

Roberts, B. W., Wood, D., & Caspi, A. (2008). The development of personality traits in adulthood. In O. P. John, R. W. Robins, & L. A. Pervin (eds), *Handbook of personality: Theory and research*, 3rd ed. (pp. 375–398). The Guilford Press.

Skodol, A. E. (2016). Personality pathology and population health. *The Lancet Psychiatry*, *3*(7), 595–596. https://doi.org/10.1016/S2215-0366(16)30084-0

Van Der Maas, H. L. J., Dolan, C. V., Grasman, R. P. P. P., Wicherts, J. M., Huizenga, H. M., & Raijmakers, M. E. J. (2006). A dynamical model of general intelligence: The positive manifold of intelligence by mutualism. *Psychological Review*, *113*(4), 842–861. https://doi.org/10.1037/0033-295X.113.4.842

von Klipstein, L., Borsboom, D., & Arntz, A. (2021). The exploratory value of cross-sectional partial correlation networks: Predicting relationships between change trajectories in borderline personality disorder. *PLoS One*, *16*(7), e0254496. https://doi.org/10.1371/journal.pone.0254496

Widiger, T. A. (1993). The DSM-III-R categorical personality disorder diagnoses: A critique and an alternative. *Psychological Inquiry*, *4*(2), 75–90. https://doi.org/10.1207/s15327965pli0402_1

Widiger, T. A., & McCabe, G. A. (2020). The alternative model of personality disorders (AMPD) from the perspective of the five-factor model. *Psychopathology*, *53*(3–4), 149–156. https://doi.org/10.1159/000507378

Widiger, T. A., & Mullins-Sweatt, S. N. (2009). Five-factor model of personality disorder: A proposal for DSM-V. *Annual Review of Clinical Psychology*, *5*, 197–220. https://doi.org/10.1146/annurev.clinpsy.032408.153542

6 A Contemporary Integrative Interpersonal Theory Formulation of Self and Social Pathology

Aidan G. C. Wright and Sienna R. Nielsen

6.1 A Contemporary Integrative Interpersonal Theory Formulation of Self and Social Pathology

What is a personality disorder? That is the fundamental question this book seeks to address. A first pass at this question might focus on the primary type or domain of dysfunction captured by personality disorder diagnoses. Modern psychiatric classification schemes tend to organize psychopathology roughly along major domains of human psychological functioning. For instance, there are the affective (i.e., internalizing) disorders, thought (i.e., psychotic) disorders, and disorders of behavioral control (i.e., disinhibitory or externalizing). Patterns of diagnostic covariation reflect this same organization, at least generally so (Kotov et al., 2021; Ringwald et al., 2023). When considered from this perspective, what personality disorder diagnoses share and what distinguishes them from other disorders are self and social impairments. These include socially costly patterns of behavior that leave afflicted individuals at odds with (i.e., antagonism) and withdrawn from (i.e., detachment) others, as well as a self-architecture or identity that lacks coherence and consistency in organization of experience and goals across time and circumstances. Consistent with this, most theoretical models of personality disorders emphasize the centrality of self and social functioning to the phenomena (Bender et al., 2011; Hopwood et al., 2013; Kernberg, 1984; Livesley, 1998; Parker et al., 2004; Wright et al., 2022), and this focus is now represented formally in the International Classification of Disease–11 (WHO, 2022) and provisionally in the *Diagnostic and statistical manual of mental disorders* (APA, 2013).

Going beyond this basic description or localization of dysfunction to define what personality disorder is, how it is maintained, and, hopefully, how it is disrupted requires a more sophisticated and thorough theoretical account of adaptive and maladaptive self and social functioning. Our goal for the current chapter is to highlight the value of Contemporary Integrative Interpersonal Theory (CIIT) for understanding the core impairments in personality disorders.

We seek to build on prior articulations of CIIT for personality pathology by further elaborating the role of the self and its relation to social behavior in the interpersonal model. In CIIT the term *interpersonal* encompasses both the self and the social domains, which represent two sides of the same coin. Consistent with this perspective, at least as far back as Mead (1934), the development of the self and social experiences has been intertwined. Indeed, a growing literature across developmental (e.g., Klimstra et al., 2012), clinical (e.g., De Meulmeester et al., 2017), and cognitive disciplines (e.g., Dimaggio et al., 2008) supports this contention that the self (e.g., identity) and social aspects of interpersonal functioning may be more similar than they are distinct. They seem to rely on similar processes (e.g., Aron et al., 2022), heavily influence each other (e.g., Sebastian et al., 2008; Melamed et al., 2024), and can be evidenced in both social settings and isolation (e.g., Bleckmann et al., 2023; Sato et al., 2020). In personality disorders, self and social dysfunction seem to align, playing out pervasively across interpersonal situations – two expressions of disruption in the same system (Pincus, 2011). We begin by describing the general tenets of CIIT to illustrate how it serves as a general model of personality and psychopathology, and then use it to translate two traditional personality disorder concepts of borderline and narcissistic pathology.

CIIT has its roots in the relational psychoanalysis movement in the first half of the twentieth century, especially the work of Harry Stack Sullivan (1953). It was Timothy Leary (1957) and the Kaiser group, influenced also by contemporary quantitative methodologists (e.g., Guttman, 1954), who took Sullivan's original theoretical propositions and sought to formalize and operationalize them for use in systematic scientific inquiry. This resulting model gave rise to the interpersonal tradition in personality and clinical psychology, which has proven highly generative and had important contributions to these and other related fields every decade since (see Pincus & Ansell, 2013; Wright et al., 2023 for reviews). CIIT purposely seeks to be ecumenical and integrative, providing an overarching and flexible framework that can incorporate specifics generated by the field's many narrower theories.

6.2 The Interpersonal Situation

Contemporary Integrative Interpersonal Theory starts with the premise that interpersonal situations are the most important contexts for the expression of personality and psychopathology. This tenet of CIIT is definitional, and support for this is evident in the fact that humans are a social species and social behavior and the psychological functioning that supports it are central to our species' survival (e.g., Cacciopo et al., 2011; Fiske, 1992).

Therefore, *the "interpersonal situation" is the basic unit of personality expression*, such that personality is the recurring pattern of behavior in interpersonal situations across the lifespan (Sullivan, 1953). In CIIT, the interpersonal situation carries specific meaning and is not limited to overt social behavior in a dyadic context. It involves the individual interacting with themselves or at least one other, including the intrapsychic processes of mental construal, motivations, self-relating, and emotions as well as overt social behavior. Therefore, although overt social exchanges between two or more people are the prototypical interpersonal situation, some situations will be entirely internal, or imaginary, through humans' capacity for fantasy and recollection. It also means interpersonal situations can primarily engage the self-system in social isolation, with the individual interacting with or relating to themselves, as might be the case when managing self-criticism, striving for self-improvement, and reflecting on past and envisioning possible future selves. CIIT offers a framework for conceptualizing interpersonal and identity functioning as inextricably linked in one dynamic system, providing a clear framework for conceptualizing, tracking, and clinically treating dysfunction within this complex system.

6.3 Interpersonal Structure: Agency and Communion

Contemporary Integrative Interpersonal Theory has an empirically established, formal structural model to organize the content of interpersonal functioning (Gurtman, 1992). The two dimensions of *agency* and *communion* form the two major orthogonal axes of the interpersonal circle (see Figure 6.1), which was initially derived through observations of behavioral counts, and has since been formalized mathematically as the interpersonal circumplex (Wiggins, 1996). A circumplex structure implies that the interstitial space between (or blends of) the main axes is full of relevant content. The interpersonal circle, and agency and communion more generally, provide the organizing structure for interpersonal functioning across levels of analysis, such as the motivational, perceptual, and behavioral (Bakan, 1966). Thus, these serve as meta-constructs, and can be instantiated in more specific goals and behavioral expression aligned with them. Agency encompasses typical strivings for self-definition, competence, self-esteem, assertiveness, and control over oneself and others, as well as bids for dominance and power. It is presumed to be a bipolar construct, with passivity, submissiveness, and temerity at the opposite end. Communion encompasses typical strivings for connectedness, nurturance, sharing, and social engagement, as opposed to separation, withdrawal, coldness, and hostility. These are broad constructs, and it can be useful to describe their manifestation in specific domains, such as social behavior, in which case agency typically manifests as dominant (versus submissive) and communion as

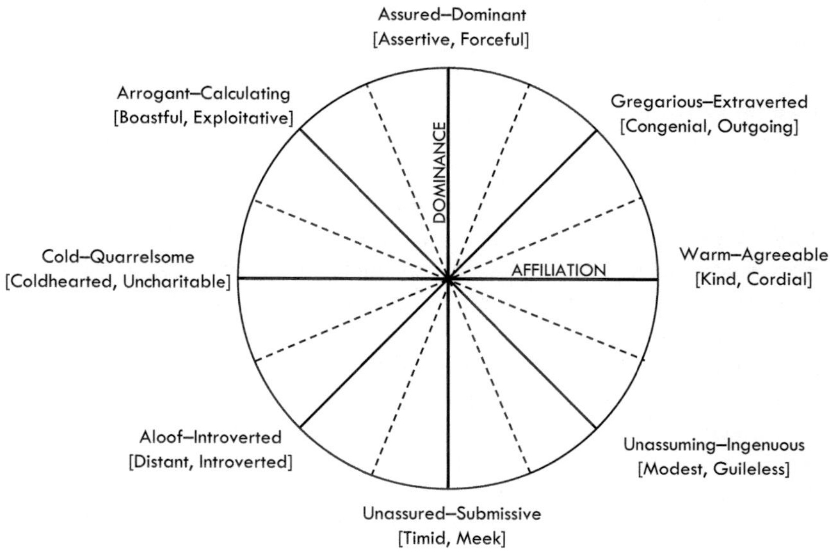

Figure 6.1 The interpersonal circumplex.

affiliative (versus detached) behavior. Other levels of expression or functioning have also been considered, such as motivations, goals, perceptions, traits, strengths, and problems (e.g., Locke, 2011).

6.4 Coordinating the Self and Social Systems

In the same way that the cardinal directions of north versus south and east versus west serve as common orienting rubrics regardless of which map is used, so too do agency and communion serve as cardinal interpersonal coordinates when going across levels and domains of functioning. For instance, the motivations that lie at the center of one's self-concept and the overt behaviors one uses to pursue those motivations can each be organized with this same framework allowing for cohesive articulations of the dynamic relation between self and social functioning. To illustrate, using a CIIT framework, we can test whether domineering social behavior in narcissistic personality disorder is linked to motivations in the moment to maintain an agentic self-concept (Kroenke et al., 2023). We can investigate instability in the borderline personality disorder self-system by tracking variability in self-construal and motivations across social and affective contexts, as well as how variability in self-construal relates to variability in social behavior (Santangelo et al., 2014; Wright et al., 2013a). Although this dynamic relation between self and social processes is integral to conceptualizations of personality disorders (Kernberg, 1984; McWilliams, 2011), bodies of research on the self-system and social-system have largely developed separately as distinct domains of functioning, with little investigation bridging them (Roche & Cain, 2021). CIIT provides guiding axes of agency and communion to investigate self and social functioning as part of one system.

Indeed, *CIIT assumes that social behavior is driven to satisfy interpersonal motivations and goals.* This was first articulated by Sullivan (1953) in terms of individuals seeking out interpersonal situations to satisfy needs for self-esteem (agentic need) and security (communal need). Individuals differ in the strength of these general motivations and they, along with the specific situational needs and contingencies, drive individual differences in social behavior. Within the broader domains of motivation, many specific goals can be accommodated that are presumed to be more proximal to the immediate needs of an individual or serve as steps towards actualization of the broader motivations (e.g., DeYoung, 2015). For instance, someone high in agentic motivations may seek professional success and acclaim, which might manifest more concretely in trying to impress a superior with the hopes of securing a promotion to ultimately be recognized by headhunters from a larger firm. Communal motivations may lead someone to seek a secure and mutual long-term relationship, which might manifest more concretely in being friendly to someone with the hopes they might ultimately want to go on a date and then ultimately become someone's significant other.

Individuals differ reliably in their dispositional levels of agentic and communal motivations (Locke, 2000). At the same time, motivations and goals are understood to be reinforced by situational contingencies, with emotions serving as innate feedback and reward signals to guide goals and behavior in the short term and shape, maintain, or reduce motivations and behaviors over the long term. What should be clear from this is that the self and social behavior vary over time and circumstances. One of the longstanding paradoxes of personality is that the individuals typically experience themselves and are experienced by others as consistent over time, even though their thoughts, feelings, and behaviors also vary substantially over time (Mischel, 2004). Thus, although noted above, we reiterate that in CIIT personality is explicitly transactional between the individual and environment such that personality is the relatively "*consistent patterning*" over situations. This has sometimes been referred to as an "interpersonal signature" (Fournier et al., 2008, 2009), making use of *if–then* or lock-and-key articulations of personality processes (e.g., Mischel & Shoda, 1995; Pincus et al., 2009).

Consistency of self and social behavior has clear implications for adaptive functioning. Accordingly, several concepts have been invoked to describe and explain individual differences in this patterning. At a basic descriptive level, Leary (1957) invoked the dimensions of stability versus instability and flexibility versus rigidity to describe relatively adaptive (stable, flexible) versus relatively maladaptive (unstable, rigid) behavioral patterns (see also Geukes et al., 2017). Although at first glance these may not seem like separable dimensions, when considerations of the interpersonal context are invoked, it can be easier to see that given a functionally consistent type of situation, goals and behavior should be similarly consistent or stable and therefore facilitate knowing what to expect or anticipate of someone. Unstable goals or behavior across functionally similar situations makes behavior unpredictable. Naturally, some spontaneity can be charming, if not the spice of life, but when it is extreme or erratic it can suggest underlying problems. This pattern of instability is the hallmark of the traditional borderline personality disorder diagnosis, and instability in emotions and behaviors in social situations has been linked with it (e.g., Russell et al., 2007). When looking across functionally different types of situations, goals and behavior should flexibly adapt to meet the shifting demands and contingencies. In contrast, when goals and behaviors are rigid and do not shift across different types of situations this too can suggest dysfunction. For instance, if a highly narcissistic individual functionally equates many different situations, seeing all of them as opportunities to get ahead and assert oneself, it can lead to interpersonal problems over time (e.g., Paulhus, 1998). Ultimately, these are useful but coarse descriptions of what are ultimately more nuanced dynamic processes that presume a transaction between the self and social context.

6.5 The Interpersonal Transaction Cycle: Social Functioning

Contemporary Integrative Interpersonal Theory has developed the interpersonal transaction cycle (Figure 6.2) to elaborate the processes contained within a typical interpersonal interaction (Carson, 1969; Kiesler, 1983). As depicted in Figure 6.2, we see that an interpersonal transaction involves an individual, Person A, behaving towards another, Person B, who construes and is impacted by the behavior of Person A, which then results in a response by Person B. Naturally, in real interactions these steps are presumed to occur quickly, implicitly, and often outside of consciousness. Elaborating these steps of the process and making them explicit facilitates detailed predictions about what supports and hinders adaptive functioning. For instance, path 1 (as labeled in the Figure 6.2) involves the impact of Person A's behavior (box 1) on how Person B's is covertly impacted (i.e., their internal subjective and automatic construal and reaction) by them (box 2), and as such is subject to accurate perception and understanding of Person A's behavior and intentions by Person B. Path 2 represents the response or behavioral selection by Person B based on their own covert impact of Person A's behavior. Here motivations and goals can insert themselves to modify behavioral selection in response to the situation.

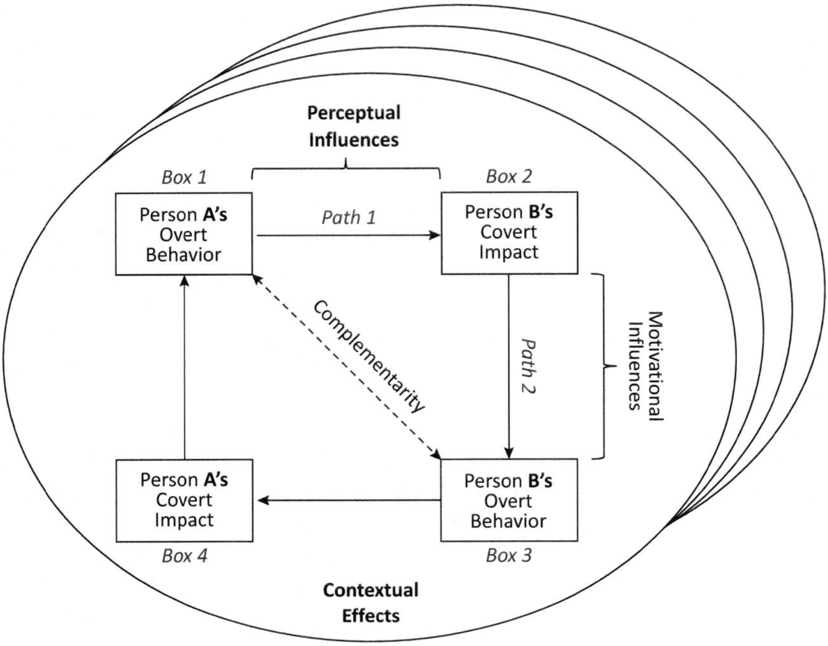

Figure 6.2 The interpersonal transaction cycle.

Interpersonal complementarity (Carson, 1969; Roche, 2022; Woods & Wright, 2024) refers to the theoretically expected patterns of interpersonal match between self and other in social situations. Originally proposed as a match between momentary behaviors, it has been extended to include situation-level (i.e., average behavior of people in a situation; Woods & Wright, 2024) and trait-level (i.e., average behavior of people) matches as well (Ansell et al., 2008). The basic premise is that all other things being equal, there should be behavioral reciprocity on dominance and matching on warmth. That is, dominance invites or compels submissiveness and vice versa, but warmth invites warmth and coldness invites coldness. When complementarity is observed, it is presumed to lead to more enjoyable interactions and positive outcomes. Yet frequently things are not equal, and differences in status or social roles can modify the expectations for these patterns (Sadler et al., 2011). Furthermore, it is not clear that complementarity is always equally rewarding, and some patterns may be counterintuitively so. For instance, in western cultures being socially outgoing is often valued, and it is easy to see how high warmth matching with high warmth would lead to harmonious interactions. It can be harder to see how matching on colder interpersonal behavior might be desirable. In this case, to the extent that one person would like space, then the other giving them that space and not intruding is ideal, even though the potential for mutual enjoyment is reduced overall – it might be a relatively good interaction, even if not the highest in the absolute sense.

Complementarity itself is dynamic and deviations from the expected patterns of complementarity often reflect bids to adjust or renegotiation the interpersonal transaction. Assuming the shift can be negotiated successfully, departures from one pattern of complementarity will give way to another and that will promote stability and good interpersonal outcomes. More to the point, Horowitz et al. (2006) have argued that complementarity is less about overt behavioral match and instead is more about satisfying one's motives. It is the motivational match with outcome that defines complementarity and the motives and behavior chosen to pursue them may or may not be aligned. For instance, when one has as a goal to control another's behavior, they can pursue that goal via assertively directing the other person to do something (alignment of goal and behavior), or they might be purposely passive hoping the other volunteers to do what is needed (misalignment of goal and behavior). How one approaches and negotiates these situational presses has implications for psychological functioning (e.g., passive aggression versus assertively voicing one's needs).

6.6 The Interpersonal Transaction Cycle: Self Functioning

According to many theories of personality (Block, 1982; DeYoung, 2015; James, 1890; Kohut, 1977; Heine et al., 2006; Swann & Hill, 1982), the self-system maintains a stable, coherent, and positive self-concept in part by aligning social behavior with personal motivations. In other words, the social situation is the context of self-expression towards maintaining a stable self-image. For example, an individual viewing themselves as caring, with core aspirations to help others, may maintain this self-concept through socially demonstrating kindness and acting warmly towards others. Situations discrepant to a caring self-concept, such as social conflicts calling for colder behavior, are potential disruptions in this self-concept, requiring compensation through (1) accommodating new beliefs about the social situation into the existing self-concept (e.g., "Sometimes being caring means navigating conflict") and/or (2) reaffirming the self-concept through social behavior (e.g., acting warmly despite conflict). Failures to flexibly compensate for discrepant social situations may result in a diminished sense of ownership and regard for the self-concept, constituting dysfunction in the self-system (McConnell et al., 2009). The social situation demanding compensation in the self-system may be an interaction with another person, groups of people, or the broader sociocultural context (McAdams & Pals, 2006). Contemporary Integrative Interpersonal Theory provides a framework for tracking the interplay of self and social processes across multiple levels of experience and expression towards understanding the breakdowns in the self-system characteristic of personality disorders.

A primary goal of the self-system is to maintain a stable sense of self, facilitating the feeling that who we are today is fundamentally the same person we were yesterday and the same person we will be tomorrow, despite changing circumstances (McAdams & Pals, 2006; Pals, 2006). Additionally, the self-system maintains the sense that we are the same person across various social contexts, despite differing social demands and constraints on our behavior (Kraus et al., 2011; McConnell & Strain, 2011; Nurius & Markus, 1990). To maintain a sense of continuity across changing social contexts, the self-system must therefore both promote consistent behavior in line with a stable self-image and flexibly accommodate some necessary and predictable variability in behavior across social contexts. Therefore, some variability in behavioral self-expression across contexts is expected for maintaining a stable self-image. Dysfunction in the self-system may occur with (1) under-adaptation to the social context through overly rigid adherence to a singular expression of the self-concept (resulting in noncomplementary social interactions) or (2) over-adaptation to the social context through over-reactivity in changes to self-regard (particularly lower self-esteem) and self-expression (Geukes et al., 2017; Hochschild Tolpin et al., 2004; Kockler et al., 2022; Vess et al., 2011; Ziegler-Hill et al., 2010).

Using language from CIIT to track motives and social behavior facilitates further investigation of reactivity in the self-system to the social situation. For example, adaptive variability in the self-concept (including traits and personality states) may be associated with appropriate adjustment to the social context, including greater complementarity in agency and communion with the interaction partner. If the self-system is maintaining a stable self-image through flexibility in expression, self-regard, motivations, and affect may stay relatively stable despite adjustment to the social context. However, maladaptive instability in the self-concept may be associated with greater reactivity to social contexts, with greater changes in the self-system (e.g., self-regard, motivations, and affect) associated with greater (more intense) or inappropriate (e.g., noncomplementary) social behavioral changes. For instance, an individual with communal motivations and maladaptive instability in the self-system may be over-reactive to an employer's dominant behavior by adopting overly detached–submissive behavior, failing to foster warmth in the interaction, leading to self-criticism (e.g., cold–dominant self-talk; Benjamin, 1993) and greater negative affect. Instability in the self-system may therefore be an outcome of over-reactivity in the self and social systems.

6.7 Bridging Contemporary Integrative Interpersonal Theory and Prior Self-System Research

Contemporary Integrative Interpersonal Theory provides a path forward for conducting new interpersonal research integrating the self-system. However, there is a rich history of self-functioning theory and research separate from the interpersonal situation, often in paradigms of personal self-reflection or narrative analysis. Contemporary Integrative Interpersonal Theory also provides a framework for bridging self-functioning literature and new research on the dynamic interpersonal system through the themes of agency and communion in our personal aspirations, life stories, and social motivations (Dunlop et al., 2023).

Psychologists and philosophers alike have long considered the experience of temporal and contextual continuity, known as the diachronic or narrative self, to be the crux of personal identity (Kierkegaard, 1941; Markus & Kunda, 1986; McAdams, 1996; Parfit, 1971; Ricoeur, 1988). A stable diachronic self provides a schema for pursuing goals and overcoming obstacles; it grounds present action in aspirations for the future and the knowledge gained from past experiences (Conway & Pleydell-Pearce, 2000). The self-system maintains this sense of continuity through processing relevant experiences into a self-defining life narrative that guides consistent behavior and decision-making (McAdams, 1996; Singer et al., 2013). These narratives are structured with themes of agency and communion associated with the individual's personal goals and motivations (McAdams et al., 1996). Difficulty constructing a coherent, positive life narrative is associated with behavioral instability and lower self-knowledge, representing frustrated efforts to maintain a stable and positive self-image (Dunlop, 2017; Uliaszek et al., 2022). However, few studies have investigated the daily life processes maintaining the diachronic self. Contemporary Integrative Interpersonal Theory proposes a framework conducive to linking narrative identity and daily life self-system maintenance processes involving social context, self-regard, self-concept, and behavior (Dunlop et al., 2023). By using the language of agency and communion, we can track motives and behaviors in narrative and momentary processes alike. Contemporary Integrative Interpersonal Theory allows for the tracking of the degree of variability in the self-system over different contexts, and how those relate to development and maintenance of the diachronic self.

6.8 General Definition of Interpersonal (Dys)Function

Defining dysfunction or impairments of personality first requires a definition of adaptive functioning. Up to this point, we have alluded to adaptive and maladaptive aspects of interpersonal functioning. From the perspective of

CIIT, adaptive personality functioning involves *a sustained ability to engage interpersonally in ways that coordinate and satisfy the agentic and communal needs of self and other, relatively consistent with one's developmental stage and sociocultural context, through the flexible, stable, and effective regulation of self, affect, and social behavior* (Wright et al., 2023). Aspects of this definition that we have not reviewed and will not elaborate due to considerations of space include the importance of considering developmental stage and sociocultural context as reference points for expectations of functioning and behavior. Similarly, a full treatment of all possible ways impairments can manifest go beyond the scope of this chapter. We will instead highlight several key impairments relevant for articulating personality pathology.

First, adaptive functioning is dynamic and therefore it is not defined by one's trait levels of dominance and affiliation. It is instead defined by the ability to flexibly coordinate and satisfy self and others' motives within interpersonal contexts. Extreme traits (i.e., very high dominance) are more likely, in a probabilistic sense, to result in situation–behavior mismatches, but the level is not definitional of dysfunction, the sustained failure to meet the demands of situations is. Additionally, appropriate behavioral selection in situations is predicated on accurate perception and construal of situations. Sullivan (1953) invoked the concept of "parataxic distortion" to explain failures to adequately construe situations, allowing one's perception and understanding to be colored or distorted by one's own motivations or fantasies.

Second, clinically relevant impairments must be sustained, not transient. Situational demands will at times call for extreme behavior, given the complexity of modern social life it is easy to misstep for any number of benign reasons, disagreements and misunderstandings occur, and so forth. To the extent that these are uncommon or the individual moves to rectify them when they occur, they do not represent dysfunction.

Third, CIIT assumes that adaptive interpersonal functioning for a social species requires some degree of mutuality. That is, it is not sufficient to satisfy one's own interpersonal needs exclusively at the expense of others' needs. At times there will be competition for scarce resources, or individuals will reach an impasse given conflicting goals that may require putting one's own needs over the other's needs, or vice versa. Again, this is natural, and so long as it is not a sustained pattern then it likely reflects reasonable resolution of the vicissitudes of social life.

Fourth, effective regulation of affect and social behavior are common features of definitions of adaptive functioning and likely do not require elaboration. However, as we alluded to above, effective regulation of the self is more complex, often involving the nuanced interface between motives, goals, perception, and construal. Additionally, it involves maintaining a consistency over time and circumstance and avoiding being buffeted about too much by life's texture.

Finally, CIIT recognizes and respects that there are extensive individual differences in dispositional levels of agentic and communal motivation, which are the result of accumulated life experience interacting with one's unique biological makeup. This means that adaptive functioning is likely to look quite different for different people.

6.9 Understanding Personality Disorder Diagnoses with Contemporary Integrative Interpersonal Theory

Like most modern personality theories, CIIT assumes that personality heterogeneity is vast and cannot be neatly summarized with a finite set of categories. The same is assumed true for interpersonal dysfunction. This is consistent with a large literature noting how poorly the 10 DSM categories do for describing personality dysfunction (Kotov et al., 2021). Whether the DSM diagnoses reflect common patterns that might serve as pragmatic heuristics or prototypes worth special attention is an interesting question, although beyond this current discussion. Rather, the tenets and methods of CIIT can be used to faithfully describe the broad individual differences in adaptive and maladaptive interpersonal patterning. We highlight this with two diagnoses, borderline and narcissistic personality disorder, both of which first entered official diagnostic schemes in 1980 and continue until today. They hold value in this context because in many respects they reflect the cardinal themes of interpersonal dysfunction mapped by the interpersonal tradition: affiliative and agentic impairments in self and social functioning.

6.9.1 Borderline: The Unstable Affiliative Pattern

In the DSM-5, borderline personality disorder is described as "a pervasive pattern of instability of interpersonal relationships, self-image, and affects" (APA, 2013, p. 663). However, the construct of "borderline" is itself variable across theorists. Perhaps the biggest distinction to be drawn is between borderline personality disorder as a defined category, as it was instantiated in the DSM, and borderline personality organization, as a level of personality dysfunction (Kernberg, 1984). Although both are highly overlapping, borderline personality organization is much broader and the borderline personality disorder category, which might best be understood as a specific manifestation of borderline organization with a particular emphasis on interpersonal themes of connectedness and attachment (Benjamin, 1996). Psychometrically, indicators of borderline personality disorder function best as indicators of general personality pathology, rather than as indicators of specific dysfunctions (Sharp et al., 2015; Wright et al., 2016) and borderline personality disorder has been shown to be interpersonally heterogeneous cross-sectionally (Wright et al.,

2013b) and longitudinally (Wright et al., 2013a). We see these findings as making a strong case for viewing the core impairments of borderline personality disorder as the core interpersonal impairments in the personality disorders generally – most notably, impairments in identity (e.g., identity diffusion, emptiness) and social relatedness (e.g., unstable relationships, hostility) or both (e.g., idealization and devaluation). Nevertheless, the emphasis on affiliative themes in interpersonal dysfunction are important from the perspective of CIIT, even if they are more complex than the more prototypical patterns associated with, for instance, the constructs of dependent and histrionic personality disorders.

Identity dysfunction in borderline personality disorder is marked by diminished connectedness to the self-image (often called identity diffusion), including feelings of emptiness and estrangement from one's true self and life experiences (Jørgensen & Bøye, 2022; Wilkinson-Ryan & Westen, 2000). Identity diffusion in borderline personality disorder is associated with temporal instability in self-knowledge, self-regard, and behaviors (Beeney et al., 2016; Santangelo et al., 2020). Although primarily associated with instability, identity diffusion is accompanied by persistent narrative themes of negative self-image, low personal agency, and frustrated communal values (Lind et al., 2020). Individuals with borderline personality disorder seem to demonstrate an over-reactive self-system. Perceived rejection, or frustrated communal motives, disproportionately influence self-esteem (Zeigler-Hill & Abraham, 2006), prompting over-compensation to avoid abandonment through disproportionate social behavior. Over-reactivity in the self-system elicits negative affect and withdrawal from interaction partners, frustrating communal goals (Bouchard et al., 2009). Further, over-reactivity in the self-system to external influences may perpetuate themes of low agency and dependence on others for identity. Inability to effectively maintain the self-system additionally stymies coherent identity formation, perpetuating identity diffusion. Using CIIT, the apparent identity and interpersonal instability in borderline personality disorder can be understood in terms of a more predictable over-reactivity in the self-system to the social context, particularly as it relates to perceptions of withdrawal that might reflect abandonment.

Specific interpersonal patterns can be further elaborated within the CIIT frameworks of the interpersonal situation and transaction cycle. Take, for instance, the DSM's borderline personality disorder diagnostic criterion of "frantic efforts to avoid real or imagined abandonment." We can imagine an individual with marked borderline pathology interacting with their significant other in a situation in which the individual expresses some hesitation about making a large and expensive purchase that holds significance for their relationship (e.g., a new and more reliable car because it is a long-distance relationship), to which the individual with borderline personality disorder responds with an angry outburst, locks themselves in the bathroom, and while arguing through the door threatens to take every bottle of pills in the medicine cabinet.

In this hypothetical example, the symptom (i.e., dramatic efforts to avoid fear of abandonment) can be translated into the transaction cycle of this interpersonal situation to raise several hypotheses about the source of the dysfunction. For example, the significant other might express real and reasonable financial concerns about making such a large purchase (box 1 in Figure 6.2), perhaps in a bid for reassurance that their partner might share the financial burden. In the context of the implications for the relationship (ability to sustain regular visits), the individual with significant borderline personality disorder might be hyper-attuned to any deviation from unequivocal and enthusiastic support for the purchase as reflective of a lack of commitment leading to a misconstrual of the significant other's behavior (distorted perception and misconstrual of path 1, perceived disaffiliation). In turn, this may elicit exquisitely painful (negative affect laden) self-states in which the individual feels helpless (low agency) and rejected (low affiliation) (box 2). Naturally, these would activate strong affiliative motives seeking to engage the significant other and shore up the relationship (path 2). However, in this example, rather than adopt the direct route to satisfy such motives (e.g., communal behavior, box 3), in the threatened self-state the individual may shift to feeling hostile (cold, dominant self-state laden with anger, path 2) leading to the outburst described above (cold dominant behavior, box 3), and thwarting the affiliative motive that was motivating the behavior. Here the initial distorted perception and misconstrual of the significant other's behavior leads to an escalation that not only threatens the relationship but potentially the physical safety of one or both individuals.

This is but one possible example of an interpersonal situation intended to illustrate how borderline features can be captured using the CIIT framework. We do not mean to suggest that in all cases the impairment manifests in the same way, although patterns like this have been captured using intensive longitudinal designs in naturalistic settings (e.g., Lazarus et al., 2018; Sadikaj et al., 2013). Rather, it highlights that the CIIT framework can flexibly handle specific aspects of psychopathology and integrate self, affect, and social behavior in coherent chains suitable for research or intervention hypotheses.

6.9.2 Narcissism: The Agentic Pattern

Contemporary perspectives on narcissism emphasize an identity organized around preoccupation on agentic concerns, particularly hierarchy, status, and social dominance (Edershile & Wright, 2022; Grapsas et al, 2020). Narcissism is a peculiar construct in that it has a large clinical descriptive and theoretical presence in the psychiatric literature, but there is very little research on narcissistic personality disorder per se (Wright & Edershile, 2018). Despite a very active literature on the broader narcissism construct in personality psychology, there is a disconnect between the bulk of empirical investigations of narcissism and clinical theories of narcissistic personality disorder, though this is changing in more recent work (e.g., Edershile & Wright, 2021b). As a result, there is ongoing debate about how narcissism should be defined (Miller et al., 2021).

Regardless of how narcissism is defined, CIIT can accommodate multiple definitions given its flexibility and the fact that narcissism is rooted in more basic interpersonal processes. To illustrate, we will use a traditional clinical conceptualization that views narcissism as a complex, if not paradoxical, construct encompassing seemingly opposite grandiose (arrogant, entitled, self-absorbed, superior) and vulnerable (inadequate, fragile, dysregulated) self-states. From this perspective, grandiosity or grandiose self-states are defensive and serve to mask or ward off core feelings of vulnerability or vulnerable self-states (Morf & Rhodewalt, 2001). That is, narcissism refers to the process of overcompensating for one's feelings of inadequacy by adopting a grandiose self-view and outward behavior. In either self-state there is a near myopic focus on oneself, and in the service of maintaining their grandiosity people with narcissistic features are willing to take advantage of and denigrate others to varying degrees, or at least show little regard for others' needs.

Contemporary Integrative Interpersonal Theory is particularly well-suited for describing the core motives, feared outcomes, and social behaviors associated with grandiose and vulnerable self-states. When in a grandiose self-state, the narcissistic individual is motivated to maintain or achieve social status (agentic motivations), and, assuming these needs are being met or are not threatened can be outwardly charming, magnanimous, and engaging (warm dominant behavior). However, when their status is perceived to be challenged in social situations, the individual is likely to respond with hostility to diminish their challenger and reassert their status. If successful, the individual will have effectively regulated their self and affect. This is typically maladaptive in its pervasiveness and misapplication of this strategy in situations where it will not be effective or socially acceptable. In such situations, when the individual fails or feels they would be unable to maintain or establish their status, then they are likely to shift into a vulnerable self-state, which is often defined by self-protective motives and behavior (cold–submissive) and negative affects, primarily shame and feelings of inadequacy, self-doubt, and resentment. Naturally, there are individual differences among narcissistic individuals in terms of how much time they spend in each of these self-states and the specific surface-level features of how they are manifested. Shifts between them can be dramatic, and lead to a fragmented sense of self and a clinical picture that is difficult to integrate (Pincus et al., 2014; Wright, 2014).

Many of the fundamental impairments in self and identity functioning articulated above for borderline personality disorder apply to severe cases of narcissism (i.e., at the borderline level of functioning; Kernberg, 1984). Research from our lab conducted among individuals in naturalistic settings confirms the fact that narcissistic self-states are contingent on the interpersonal behavior of others and relate in expected ways to one's own social behavior in the same situations (Edershile & Wright, 2021a). Similarly, individuals high in trait-level narcissism, particularly narcissistic vulnerability, show a sensitivity to perceptions of others' dominance and cold behavior and respond with stronger negative emotions and hostility (Edershile & Wright, in press). However, evidence for grandiosity serving as a response to or defense against vulnerability is weak (Edershile & Wright, 2021b).

6.10 Concluding Comments

In sum, CIIT provides a framework for guiding new research on personality disorders and integrating it with existing theory across disciplines. The guiding principles of CIIT are that (1) the interpersonal situation is the site of dysfunctional self and social processes maintaining personality disorders, (2) both self and social processes can be organized on axes of agency and communion, and (3) self and social processes can be investigated in relation to each other across contexts and time scales. Although interpersonal theory has historically emphasized the social-system in the interpersonal transaction cycle, we highlight in this chapter that he self-system is an under-researched but critical aspect of understanding personality pathology. We demonstrate in our examples of self and social dysfunction in narcissistic personality disorder and borderline personality disorder how the guiding principles of CIIT can integrate research on the self-system into a more comprehensive understanding of the full interpersonal system.

References

American Psychiatric Association. (2013). *Diagnostic and statistical manual of mental disorders* (5th ed.). American Psychiatric Association.

Ansell, E. B., Kurtz, J. E., & Markey, P. M. (2008). Gender differences in interpersonal complementarity within roommate dyads. *Personality and Social Psychology Bulletin*, *34*(4), 502–512.

Aron, A., Lewandowski, G., Branand, B., Mashek, D., & Aron, E. (2022). Self-expansion motivation and inclusion of others in self: An updated review. *Journal of Social and Personal Relationships*, *39*(12), 3821–3852.

Bakan, D. (1966). *The duality of human existence: Isolation and communion in Western man*. Beacon.

Beeney, J. E., Hallquist, M. N., Ellison, W. D., & Levy, K. N. (2016). Self–other disturbance in borderline personality disorder: Neural, self-report, and performance-based evidence. *Personality Disorders: Theory, Research, and Treatment*, *7*(1), 28–39.

Bender, D. S., Morey, L. C., & Skodol, A. E. (2011). Toward a model for assessing level of personality functioning in DSM-5, Part I: A review of theory and methods. *Journal of Personality Assessment*, *93*, 332–346.

Benjamin, L. (1993). Every psychopathology is a gift of love. *Psychotherapy Research*, *3*(1), 1–24.

Benjamin, L. S. (1996). *Interpersonal diagnosis and treatment of personality disorders*. Guilford.

Bleckmann, E., Lüdtke, O., Mueller, S., & Wagner, J. (2023). The role of interpersonal perceptions of social inclusion and personality in momentary self-esteem and self-esteem reactivity. *European Journal of Personality*, *37*(2), 187–206.

Block, J. (1982). Assimilation, accommodation, and the dynamics of personality development. *Child Development*, *53*, 281–295.

Bouchard, S., & Sabourin, S. (2009). Borderline personality disorder and couple dysfunctions. *Current Psychiatry Reports*, *11*(1), 55–62.

Cacioppo, J. T., Hawkley, L. C., Norman, G. J., & Berntson, G. G. (2011). Social isolation. *Annals of the New York Academy of Sciences*, *1231*(1), 17–22.

Carson, R. C. (1969). *Interaction concepts of personality*. Aldine Publishing Co.

Conway, M. A., & Pleydell-Pearce, C. W. (2000). The construction of autobiographical memories in the self-memory system. *Psychological Review*, *107*(2), 261–288.

De Meulemeester, C., Lowyck, B., Vermote, R., Verhaest, Y., & Luyten, P. (2017). Mentalizing and interpersonal problems in borderline personality disorder: The mediating role of identity diffusion. *Psychiatry Research*, *258*, 141–144.

DeYoung, C. G. (2015). Cybernetic big five theory. *Journal of Research in Personality*, *56*, 33–58.

Dimaggio, G., Lysaker, P. H., Carcione, A., Nicolò, G., & Semerari, A. (2008). Know yourself and you shall know the other … to a certain extent: Multiple paths of influence of self-reflection on mindreading. *Consciousness and Cognition*, *17*(3), 778–789.

Dunlop, W. L. (2017). Situating self-concept clarity in the landscape of personality. In J. Lodi-Smith & K. G. DeMarree (eds), *Self-concept clarity: Perspectives on assessment, research, and applications*, pp. 19–41. Springer.

Dunlop, W. L., Lind, M., & Hopwood, C. J. (2023). Synthesizing contemporary integrative interpersonal theory and the narrative identity approach to examine personality dynamics and regulatory processes. *Journal of Personality*, *91*(4), 963–976.

Edershile, E. A., & Wright, A. G. C. (2021a). Grandiose and vulnerable narcissistic states in interpersonal situations. *Self and Identity*, *20*(2), 165–181.

Edershile, E. A., & Wright, A. G. C. (2021b). Fluctuations in grandiose and vulnerable narcissistic states: A momentary perspective. *Journal of Personality and Social Psychology*, *120*(5), 1386–1414.

Edershile, E. A., & Wright, A. G. C. (2022). Narcissism dynamics. *Social and Personality Psychology Compass*, *16*(1), e12649.

Edershile, E. A., & Wright, A. G. C. (in press). Narcissism's effect on interpersonal regulation. *Personality Disorders: Theory, Research, and Treatment*. https://osf.io/preprints/psyarxiv/xza6c

Fiske, A. P. (1992). The four elementary forms of sociality: Framework for a unified theory of social relations. *Psychological Review, 99*(4), 689–723.

Fournier, M. A., Moskowitz, D. S., & Zuroff, D. C. (2008). Integrating dispositions, signatures, and the interpersonal domain. *Journal of Personality and Social Psychology, 94*(3), 531–545.

Fournier, M., Moskowitz, D. S., & Zuroff, D. (2009). The interpersonal signature. *Journal of Research in Personality, 43*, 155–162.

Geukes, K., Nestler, S., Hutteman, R., Dufner, M., Küfner, A. C., Egloff, B., . . . & Back, M. D. (2017). Puffed-up but shaky selves: State self-esteem level and variability in narcissists. *Journal of Personality and Social Psychology, 112*(5), 769–786.

Grapsas, S., Brummelman, E., Back, M. D., & Denissen, J. J. (2020). The "why" and "how" of narcissism: A process model of narcissistic status pursuit. *Perspectives on Psychological Science, 15*(1), 150–172.

Gurtman, M. B. (1992). Construct validity in interpersonal personality measures: The interpersonal circumplex as a nomological net. *Journal of Personality and Social Psychology, 63*, 105–118.

Guttman, L. (1954). A new approach to factor analysis: The Radex. In P. F. Lazarsfeld (ed.), *Mathematical thinking in the social sciences*, pp. 258–348. Free Press.

Heine, S. J., Proulx, T., & Vohs, K. D. (2006). The meaning maintenance model: On the coherence of social motivations. *Personality and Social Psychology Review, 10*(2), 88–110.

Hochschild Tolpin, L., Cimbolic Gunthert, K., Cohen, L. H., & O'Neill, S. C. (2004). Borderline personality features and instability of daily negative affect and self-esteem. *Journal of Personality, 72*(1), 111–138.

Hopwood, C. J., Wright, A. G. C., Ansell, E. B., & Pincus, A. L. (2013). The interpersonal core of personality pathology. *Journal of Personality Disorders, 27*(3), 271–295.

Horowitz, L. M., Wilson, K. R., Turan, B., Zolotsev, P., Constantino, M. J., & Henderson, L. (2006). How interpersonal motives clarify the meaning of interpersonal behavior: A revised circumplex model. *Personality and Social Psychology Review, 10*(1), 67–86.

James, W. (1890). *The principles of psychology*. H. Holt and Company.

Jørgensen, C. R., & Bøye, R. (2022). How does it feel to have a disturbed identity? The phenomenology of identity diffusion in patients with borderline personality disorder: A qualitative study. *Journal of Personality Disorders, 36*(1), 40–69.

Kernberg, O. F. (1984). *Severe personality disorders: Psychotherapeutic strategies*. Yale University Press.

Kierkegaard, S. (1941). *The sickness unto death*. Princeton University Press.

Kiesler, D. J. (1983). The 1982 interpersonal circle: A taxonomy for complementarity in human transactions. *Psychological Review, 90*, 185–214.

Klimstra, T. A., Luyckx, K., Germeijs, V., Meeus, W. H., & Goossens, L. (2012). Personality traits and educational identity formation in late adolescents: Longitudinal associations and academic progress. *Journal of Youth and Adolescence, 41*, 346–361.

Kockler, T. D., Santangelo, P. S., Eid, M., Kuehner, C., Bohus, M., Schmaedeke, S., & Ebner-Priemer, U. W. (2022). Self-esteem instability might be more characteristic of borderline personality disorder than affective instability: Findings from an e-diary study with clinical and healthy controls. *Journal of Psychopathology and Clinical Science*, *131*(3), 301.

Kohut, H. (1977). *The restoration of the self*. University of Chicago Press.

Kotov, R., Krueger, R. F., Watson, D., Cicero, D. C., Conway, C. C., DeYoung, C. G., Eaton, N. R., Forbes, M. K., Hallquist, M. N., Latzman, R. D., Mullins-Sweatt, S. N., Ruggero, C. J., Simms, L. J., Waldman, I. D., Waszczuk, M. A., & Wright, A. G. C. (2021). The Hierarchical Taxonomy of Psychopathology (HiTOP): A quantitative nosology based on consensus of evidence. *Annual Review of Clinical Psychology*, *17*, 83–108.

Kraus, M. W., Chen, S., & Keltner, D. (2011). The power to be me: Power elevates self-concept consistency and authenticity. *Journal of Experimental Social Psychology*, *47*(5), 974–980.

Kroencke, L., Kuper, N., Mota, S., Geukes, K., Zeigler-Hill, V., & Back, M. D. (2023). Narcissistic status pursuit in everyday social life: A within-person process approach to the behavioral and emotional dynamics of narcissism. *Journal of Personality and Social Psychology*, *125*(6), 1519–1541.

Lazarus, S. A., Scott, L. N., Beeney, J. E., Wright, A. G. C., Stepp, S. D., & Pilkonis, P. A. (2018). Borderline personality disorder symptoms and affective responding to perceptions of rejection and acceptance from romantic versus non-romantic partners. *Personality Disorder: Theory, Research, and Treatment*, *9*(3), 197–206.

Leary, T. (1957). *Interpersonal diagnosis of personality*. Ronald Press.

Lind, M., Adler, J. M., & Clark, L. A. (2020). Narrative identity and personality disorder: An empirical and conceptual review. *Current Psychiatry Reports*, *22*, 1–11.

Livesley, W. J. (1998). Suggestions for a framework for an empirically based classification of personality disorder. *Canadian Journal of Psychiatry*, *43*, 137–147.

Locke, K. D. (2000). Circumplex scales of interpersonal values: Reliability, validity, and applicability to interpersonal problems and personality disorders. *Journal of Personality Assessment*, *75*(2), 249–267.

Locke, K. D. (2011). Circumplex measures of interpersonal constructs. In L. M. Horowitz & S. Strack (eds.), *Handbook of interpersonal psychology*, pp. 313–324. Wiley.

Markus, H., & Kunda, Z. (1986). Stability and malleability of the self-concept. *Journal of Personality and Social Psychology*, *51*(4), 858–866.

McAdams, D. P. (1996). Narrating the self. In G. M. Kenyon, J. E. Birren, J.-E. Ruth, J. J. F. Schroots, & T. Svensson (eds), *Aging and biography: Explorations in adult development*, pp. 131–148. Springer.

McAdams, D. P., & Pals, J. L. (2006). A new Big Five: Fundamental principles for an integrative science of personality. *American Psychologist*, *61*(3), 204–217.

McAdams, D. P., Hoffman, B. J., Day, R., & Mansfield, E. D. (1996). Themes of agency and communion in significant autobiographical scenes. *Journal of Personality*, *64*(2), 339–377.

McConnell, A. R., & Strain, L. M. (2011). Content and structure of the self-concept. In C. Sedikides & S. Spencer (eds), *The self*, pp. 51–73. Psychology Press.

McConnell, A. R., Rydell, R. J., & Brown, C. M. (2009). On the experience of self-relevant feedback: How self-concept organization influences affective responses and self-evaluations. *Journal of Experimental Social Psychology*, *45*(4), 695–707.

McWilliams, N. (2011). *Psychoanalytic diagnosis: Understanding personality structure in the clinical process*. Guilford Press.

Mead, G. H. (1934). *Mind, self, and society from the standpoint of a social behaviorist.* University of Chicago Press.

Melamed, D. M., Botting, J., Lofthouse, K., Pass, L., & Meiser-Stedman, R. (2024). The relationship between negative self-concept, trauma, and maltreatment in children and adolescents: A meta-analysis. *Clinical Child and Family Psychology Review, 27*(1), 220–234.

Miller, J. D., Back, M. D., Lynam, D. R., & Wright, A. G. C. (2021). Narcissism today: What we know and what we need to learn. *Current Directions in Psychological Science, 30*(6), 519–525.

Mischel, W. (2004). Toward an integrative science of the person. *Annual Review of Psychology, 55*, 1–22.

Mischel, W., & Shoda, Y. (1995). A cognitive-affective system theory of personality: Reconceptualizing situations, dispositions, dynamics, and invariance in personality structure. *Psychological Review*, 102(2), 246–268.

Morf, C. C., & Rhodewalt, F. (2001). Unraveling the paradoxes of narcissism: A dynamic self-regulatory processing model. *Psychological Inquiry, 12*(4), 177–196.

Nurius, P. S., & Markus, H. (1990). Situational variability in the self-concept: Appraisals, expectancies, and asymmetries. *Journal of Social and Clinical Psychology, 9*(3), 316–333.

Pals, J. L. (2006). Narrative identity processing of difficult life experiences: Pathways of personality development and positive self-transformation in adulthood. *Journal of Personality, 74*(4), 1079–1110.

Parfit, D. (1971). Personal identity. *The Philosophical Review, 80*(1), 3–27.

Parker, G., Hadzi-Pavlovic, D., Both, L., Kumar, S., Wilhelm, K., & Olley, A. (2004). Measuring disordered personality functioning: To love and work reprised. *Acta Psychiatrica Scandinavica, 110*, 230–239.

Paulhus, D. L. (1998). Interpersonal and intrapsychic adaptiveness of trait self-enhancement: A mixed blessing? *Journal of Personality and Social Psychology, 74*(5), 1197–1208.

Pincus, A. L. (2011). Some comments on nomology, diagnostic process, and narcissistic personality disorder in the DSM-5 proposal for personality and personality disorders. *Personality Disorders: Theory, Research, and Treatment, 2*, 41–53.

Pincus, A. L., & Ansell, E. B. (2013). Interpersonal theory of personality. In J. Suls & H. Tennen (eds.), *Handbook of psychology Vol. 5: Personality and social psychology* (2nd ed.), pp. 141–159. Wiley.

Pincus, A. L., Ansell, E. B., Pimentel, C. A., Cain, N. M., Wright, A. G. C., & Levy, K. N. (2009). The initial development and derivation of the Pathological Narcissism Inventory. *Psychological Assessment, 21*(3), 365–379.

Pincus, A. L., Cain, N. M., & Wright, A. G. C. (2014). Narcissistic grandiosity and narcissistic vulnerability in psychotherapy. *Personality Disorders: Theory, Research, and Treatment, 5*(4), 439–443.

Ricoeur, P. (1988). The human being as the subject matter of philosophy. *Philosophy & Social Criticism, 14*(2), 203–215.

Ringwald, W. R., Forbes, M. K., & Wright, A. G. C. (2023). Meta-analysis of structural evidence for the Hierarchical Taxonomy of Psychopathology (HiTOP) model. *Psychological Medicine*, *53*(2), 533–546.

Roche, M. J. (2022). Tethering theory to timescale: Advances in measuring interpersonal complementarity and covariation. *Journal of Research in Personality*, *99*, 104264.

Roche, M. J., & Cain, N. M. (2021). Interpersonal theory and personality processes. In J. F. Rauthmann (ed.), *The handbook of personality dynamics and processes*, pp. 669–688. Academic Press.

Russell, J. J., Moskowitz, D. S., Zuroff, D. C., Sookman, D., & Paris, J. (2007). Stability and variability of affective experience and interpersonal behavior in borderline personality disorder. *Journal of Abnormal Psychology*, *116*, 578–588.

Sadikaj, G., Moskowitz, D. S., Russell, J. J., Zuroff, D. C., & Paris, J. (2013). Quarrelsome behavior in borderline personality disorder: Influence of behavioral and affective reactivity to perceptions of others. *Journal of Abnormal Psychology*, *122*(1), 195–207.

Sadler, P., Ethier, N., & Woody, E. (2011). Interpersonal complementarity. In L. M. Horowitz & S. Strack (eds), *Handbook of interpersonal psychology*, pp. 123–142. Wiley.

Santangelo, P., Bohus, M., & Ebner-Priemer, U. W. (2014). Ecological momentary assessment in borderline personality disorder: A review of recent findings and methodological challenges. *Journal of Personality Disorders*, *28*(4), 555–576.

Santangelo, P. S., Kockler, T. D., Zeitler, M. L., Knies, R., Kleindienst, N., Bohus, M., & Ebner-Priemer, U. W. (2020). Self-esteem instability and affective instability in everyday life after remission from borderline personality disorder. *Borderline Personality Disorder and Emotion Dysregulation*, *7*, 1–20.

Sato, M., Fonagy, P., & Luyten, P. (2020). Rejection sensitivity and borderline personality disorder features: The mediating roles of attachment anxiety, need to belong, and self-criticism. *Journal of Personality Sisorders*, *34*(2), 273–288.

Sebastian, C., Burnett, S., & Blakemore, S. J. (2008). Development of the self-concept during adolescence. *Trends in Cognitive Sciences*, *12*(11), 441–446.

Sharp, C., Wright, A. G. C., Fowler, J. C., Freuh, C., Allen, J. G., Oldham, J., & Clark, L. A. (2015). The structure of personality pathology: Both general ('g') and specific ('s') factors? *Journal of Abnormal Psychology*, *124*(2), 387–398.

Singer, J. A., Blagov, P., Berry, M., & Oost, K. M. (2013). Self-defining memories, scripts, and the life story: Narrative identity in personality and psychotherapy. *Journal of Personality*, *81*(6), 569–582.

Sullivan, H. S. (1953). *The interpersonal theory of psychiatry*. Norton.

Swann, W. B., & Hill, C. A. (1982). When our identities are mistaken: Reaffirming self-conceptions through social interaction. *Journal of Personality and social Psychology*, *43*(1), 59–66.

Uliaszek, A. A., Fournier, M. A., Southward, M. W., Al-Dajani, N., & Quitasol, M. (2022). Bridging development and disturbance: A translational approach to the study of identity. *Personality Disorders: Theory, Research, and Treatment*, *13*(5), 460–473.

Vess, M., Arndt, J., & Schlegel, R. J. (2011). Abstract construal levels attenuate state self-esteem reactivity. *Journal of Experimental Social Psychology*, *47*(4), 861–864.

Wiggins, J. S. (1996). An informal history of the interpersonal circumplex tradition. *Journal of Personality Assessment*, *66*(2), 217–233.

Wilkinson-Ryan, T., & Westen, D. (2000). Identity disturbance in borderline personality disorder: An empirical investigation. *American Journal of Psychiatry, 157*(4), 528–541.
World Health Organization (2022). International Classification of Diseases, Eleventh Revision (ICD-11). https://icd.who.int/browse11.
Woods, W. C., & Wright, A. G. C. (2024). Approaches to modeling interpersonal complementarity in intensive longitudinal data. *Journal of Research in Personality, 111*, 104512.
Wright, A. G. C. (2014). Integrating trait and process based conceptualizations of pathological narcissism in the DSM-5 era. In A. Besser (ed.) *Handbook of psychology of narcissism: Diverse perspectives*, pp. 153–174. Nova Science Publishers.
Wright, A. G. C., & Edershile, E. A. (2018). Issues resolved and unresolved in pathological narcissism. *Current Opinion in Psychology, 21*, 74–79.
Wright, A. G. C., Hallquist, M. N., Beeney, J. E., & Pilkonis, P. A. (2013a). Borderline personality pathology and the stability of interpersonal problems. *Journal of Abnormal Psychology, 122*(4), 1094–1100.
Wright, A. G. C., Hallquist, M. N., Morse, J. Q., Scott, L. N., Stepp, S. D., Nolf, K. A., & Pilkonis, P. A. (2013b) Clarifying interpersonal heterogeneity in borderline personality disorder using latent mixture modeling. *Journal of Personality Disorders, 27*(2), 125–143.
Wright, A. G. C., Hopwood, C. J., Skodol, A. E., & Morey, L. C. (2016). Longitudinal validation of general and specific structural features of personality pathology. *Journal of Abnormal Psychology, 125*(8), 1120–1134.
Wright, A. G. C., Pincus, A., & Hopwood, C. J. (2023). Contemporary integrative interpersonal theory: Integrating structure, dynamics, temporal scale, and levels of analysis. *Journal of Psychopathology and Clinical Science, 132*(3), 263–276.
Wright, A. G. C., Ringwald, W. R., Hopwood, C. J., & Pincus, A. L. (2022). It's time to replace the personality disorders with the interpersonal disorders. *American Psychologist, 77*(9), 1085–1099.
Zeigler-Hill, V., & Abraham, J. (2006). Borderline personality features: Instability of self–esteem and affect. *Journal of Social and Clinical Psychology, 25*(6), 668–687.
Zeigler-Hill, V., Myers, E. M., & Clark, C. B. (2010). Narcissism and self-esteem reactivity: The role of negative achievement events. *Journal of Research in Personality, 44*(2), 285–292.

7 The Inflexible Self and Lived Time

A Phenomenological Approach to Personality Disorders

Anna Sterna, Marcin Moskalewicz, Philipp Schmidt-Boddy, and Thomas Fuchs

7.1 Phenomenological Approach to Personality Disorders: Inflexibility as *Weakened Capability to Elude Recurrence*

Alterations of lived time have been placed at the phenomenal core of various psychiatric diagnoses (Fuchs, 2010; Kent et al., 2023; Moskalewicz & Fuchs, 2023; Moskalewicz & Messas, 2022; Moskalewicz & Schwartz, 2020). As far as personality disorders are concerned, the discourse leans heavily on insights derived from analyses of borderline personality disorder (BPD), an approach that has been criticized for establishing a specific and ultimately distorting category of (B)PD (Lind et al., 2020). In this respect, the primary phenomenological theses concern the qualities of immediacy (Fuchs, 2007a), instantaneity (Stanghellini & Mancini, 2018), affective over-identification (Schmidt, 2020b), and rupture (Schmidt & Fuchs, 2021), which all result in a discontinuity of the passage of time (Sterna & Moskalewicz, 2022). These phenomena appear to be closely tied to the emotional over-reactivity specific to the BPD gestalt (Schmidt, 2020a, 2022), but not to all PD.

Given this specificity, it is important to remain cautious when describing the temporal characteristics of personality disorder more generally. This chapter aims to describe the temporal structures involved in personality disorder from a more cross-typological perspective by shedding light on what has been psychopathologically named as *inflexibility* (DSM-5, section II), which is associated with a *disturbed self-directedness* (DSM-5, section III). By looking at the life-world in personality disorder, we argue that these are temporally grounded phenomena in which inflexibility can be understood as being stuck in repetitive, past–present cycles, whereas diminished self-directedness, relatedly, refers to a blurred sense of futurity.

A phenomenology-inspired taxonomy distinguishes between a macro-layer of temporality, referring to the explicit integration of the distinct and distinguishable in the mind dimensions of past, present, and future, and implicit, micro-layer of temporality, which is constituted by the so-called retention, presentation, and protention (Kent et al., 2023). In the case of the latter phenomenological concepts, one cannot clearly distinguish between their temporal situatedness in terms of past, present, and future, with retention sometimes being referred to as immediate past and protention as immediate future. Although disturbances in the micro-layer are considered more severe and have often been ascribed to schizophrenia and related disorders (Sul, 2022), we contend that the temporal specificity of personality disorder lies rather in an imbalanced macro-layer. Macro-layers seem to be organized in a way that the past and present are repetitively close-cycled, so that the future dimension, which enables the future extension of oneself and existential becoming, becomes unattainable. This results in an endangered temporal continuity manifested as a lack of *self-cohesion* (DSM-5; Silverstein, 2007). This model extends the often-used micro–macro temporal phenomenological framework by combining it with the characteristics of rhythm or repetitiveness (Fuchs, 2020). Seen from this angle, PD temporality appears as deeply entangled in the circular time of *zoe* (i.e., life in the biological sense), and with a limited capacity to build a more temporarily linear *bios* (i.e., life in the biographical sense), in which self-experience is built around creating and appropriating novelty instead of repeating the same pattern (Fuchs, 2018; Moskalewicz, 2024, pp. 93–94).

That said, considering the heterogeneity of personality disorders, apart from the core temporal characteristics, some may exhibit symptoms of micro-layer disturbances. For instance, high impulsivity (disinhibition dimension, DSM-5) may be hypothesized to stem from the deeper, more immediate and less-controllable acceleration of micro-layer flow whereas deceleration may occur with high negative affectivity. However, this chapter delineates the structural temporal gestalt of all personality disorders, leaving type- or dimension-specific particulars for future research.

We assume that flexibility is contingent upon a more general capability of changing oneself over time. Flexibility, then, is conditioned by the ability to navigate and integrate different kinds of temporal horizons. In the experience of personality disorder, this dynamic is hindered, translating into a felt sense of *stuckness in oneself*, which encompasses both the interpersonal dimension and self-experience. Inflexibility in interpersonal interactions and low self-directedness, we suggest, have their root in the structure of lived time, which remains organized according to recurring patterns that constitute inevitable cycles. This perspective aligns with the classification manuals' stance that *self-impairment* lies at the core of personality disorder (DSM-5, section III). Lack of future openness, along with over-arching past–present loops, co-constitute repetitions and are responsible for a sense that *going further* is unreachable. Specifically, this impairment may pertain to a weakness in narrative self-synthesis, which cannot effectively unite one's historicity and project oneself into the future as intended (Fuchs, 2013; Schmidt & Fuchs, 2021).

To characterize inflexibility and circular patterns of lived temporality in personality disorder in more detail, we address five interrelated temporal topoi – *repetitiveness of interpersonal patterns*, *affective rigidity*, *reification of self-experience*, *lack of future openness*, and *the feeling of being stuck*. Suggesting that the phenomena relating to these five topoi together constitute a *weakened capability to escape from the disturbing cycles*, we provide section-by-section glimpses of felt inflexibility in the top-down manner: from the interpersonal dimension, through affectivity, until reaching the self-issues that form the kernel of personality disorder. We illustrate them with selected lived experience reports taken from our clinical practice and research.

7.1.1 Topos 1: Repetitiveness of Interpersonal Patterns

The first temporal aspect we discuss refers to the cyclicity of interpersonal patterns prevalent across personality disorders. Although their interpersonal life-worlds may differ considerably, there is a salient aspect common to all of them: the interpersonal life-world of people with personality disorder is organized in accordance with a certain, specific *leitmotif*. For instance, in the case of avoidant personality disorder the experience of being lonely and longing for intimacy is central from one's very youth (Sørensen et al., 2020). For those with narcissistic personality disorder the topic of external admiration and the prevention of humiliation is in the foreground (Kernberg, 2007), whereas in borderline personality disorder efforts are made to avoid any sense of abandonment (Dibenedetti et al., 2023). Finally, those with obsessive-compulsive personality disorder remain focused on their productivity while excluding interpersonal needs (Dimaggio et al., 2011).

Being concerned with such leitmotifs evidently does not only lead to certain behavioral repetitions, for example, seeking contexts of high attention typical of histrionic personality disorder (Wakefield, 2008). These themes also determine how a person cyclically experiences self, world, and others in general. The recurring nature of interpersonal patterns thus refers rather to rigid self–other mental representations and their potential to behaviorally shape one's intersubjective world, which precludes development.

In personality disorder, this may also show in a heightened external locus of control. Instead of engaging in a reflection on how one perceives the world, those with PD take the world as it appears to them at face value. Whatever change may be desired, it is one that is always to be made in the world, rather than in one's attitude toward a given situation. In clinical work with personality disorder, one can easily spot a position of constant *waiting for the world to change*, each new relationship begins with the initial hope that this time it will go far differently. Yet, when the realization comes that *I was abandoned again, humiliated, unnoticed, or the only righteous one more time*, the impression of being stuck in one's fate arises. Interpersonal experiences are painfully persistent and recurring. Questioning one's own way of perceiving and interacting with others is unavailable because the locus of this consistency is denoted *out there*, in the qualities of the world or others. The core belief in paranoid personality disorder, for example, is that *this world is so dangerous, or others are duplicitous, therefore I have to maintain a certain level of distrust.* Young et al. (2003) attribute this repetitiveness to the human drive for consistency. In personality disorder, it can give rise to a feeling of "rightness" about others, further petrifying the pattern of experiencing and interacting with them.

This appears as an auto-reifying mechanism (co-constitutive of, but not equal to self-reification), wherein the lived anticipation of a perpetual interpersonal schema, aligned with a highly selective focus on consistency, establishes favorable conditions for schema confirmation. The anticipatory over-focus on consistency, along with a pre-reflective selection of people of certain dispositions, "willing" to join the scene, translates into a world-experience in which the expected interpersonal *future holds little novelty* as if predetermined for repetition. The world is therefore felt as being construed in a well-defined, stiff manner, as if one's lived space was designed to reciprocally reinforce one's core beliefs (Fuchs, 2007b).

The lack of natural changeability embedded in the cognitive-affective *sameness* of the self–other perspective constrains interpersonal dynamics to the repetitive, single scene. Even in the borderline case, recognized as having high volatility, lived experience is so perpetual that it resembles the first-person quality of what some have described as *drifting into the swamp* (Sterna & Moskalewicz, 2022). This metaphor indicates the lack of agency regarding the inevitability of repetitions. One's experienced freedom is then limited. In Blankenburg's terms, freedom is a capacity to act as the creative agent, instead of being a supporting actor in an externally created scenery (Blankenburg, 1987). One of the individuals with personality disorder reflected it as follows: "My whole life no one cared about me (. . .) so many years, the same pattern repeats itself, people react to me in the same way again and again."[1]

The possibility of change would require adopting the stance of the *other* toward *oneself*, the moment of decentering, de-identifying with one's world-view, gaining insight into the selective and subjective nature of one's life-scenario. However, people with personality disorder struggle with this precise capability of perspective-taking.

[1] All the quotes included were extracted from semi-structured interviews conducted by Anna Sterna in 2023 with PD individuals in one of the Polish psychiatric hospitals.

Above, we delved into the qualities of stiffened interpersonal patterns, which are pre-reflectively enacted and, therefore, repeated. This, along with diminished reflexivity and experiential avoidance, can possibly constrain two aspects of one's ability to change: (1) to adopt an alternative self–other view, and (2) to allow experiences that conflict with one's previous self–other view.

7.1.2 Topos 2: Affective Rigidity

This section delves into the aspect of rigid affectivity, a constituent of lived inflexibility intertwined with interpersonal repetitiveness. Proneness to affective responses of a certain color is discussed regarding borderline personality disorder in relation to anger and dysphoria (Stanghellini & Mancini, 2018) or regarding narcissistic personality disorder and shame (Di Sarno et al., 2020). On the other hand, perceived ineffectiveness of one's regulatory strategies is reported in, for example, obsessive-compulsive personality disorder (Steenkamp et al., 2015) and BPD (Schmidt, 2022). Below, we explore how the diminished intrapersonal variance of lived affect, coupled with a restricted repertoire of regulative strategies, places individuals with personality disorders in a position where personal development is felt as inhibited.

Interpersonal schema and mental representations, delineated in the preceding section, seem to operate as filters or organizers of information. As information reduction constitutes schemas' main functionality, they delimit patterns of interpretation, subsequently decreasing the variance of affective responses. This reduction is sensed as an over-representation of a certain affective context, retrospectively summoning a sense of a negativity-biased past (Zajenkowski et al., 2021). For example, an individual with BPD may have a limited capability to interpret a partner's need for aloneness in terms other than as a sign of abandonment. Along with interpretation the frequency of felt despair increases, causing one to feel rejected *again*. In this manner, past and present affective contexts become indistinguishable, resulting in a felt sense of situational and, therefore, reactional *sameness*, precluding effective adjustment of response to present stimuli. This may stem from a traumatic heritage attributed as PD background, where the past affective patterns are repeated instead of remembered (Boschan, 1990; Freud, 1920).

Another facet of affective rigidity refers to emotion regulation strategies. Across personality disorders, both: interpretative patterns described above and compensatory mechanisms are limited constituting schemas, namely "themes" organizing information about oneself and others used to process any experience (Young & Lindemann, 1992). Others would call it an individually organized set of defense mechanisms (Bowins, 2010). Soon after a situation has been interpreted as abandonment, a regulative strategy or defense mechanism needs to be adopted – for instance, the partner's devaluation and the anger that it has triggered. Then rigidity here is felt as a recurrence of coping strategies toward reverberating interpersonal situations, as if one had only access to *limited affective repertoires*.

It seems that the lived effect of the abovementioned affective rigidity is a felt sense of disharmonious personal growth. While one gradually acquires social competencies and can observe their accumulation (e.g., goes to work even though feeling anxious about interactions) or reaches developmental milestones (e.g., starts a family), simultaneously their affective repertoire is felt as petrified rather than developed. One of the common complaints of individuals with personality disorder is that their affective reactions are personally felt as inadequate. Consider a socially respected person diagnosed with narcissism, whose self-esteem collapses entirely after a mild critique, or who reacts with intense shame every time there is need for partial self-disclosure, or an individual with avoidant personality disorder, who, regardless of their professional competencies, reacts with intense anxiety when required to interact with strangers. Disharmony between one's emotional and, for example, professional competencies constitutes a felt sense of *immaturity* – "I am almost 40, but sometimes I feel like 5 year old, I hate it!", as one of the individuals with PD put it. Immaturity of this kind may be understood as an effect of experiential cognition–affection inconsistency or lack of an integration of different self-states, of possibly traumatic origin. Nosologically speaking, it seems to differentiate symptom severity. When personality disorder symptoms are mild, dysregulation of self-states occurs on the occasion of intense stress. In severe cases, it affects all aspects of functioning (DSM-5). Felt inconsistency significantly impacts both self-knowledge and self-understanding (Schmidt & Fuchs, 2021), giving rise to doubts about inner reliability or sense of one's multiplicity, a concept explored in various psychotherapeutic modalities (e.g., Fisher, 2017; Young et al., 2003). "Actually, I don't know who I am (. . .) I do things that surprise me. Or sometimes my reactions just shock me."

The lived paradox lies in the fact that, although certain social skills may objectively be acquired and developed over time, there are aspects that structurally *remain the same*, stay undeveloped, with new material failing to integrate (Kernberg, 2007). For instance a sense of being over-reliant, compulsively seeking a reference person in dependent personality disorder, although having the ability to make independent decisions at work. Another paradox refers to one's lived sense of moving in a cycle – when I realize that I reacted *as usual* again, I can feel vertically consistent, identified with my personal history of over-reactivity to critique, but at the same time this does not horizontally align with other areas of functioning, leaving me in a sense of incoherence, characteristic for personality disorder. This quality of *remaining the same* seems parallel to trauma's repercussions – as if the traumatized region, for example the sense of absolute worthlessness in narcissism, becomes perpetually trapped in the recurring present, affectively resurfacing whenever evoked by ongoing life occurrences (Stolorow, 2003). Now, with the growing incorporation of the embodied aspect into the conceptualization of various psychopathologies, it is understood that this kind of trauma residue may possess a non-verbal, intrinsic character as well (Van der Kolk, 1998) and enhance affective rigidity.

7.1.3 Topos 3: Reification of Self-Experience

The question to what extent self-flexibility should be considered normative remains at issue (C. R. Cloninger et al., 2017; Tyrer, 2005), although – as Jaspers put it – personality should be considered as a constant self-creation in time (Jaspers, 1997, p. 430). Following Blankenburg (1987), freedom's essence lies not in fulfillment but in the possibility of change. Therefore, personal freedom does not have to be consumed in the sense that my personality *is changing*; instead it relies on a felt sense, that my personality *is changeable*. Just the opposite – the personality disorder's first-person self-experience holds the quality of a lost ability to self-transform, felt as being stuck in oneself (despite possible surface changeability of, e.g., social roles or affects).

Previously, we explored how interpersonal patterns and unchanging beliefs about self–others mutually confirm each other, influencing one's disposition toward the world. In the obsessive-compulsive personality disorder case, for example, no matter how adaptive and feedback-grounded elasticity would be, the urge for scrupulousness persists, uncorrectable as it were. There appears to be a twofold causality at play here. Due to interpersonal loops one can experientially lack the material for integrating new knowledge about oneself (as we indicated in *the repetitiveness of interpersonal patterns* and *affective rigidity* sections), but when a new interpersonal context unfolds, it cannot be incorporated into the self either. Imagine an individual with avoidant personality disorder who habitually avoids interactions due to fear of being harmed or judged as interpersonally unskilled. Even if, on a rare occasion, they attend a team-building event at work and get feedback on being skillful, this is likely to be externally attributed or undermined. Paradoxically, this situation represents lived over-cohesion, in which one's drive for consistency dominates the internal discourse by excluding potentially transformative experiences: "There were probably some situations that said that I'm not a nobody, I'm not that insignificant, but I assume that in the midst of all this, I simply don't remember it now. I was just confirming it."

Even in the case of BPD, where self-discontinuity and fragmentation are highly symptomatic, this paradox can be discerned. Referred fragmentation occurs in terms of a certain repertoire – as if the access to different modes of functioning was limited. Therefore, in BPD, swinging is used as a popular metaphor describing the closed-circuit nature of alternating self-states' over-identification and the fairly restricted experiential possibilities associated with them.

In this way, one is set into a static *being-as-such*, instead of dynamic, natural changeability and inconclusiveness (Jaspers, 1997). There appears to be an inaccessibility of a Jungian transcendent function (Gildersleeve, 2015), which makes those with personality disorder feel stuck in their *personas*, lacking actuality and capability for psychological growth. Kraus terms it *sclerosis-identity* (Kraus, 1991), posing a sense of fixation on identity, and an inability to deviate from its characteristics. In other words, personality disorder symptomatology may intrinsically posit a negation of possibilities of alternative being (Doerr-Zegers, 2008), establishing a *self which is being over-identified with itself*, and therefore stuck. Even though this stuckness shares punctual character with, for example, psychotic standstill (Moskalewicz, 2016), it is rooted in a past–present closed-cyclicity intertwined with locked futurity, and not in a lack of time. It is more located on the personal level and refers to the inability of experiencing possibilities in ways that would allow an individual to choose itself in a Sartrean fashion or to shape itself actively according to genuine self-interpretations, as Heidegger might have it (Han-Pile, 2009). The quality of immersion and absorption into a specific state of being preclude self-transcendence and undermine any sense of existential freedom or self-choice (Pearl, 2013).

7.1.4 Topos 4: Lack of Future Openness

The concept of futurity refers to how the future (regardless of what shape it will eventually take upon happening) is lived in the present. Reflectively, the image of the future in personality disorder is often vague, blurred, emotionally distant, or anxiety-provoking (Sterna & Moskalewicz, 2022). This specificity may mirror negative past experiences, manifesting as an over-general memory (lacking specific events, providing loose narrative instead) linked to an over-general future experience (Bech et al., 2015).

Inherently across PD, there is a lack of motivational drive and *appetitive tension* toward the future (Fuchs, 2013), which diagnostically corresponds to low *self-directedness* (Skodol et al., 2011). Motivational drive refers to meaningful, creatively deposited goals or desired self-projections, in contrast to a future that is passively experienced and determined, into which one can only *stumble* (Fuchs, 2007a). Low self-directedness is one of the most consistent characteristics of all personality disorders, even for obsessive-compulsive personality disorder, regardless of symptoms' severity (R. Cloninger, 2000). Self-directedness merges both externally directed abilities such as planning and internally directed abilities such as limiting one's impulsivity, and should be distinguished from the self-centeredness common in PD. In personality disorder the sense of futurity is constructed only as a thesis or antithesis of the past; there is no tangible future, only past-like future repetitions and, therefore, lived cyclicality. This kind of futurity reflects an *as-is* mode, stating what is already known, rather than an *as-if* mode, hypothesizing about what is unknown (Märtsin, 2019). Such lived cyclicality is more subtle than the well-known cycles in addiction (Moskalewicz, 2016; Moskalewicz & Messas, 2022), which are more behavioral and tangible in terms of recurring rounds of craving, using, and guilt. In personality disorder it is predominantly self-experience and interpersonal patterns that are reverberating. A man in his thirties, whose life was marked by unexpected losses and who described himself as constantly struggling to survive in the past, summarized it as: "I'm actually afraid of the future. I don't know what will happen. I don't know if I will be there . . . (. . .) In fact, these [past, present, future] are separate things for me – I just live, time is passing by and that's it."

The twofold paradox concealed in the quote mirrors the pre-reflective sense of emotional detachment and passivity toward the unknown, coupled with a reflective sense of insecurity projected into the future as if it was already determined. This aligns with Derrida's concept of the temporality of trauma, suggesting that the traumatizing power does not lie in hypervigilance about the recurrence of *what-has-happened* but in apprehension that *worse-is-to-come* (Derrida, 2005, pp. 104–105).

The lack of future openness is intertwined with repetitive interpersonal scenarios and an inability to self-transcend, which in classical phenomenological psychopathology was considered the existential core of neurotic disorders (Binswanger, 1968; Straus, 1930; Von Gebsattel, 1954). Future openness discloses alternatives and possibilities. If these are hindered, one cannot manage one's relationships differently or assert that one has really chosen oneself. Instead, one stays undifferentiated, as Heidegger put it, which resembles the state of *being without having chosen to do so* (Han-Pile, 2009), stuck in repetitions without a future way out.

7.1.5 *Topos 5: Feeling of* Being Stuck *in the Lived Passage of Time*

The indispensable condition for a felt sense of the passage of time is the ability to observe the sequence of ongoing changes (Wyllie, 2005). Perspectives on oneself and the world, along with behavioral patterns, must be acknowledged as evolving over time, contributing to a sense of narrative self-development. We argued that the core of personality disorder stability in time may lie in a unique, lived, past–present temporal cycle. In line with a blocked sense of futurity, this temporal situation invokes the experience of *being stuck in time*, where the sense of personal development appears inhibited and nothing progresses beyond the current state.

While discussing the temporality of narcissism, Kernberg posits this quality as the *destruction of time* (Kernberg, 2007). Elsewhere, Green (2009) refers to it as the *murder of time*. Both metaphors indicate that nothing new is occurring aside from a constant escape from a sense of inferiority and humiliation, and a continuous search for external sources of self-appraisal. This perpetuity does not refer only to narcissistic or borderline personality. Recent phenomenological insights into avoidant personality disorder suggest that their lives are dominated by the oscillating movement between a longing to connect with others and a fear of intimacy (Sørensen et al., 2019).

However, it would be an over-simplification to say that, in personality disorder, lived time is explicitly annihilated. Rather, its passage is retrospectively assessed as inhibited, giving rise to a felt sense of an unlived life facing the finitude. This applies also to the paradoxical situation of individuals with obsessive-compulsive personality disorder – although being explicitly over-focused on time management and productivity, taking the bigger picture, they get stuck in repetitions and detailed structures, instead of developing, progressing in time (Hashemi Mofrad et al., 2018). One of Boschan's patients with personality disorder described this position as follows:

> And there were things that could only be endured by putting myself inside, isolating myself completely, turning into a stone. And of course, I did this so many times, and spent so much time that way, that I now feel that I lack big chunks of life which I did not live; like a book from which lots of pages have been torn, and cannot any longer be read continuously. (Boschan, 1990, p. 345)

The necessary condition for temporalizing oneself is to actively lead one's life, whereas failing to do so results in passive exposure to the domination of explicit time (Fuchs, 2013, p. 81). This inactive exposure appears to be characteristic of PDs, transcending typological distinctions, uniting them in a shared experience of passivity, expressed as ineffectiveness (Gutiérrez et al., 2008) and low self-directedness.

Consequently, this position can be perceived as a trap, in which one, devoid of agency, exteriorizing locus of control, may have a sense of powerlessness (Gilbert et al., 2011). This resembles other psychiatric conditions (Maiese, 2018); however, the uniqueness of personality disorder appears to refer to the completeness and intrinsicness of this quality in one's narrative self. Explicitly, this may be experienced as a sense of temporal sparsity (living 40 years without feeling that much time has passed; Kernberg, 2007) or density – living 20 feeling as if 40 has already elapsed. However, regardless of whether life is perceived as dense or sparse, the key lies in a felt sense that it is not the agent who undergoes these changes. This concept aligns more closely with

Berdyaev's existential time, which is founded upon one's sense of personal, inward change (Gordon, 2012), inhibited in personality disorders due to its cognitive, behavioral, and emotional rigidity over time.

The passivity referred to extends beyond a simple retrospective assessment of one's life while reflecting upon its finitude. It also encompasses determinism of the future, as discussed earlier, in terms of a lack of future openness. Here, we align with Wyllie's hypothesis that the essential condition for one's sense of the future is to perceive it as an open absence, contrasting with the static present (Wyllie, 2005). In personality disorder, this intriguing *openness* is replaced by a sense of *sameness* (as distinguished from psychotic, atemporal *eternity*). Therefore, lack of self-direction rooted in a disrupted sense of agency may inevitably imply a subtle sense of purposeless or meaninglessness of life, which has some empirical evidence across personality disorders (Steen et al., 2024). "I feel like I'm not the main character in my own life. I feel like I'm the secondary one. I just don't feel like the main character in my own story. I just don't see myself existing."

This way of living oneself also has significant ramifications for a felt happiness. An overview of one's life, that is, a reflection on one's history and its development, is an essential element of satisfaction with how things have run and how one contributed to them through one's engagements. Husserl takes it to be a central cornerstone of the phenomenon of happiness (Cavallaro & Heffernan, 2019), but feeling stuck also impinges on happiness in a different way. Some phenomenologists have emphasized that happiness is distinct to mere enjoyment, which they take to be restricted to things given in the present (Klein & Schmidt, 2024). Happiness sometimes also refers to the present moment, as if past and future were fully irrelevant to what is now, which may acclaim the central locus of meaning. Yet, more profound, comprehensive forms of happiness have a self-transcendent character. They involve not only the idea that one's current state is the result of prior fulfilment of intentions, but also contain an optimism toward the future, experienced as an imperishable *promise* of complete satisfaction. No matter the life circumstances, the happy in this sense experience the future as something in which satisfaction and fulfilment remain possible. This kind of human happiness is fundamentally anticipatory in that the happy await their future with gratitude, openness, hope, and an abiding striving toward ultimate fulfillment. This deep and existential form of happiness is less a passive state than an active temporal attitude. But given personality disorder's style of experiencing themselves as stuck in predictable time, with inflexible and unfulfilling interpersonal patterns, this temporal attitude is precisely made impossible. Most importantly, in PD, it is experienced *as* impossible, rendering the mode of being of individuals with personality disorder one of *existential frustration*. Whatever lusts and pleasures they are capable of, the desire for personal flourishing is fundamentally experienced as infinitely unfulfilled.

7.2 Summary

Developing a phenomenological perspective on the ways in which selfhood is experienced in personality disorder, this chapter explored the structure of temporality inherent to experiences of self, others, and the world. It examined how disturbances of lived temporality may underlie the inflexible personality structures associated with PD. It departed from more reflectively accessible and explicit manifestations of inflexibility and proceeded towards more implicit layers:

- As topos 1, we identified the *repetitiveness of interpersonal patterns*. PD individuals often experience a limited and unchangeable repertoire of behavioral possibilities toward others, which contributes to the recurrence of experiences. Behavioral repertoires and reactions from others often go hand in hand and determine how individuals experience themselves and others.
- Relatedly, topos 2 concerned *affective rigidity*, referring to limited sets of emotions and affective stances that can be authentically felt by individuals in personality disorder. This also involves recurring, not seldom, maladaptive emotion regulation strategies that also translate into the cyclicality of temporal experience. With recurring interpersonal interactions that follow certain schemes and the affects that accompany and trigger them, certain self-experiences are more likely to ensue.
- We discussed the associated *reification of self-experience* as topos 3, which refers to the lost ability to self-transcend and transform oneself. This ability is crucial in the development of selfhood across lifetime. We described such a development as flattened, and concomitantly the self as immutable and unalterable.
- Closely related to this is a general *lack of future openness*, which we discussed as topos 4. Because patterns repeat themselves and are anticipated, the future is experienced as an infinite recurrence of the same that cannot be fled from.
- As we discussed in topos 5, this ultimately translates into a general *sense of being stuck*. Lived time that is normally dynamic and full of chances transforms into an inevitable cage in which individuals will hardly ever feel at home. At the bottom of personality disorder inflexibility lies a temporality that implies an existential frustration with no hope of deeper fulfillment.

Acknowledgments

Anna Sterna is a participant in STER Internationalization of Doctoral Schools Program from NAWA Polish National Agency for Academic Exchange No. PPI/STE/2020/1/00014/DEC/02. NAWA is only a founder of the doctoral scholarship and has no role either in data collection or chapter preparation. Anna Sterna's research was financed from the large research grant from statutory funding for young researchers – doctoral students for 2022.

Anna Sterna's and Marcin Moskalewicz's research on temporal experience was funded by National Science Center in Poland (No. 2021/42/E/HS1/00106); Marcin Moskalewicz was also supported by the Alexander von Humboldt Stiftung.

Thomas Fuchs and Philipp Schmidt-Boddy were supported by the German Research Foundation (Deutsche Forschungsgemeinschaft, DFG projects nr. 513696000 and 446126658).

References

Bech, M., Elklit, A., & Simonsen, E. (2015). Autobiographical memory in borderline personality disorder – A systematic review. *Personality and Mental Health*, *9*, 162–171. https://doi.org/10.1002/pmh

Binswanger, L. (1968). *Being-in-the-World* (J. Needleman, ed.). Harper & Row.

Blankenburg, W. (1987). The dialectics of "freedom" and "unfreedom" in the psychiatric view. In A. T. Tymaniecka (ed.), *Morality within the life- and social world: Interdisciplinary phenomenology of the authentic life in the "moral sense"* (pp. 409–423). Springer Netherlands.

Boschan, P. J. (1990). Temporality and narcissism. *International Reviews of Psycho-Analysis*, *17*, 337–349.

Bowins, B. (2010). Personality disorders: A dimensional defense mechanism approach. *American Journal of Psychotherapy*, *64*(2), 153–169.

Cavallaro, M., & Heffernan, G. (2019). From happiness to blessedness: Husserl on eudaimonia, virtue, and the best life. *Horizon*, *8*(2), 353–389.

Cloninger, C. R., Svrakic, D. M., Lester, N. C., Lecic-Tosevski, D., Koldobsky, N., & Botbol, M. (2017). Personality disorders. In J. E. Mezzich, M. Botbol, G. N. Christodoulou, C. R. Cloninger, & I. M. Salloum (eds), *Person centered psychiatry* (pp. 427–444). Springer International Publishing.

Cloninger, R. (2000). A practical way to diagnosis personality disorders. *Journal of Personality Disorders*, *14*(2), 99–108.

Derrida, J. (2005). *Rogues: Two essays on reason*. Stanford University Press.

Di Sarno, M., Zimmermann, J., Madeddu, F., Casini, E., & Di Pierro, R. (2020). Shame behind the corner? A daily diary investigation of pathological narcissism. *Journal of Research in Personality*, *85*, 103924. https://doi.org/10.1016/J.JRP.2020.103924

Dibenedetti, D., Kosa, K., Waters, H. C., & Oberdhan, D. (2023). Understanding patients' experiences with borderline personality disorder: Qualitative interviews.

Neuropsychiatric Disease and Treatment, *19*, 2115–2125. https://doi.org/10.2147/NDT.S423882

Dimaggio, G., Carcione, A., Salvatore, G., Nicolò, G., Sisto, A., & Semerari, A. (2011). Progressively promoting metacognition in a case of obsessive-compulsive personality disorder treated with metacognitive interpersonal therapy. *Psychology and Psychotherapy: Theory, Research and Practice*, *84*(1), 70–83. https://doi.org/10.1348/147608310X527240

Doerr Zegers, O. (2008). Personality disorders from a phenomenological perspective. *Actas Españolas de Psiquiatria*, *36*(1), 10–19.

Fisher, J. (2017). *Healing the fragmented selves of trauma survivors*. Routledge.

Freud, S. (1920). *Beyond the pleasure principle* (XVIII). Hogarth Press.

Fuchs, T. (2007a). Fragmented selves: Temporality and identity in borderline personality disorder. *Psychopathology*, *40*(6), 379–387. https://doi.org/10.1159/000106468

Fuchs, T. (2007b). Psychotherapy of the lived space: A phenomenological and ecological concept. *American Journal of Psychotherapy*, *61*(4), 423–439.

Fuchs, T. (2010). Phenomenology and psychopathology. In S. Gallagher & D. Schmicking (eds), *Handbook of phenomenology and cognitive science*, 546–573. Springer.

Fuchs, T. (2013). Temporality and psychopathology. *Phenomenology and the Cognitive Sciences*, *12*(1), 75–104. https://doi.org/10.1007/s11097-010-9189-4

Fuchs, T. (2018). The cyclical time of the body and its relation to linear time. *Journal of Cosciousness Studies*, *25*(7–8), 47–65.

Fuchs, T. (2020). Time, the body, and the other in phenomenology and psychopathology. In C. Tewes & G. Stanghelleni (eds), *Time and body* (pp. 12–40). Cambridge University Press.

Gilbert, T., Farrand, P., & Lankshear, G. (2011). "I don't want to live like this anymore": Disrupted habitus in young people "at risk" of diagnosis of personality disorder. *Youth & Society*, *45*(3), 347–364. https://doi.org/10.1177/0044118X11417979

Gildersleeve, M. (2015). Unconcealing Jung's transcendent function with Heidegger. *Humanistic Psychologist*, *43*(3), 297–309. https://doi.org/10.1080/08873267.2014.993074

Gordon, S. (2012). Existential time and the meaning of human development. *Humanistic Psychologist*, *40*(1), 79–86. https://doi.org/10.1080/08873267.2012.643691

Green, A. (2009). From the ignorance of time to the murder of time. From the murder of time to the misrecognition of temporality in psychoanalysis. In L. Glocer Fiorini & J. Canestri (eds), *The experience of time. Psychoanalytic perspectives* (pp. 1–21). Karnac.

Gutiérrez, F., Navinés, R., Navarro, P., García-Esteve, L., Subirá, S., Torrens, M., & Martín-Santos, R. (2008). What do all personality disorders have in common? Ineffectiveness and uncooperativeness. *Comprehensive Psychiatry*, *49*(6), 570–578. https://doi.org/10.1016/J.COMPPSYCH.2008.04.007

Han-Pile, B. (2009). Freedom and the "choice to choose oneself" in *Being and Time*. In M. Wrathall (ed.), *The Cambridge Companion to Heidegger's Being and Time* (pp. 291–319). Cambridge University Press.

Hashemi Mofrad, S., Sadat Jazayeri, R., Fatehizade, M., Etemadi, O., & Abedi, M. (2018). Analyzing difficulties in family life of women with symptoms analyzing difficulties in family life of women with symptoms obsessive-compulsive personality disorder (OCPD): A qualitative research analyzing difficulties in family life of women with symptoms. *Revista Publicando*, *5*(15), 230–260.

Jaspers, K. (1997). *General psychopathology* (Vol. 2). Johns Hopkins University Press.

Kent, L., Nelson, B., & Northoff, G. (2023). Can disorders of subjective time inform the differential diagnosis of psychiatric disorders? A transdiagnostic taxonomy of time. *Early Intervention in Psychiatry*, *17*(3), 231–243. https://doi.org/10.1111/EIP.13333

Kernberg, O. F. (2007). The destruction of time in pathological narcissism. *International Journal of Psychoanalysis*, *89*, 299–312.

Klein, M., & Schmidt, P. (2024). Über Erfüllung: Genuss und Glück bei Stephan Strasser und Thomas von Aquin. *Deutsche Zeitschrift Für Philosophie*, *72*(3), 413–431.

Kraus, A. (1991). Methodological problems with the classification of personality disorders: The significance of existential types. *Journal of Personality Disorders*, *5* (1), 82–92.

Lind, M., Adler, J. M., & Anna Clark, L. (2020). Narrative identity and personality disorder: An empirical and conceptual review. *Current Psychiatry Reports*, *22*, 67. https://doi.org/10.1007/s11920-020-01187-8

Maiese, M. (2018). Getting stuck: Temporal desituatedness in depression. *Phenomenology and the Cognitive Sciences*, *17*(4), 701–718. https://doi.org/10.1007/S11097-017-9538-7/METRICS

Märtsin, M. (2019). Beyond past and present: Meaning making, narrative self and future-orientation. *Integrative Psychological and Behavioral Science*, *53*(4), 669–678. https://doi.org/10.1007/s12124-019-09488-1

Moskalewicz, M. (2016). Disturbed temporalities. Insights from phenomenological psychiatry. *Time and Society*, *25*(2), 234–252. https://doi.org/10.1177/0961463X15577257

Moskalewicz, M. (2024). *Hannah Arendt's ambiguous storytelling: Temporality, judgment, and the philosophy of history*. Bloomsbury Academic.

Moskalewicz, M., & Fuchs, T. (2023). Psychotic disorders of space and time – A contribution of Erwin W. Straus. *Frontiers in Psychiatry*, *14*, 1150005. https://doi.org/10.3389/FPSYT.2023.1150005/BIBTEX

Moskalewicz, M., & Messas, G. (2022). Lived future in addiction. *SUCHT*, *68*(2), 83–88. https://doi.org/10.1024/0939-5911/A000762

Moskalewicz, M., & Schwartz, M. A. (2020). Temporal experience in mania. *Phenomenology and the Cognitive Sciences*, *19*, 291–304. https://doi.org/10.1007/S11097-018-9564-0/METRICS

Pearl, J. (2013). The temporal foundation of the self and the other: A phenomenological reading of narcissism. *Pastoral Psychology*, *62*(4), 533–544. https://doi.org/10.1007/S11089-012-0474-8/METRICS

Schmidt, P. (2020a). Nobody? Disturbed self-experience in borderline personality disorder and four kinds of instabilities. In G. Stanghellini & C. Tewes (eds), *Time and body: Phenomenological and psychopathological approaches* (pp. 206–229). Cambridge University Press.

Schmidt, P. (2020b). Störungen des Selbst in der Borderline-Persönlichkeit. Der Zusammenhang von Affekt und Identitätserleben. In T. Fuchs & T. Breyer (eds), *Selbst und Selbststörungen* (pp. 165–193). Karl Alber.

Schmidt, P. (2022). Affective instability and emotion dysregulation as a social impairment. *Frontiers in Psychology*, *13*, 666016. https://doi.org/10.3389/fpsyg.2022.666016

Schmidt, P., & Fuchs, T. (2021). The unbearable dispersal of being: Narrativity and personal identity in borderline personality disorder. *Phenomenology and the Cognitive Sciences*, *20*(2), 321–340. https://doi.org/10.1007/s11097-020-09712-z

Silverstein, M. L. (2007). *Disorders of the self: A personality-guided approach* (T. Millon, ed.). American Psychological Association.

Skodol, A. E., Bender, D. S., Oldham, J. M., Clark, L. A., Morey, L. C., Verheul, R., Krueger, R. F., & Siever, L. J. (2011). Proposed changes in personality and personality disorder assessment and diagnosis for DSM-5 part II: Clinical application. *Personality Disorders: Theory, Research, and Treatment*, *2*(1), 23–40. https://doi.org/10.1037/a0021892

Sørensen, K. D., Råbu, M., Wilberg, T., & Berthelsen, E. (2019). Struggling to be a person: Lived experience of avoidant personality disorder. *Journal of Clinical Psychology*, *75*(4), 664–680. https://doi.org/10.1002/jclp.22740

Sørensen, K. D., Wilberg, T., Berthelsen, E., & Råbu, M. (2020). Subjective experience of the origin and development of avoidant personality disorder. *Journal of Clinical Psychology*, *76*(12), 2232–2248. https://doi.org/10.1002/jclp.23013

Stanghellini, G., & Mancini, M. (2018). The life-world of persons with borderline personality disorder. In G. Stanghellini, M. Broome, A. Raballo, A. V. Fernandez, P. Fusar-Poli, & R. Rosfort (eds), *The Oxford handbook of phenomenological psychopathology* (pp. 664–681). Oxford University Press.

Steen, A., Braam, A., Berghuis, H., & Glas, G. (2024). Meaning in life in personality disorder: An empirical approach considering self-direction, self-transcendence and spiritual/religious worldviews. *Journal of Spirituality in Mental Health*, 26, 202–217. https://doi.org/10.1080/19349637.2023.2199172

Steenkamp, M., Suvak, M., & Shea, T. (2015). Emotional functioning in obsessive-compulsive personality disorder: Comparison to borderline personality disorder and healthy controls. *Journal of Personality Disorders*, *29*(6), 1–15. https://doi.org/10.1521/pedi_2014_28_174

Sterna, A., & Moskalewicz, M. (2022). "As if there are two of us": The battle of borderline personality disorder diagnosis in lived time. *Psychopathology*, *56*(4), 239–250. https://doi.org/10.1159/000527028

Stolorow, R. D. (2003). Trauma and temporality. *Psychoanalytic Psychology*, *20*(1), 158–161. https://doi.org/10.1037/0736-9735.20.1.158

Straus, E. (1930). Zugleich eine Historiologische Deutung des psychischen Traumas und der Renten-Neurose. Springer.

Sul, J. R. (2022). Schizophrenia, temporality, and affection. *Phenomenology and the Cognitive Sciences*, *21*(4), 927–947. https://doi.org/10.1007/s11097-021-09757-8

Tyrer, P. (2005). Temporal change: The third dimension of personality disorder. *Journal of Personality Disorders*, *19*(5), 573–580.

Van der Kolk, B. (1998). Trauma and memory. *Psychiatry and Clinical Neurosciences*, *52*(S1), S52–S64. https://doi.org/10.1046/J.1440-1819.1998.0520S5S97.X

Von Gebsattel, V. E. (1954). *Prolegomena einer medizinischen Anthropologie. Ausgewählte Aufsätze*. Springer.

Wakefield, J. C. (2008). The perils of dimensionalization: Challenges in distinguishing negative traits from personality disorders. *Psychiatric Clinics of North America*, *31* (3), 379–393. https://doi.org/10.1016/j.psc.2008.03.009

Wyllie, M. (2005). Lived time and psychopathology. *Philosophy, Psychiatry & Psychology*, *12*(3), 173–185.

Young, J. E., Klosko, J. S., & Weishaar, M. E. (2003). *Schema therapy. A practitioner's guide*. The Guilford Press.

Young, J. E., & Lindemann, M. D. (1992). An integrative schema-focused model for personality disorders. *Journal of Cognitive Psychotherapy*, *6*(1), 11–23.

Zajenkowski, M., Rogoza, R., Maciantowicz, O., Witowska, J., & Jonason, P. K. (2021). Narcissus locked in the past: Vulnerable narcissism and the negative views of the past. *Journal of Research in Personality*, *93*, 104123. https://doi.org/10.1016/J.JRP.2021.104123

8 Psychopharmacology and Personality Disorder

Treatment or Enhancement?

Stefan Jerotic and Milutin Kostic

8.1 Overview of the Concept of Personality Disorder and Implications for the Use of Medication

Personality disorders are recognized as a class of mental disorders characterized by pervasive and inflexible patterns of inner experience and behavior that deviate markedly from the expectations of one's culture (World Health Organization, 2019). These patterns were mostly viewed as typically stable over time and cause significant distress and impairment in personal, social, and occupational functioning, although recent studies have put this view in question (d'Huart et al., 2023; Yang et al., 2022).

To fully understand the debate surrounding the use of medication for personality disorders, it is essential to consider the different conceptual models used to approach them. Zachar (2011) has outlined six models, each of which has implications for how we view the use of medication as an intervention. The *vulnerability model* suggests that personality disorders increase the risk of developing other disorders such as depression or substance abuse. In this case, medication could be used to mitigate this risk, similar to how hypertension medication reduces the risk of stroke or heart attack. The *pathoplasticity model* posits that personality disorder affects the course and outcome of other psychiatric disorders. Medication could potentially address this issue by targeting both the personality disorder and comorbid conditions. The *spectrum model* considers some personality disorders to be part of a broader spectrum. For example, schizotypal personality disorder is considered by some to be a part of the schizophrenia spectrum, for which the mainstay of treatment is psychopharmacology. The *decline-in-functioning model* compares personality disorder symptoms to psychological scars caused by emotional trauma, which are linked to a decline in functioning. Medication could be effective in treating traumatic psychological injury, which may also apply to personality disorders. The *impairment–distress model* views personality disorders as directly associated with clinically significant distress or impairment in important areas of functioning. Rather than identifying a specific treatment target, this model raises the central question of whether medication can alleviate distress. Finally, the *capacity-failure model* suggests that personality disorders represent a failure of adaptive psychological capacities. Medication could be used to restore these functions to their evolutionary designed track. By considering these different models, we can better understand the role that medication may play in treating personality disorders.

8.2 Arguments for the Use of Medication for Personality Enhancement

In the bioethical enhancement discourse, several proponents have asserted that the notions of health and illness are heavily contested. Hence, using them as a foundation to differentiate between treatment and enhancement is deemed impractical (Schermer, 2015). Consequently, the use of medication for personality disorders can be argued for, regardless of whether we dismiss criticisms regarding the validity of the disorder (and its pharmacotherapy) or acknowledge the lack of validity (i.e., using medication for personality enhancement). In the next section, we will explore the arguments for using medication in the treatment of personality disorders.

One argument supporting the use of medication for personality disorders is that there may be underlying biological disturbances contributing to behavioral and emotional difficulties. Peter Kramer's book *Listening to Prozac* discusses the idea that certain psychological traits, like panic sensitivity, may have a biological basis (Kramer, 1994). This perspective suggests that individuals with personality disorders may also have neurobiological disturbances contributing to their difficulties. In addition, recent evidence suggests that antidepressants can be effective in treating minor disorders, which can still cause significant disability (Stein, 2012). This is particularly relevant for personality disorders, which are known to be associated with significant disability (Skodol et al., 2002).

Personality disorder symptoms are often complex and multifaceted, with secondary disturbances that can have a significant impact on a person's life. For instance, studies have shown that selective serotonin reuptake inhibitors (SSRIs) can be effective in reducing impulsivity in individuals with personality disorders, and this treatment approach can also improve their ability to adapt to social situations and decrease feelings of guilt and shame (Cameron et al., 2021). This is particularly relevant for individuals with borderline personality disorder, where social isolation can be a significant problem. Instead of focusing solely on reducing impulsive behaviors, treatment should also aim to address mood disturbances, such as guilt and shame, that may hinder social connection. These treatment approaches are in line with Meehl's belief that people should not accept a limited capacity for pleasure (or in this case, suffer from guilt, shame and social disconnectedness), but should seek effective treatments such as medication (cited in Kramer, 1994).

Moreover, data from several studies, including one meta-analysis, have shown that classes of drugs such as antidepressants, mood stabilizers, and antipsychotics exert a beneficial effect on various core symptoms of borderline personality disorder, such as affective instability, anger, impulsiveness, and benefit to the improvement of interpersonal relationships and global functioning (Nosè et al., 2006). Although there is some debate over how specifically affective instability is associated with borderline personality disorder, many researchers agree that it is a persistent (i.e., stable) trait (Zachar, 2015). Given the evidence supporting the efficacy of medication in treating these symptoms, it is worth considering whether medication should be used as a treatment option for affective instability in borderline personality disorder.

While there may be debate about the validity of personality disorder as a diagnosis, there are still compelling reasons to consider medication as a form of personality enhancement. One common alternative to medication is psychotherapy, which is often presented as a way to help people achieve psychological well-being regardless of whether they have a diagnosis of a mental disorder. However, both psychotherapy and medication can exert their effects on both the psychological and biological aspects of human existence. Psychotherapy typically aims to help individuals change their thoughts and behaviors, which can lead to changes in brain function and neurochemistry. Meanwhile, medication can alter neurochemistry directly, which may bring about changes in thoughts, emotions, and behaviors. Given that both interventions can impact the neurobiological basis of personality and behavior, it is worth questioning why medication is often viewed as a more controversial form of intervention compared to psychotherapy. In fact, psychotherapy has been criticized in the past for promoting conformity to societal norms, and now similar arguments are made about psychotropic medication (Kramer, 1994). It is also worthwhile noting that there are adverse effects in both cases, and that psychotherapy may cause emotional discomfort or distress in the short term, and there is a risk of adverse effects such as therapist–patient boundary violations or re-traumatization in some cases. Furthermore, in one of the most widely used and empirically supported psychotherapies for borderline personality disorder, dialectical behavior therapy (DBT), emotion dysregulation is considered a central biological predisposing factor (Neacsiu et al., 2014). Dialectical behavior therapy focuses on enhancing emotion regulation skills, specifically addressing rapid mood shifts and impulsivity. It's noteworthy that these are the same targets as those aimed for by pharmacological interventions.

However, unlike pharmacological treatment, DBT is typically not viewed as problematic.

Bortolotti argues that medical care should be considered as a viable solution to problems that individuals face, regardless of whether these problems are deemed pathological. While it is commonly believed that the identification of disorders is essential in determining the need for medical care, this notion is rooted in the assumption that medicine's primary objective is to prevent and treat disorders (Bortolotti, 2020). However, even for conditions such as delusions in schizophrenia, which are considered paradigmatic cases for psychiatry, a careful analysis reveals that there is no clear distinction between distressing beliefs that constitute medical problems and unusual beliefs that are issues of daily living. In the same vein, we can apply this reasoning to personality disorders. Even if we reject the concept of personality disorder as a legitimate mental illness, providing medication to struggling individuals can still be viewed as a legitimate means of addressing problems in living. Medication has the potential to alleviate the negative effects of these problems without implying that the individual is abnormal or disordered. This means that "my problem in living has a medical solution, or at least that medical intervention can alleviate some of the negative effects of my problem in living" (Bortolotti, 2020). There are many such examples of using medicine and medical care, without having an "illness," from pregnancy to using estrogen in menopause, or treating isolated insomnia in the elderly (Kramer, 1994), to routine vaccination and fluoride supplementation (Stein, 2012). Ultimately, medication has the potential to alleviate the negative effects of problems in living without stigmatizing individuals as disordered or abnormal.

There is also the pragmatic approach, which considers that it is almost irrelevant how good or bad the practice of medicating personality disorders is, be it for treatment or personality enhancement. The fact is that since we have existed humans have used substances to alleviate unpleasant feelings. Alcohol and illicit drugs being all present and part of the culture, and completely devoid of psychiatric influence, as we write this. In this regard, one can argue that it would be wise to use guidance from psychiatrists to navigate through these experiences when there is such a need, in a safer and controlled environment. This could be said to be especially relevant for personality disorders where substance abuse is often one of the manifestations of the condition.

8.3 Criticisms of the Use of Medication for Personality Enhancement

Biological dysfunction as a basis of impairment in personality disorders may exist, but also, it may not. So far, no robust findings exist. Also, if a person feels better with a drug, this doesn't mean that this person has the deficit in the very system that the drug is targeting. Most people will have a positive feeling from taking cocaine or heroin, but that does not mean that there is lack of dopamine or opioids in the person taking the drug. Subsequently the serotonin hypothesis has all but been abandoned for depression, but that does not mean that antidepressants, which are posited to exert some of their effects via the serotonergic system, don't have short-term positive effects for some patients. The problem when this is the case, with regard to any psychotropic taken for personality disorder or personality enhancement, is the long-term effects of such an approach. Considering that in psychiatry there are no causal treatments, only symptomatic, most treatments used in this regard are used long term, or even life-long. Such use may disrupt the physiological homeostasis of the brain and lead to negative consequences in the long run.

There may be several negative consequences. One is the adverse effects of medication, which in the long term might cause more harm than good. It is important to note here that most studies into the efficacy of psychiatric treatments are short term. Namely, over 75 percent of randomized controlled trials (RCTs) for antidepressants, for instance, are 6–8 weeks, but almost never longer than 16 weeks (Stone et al., 2022). Conducting long-term studies presents significant challenges in terms of resources and methodology, and there is a lack of sufficient incentive to pursue such studies (Kramer, 2016). With time, adverse effects may pile up, while positive effects on the contrary may diminish. Overall, long-term risks of many psychotropic agents are still not well understood (Cartwright et al., 2016; Pozzi et al., 2022). One historic fact is that, for instance, first-generation antipsychotics may inflict life-long damage in the form of tardive dyskinesia, but many psychiatrists were slow to acknowledge this, or in active denial (Munetz & Schulz, 1986).

Another concern is the risk of addiction or withdrawal symptoms. In some cases, these symptoms may be so severe that the patient is unable to stop taking the medication. Additionally, there is a risk that the physician and the patient may mistake these symptoms for a relapse, leading to prolonged or even chronic drug use (Hengartner & Plöderl, 2021). Both physicians and patients have only limited knowledge about this problem and training for medically supervised deprescribing, or slow tapering, is in its infancy.

The third concern is related to psychological factors. Studies suggest that attributing a disorder primarily to biological causes, such as in depression, may lead to feelings of pessimism (Lebowitz, 2019; Lebowitz & Ahn, 2015). Patients may view the disorder as an intrinsic part of themselves, which can hinder their belief in the possibility of recovery even if their social circumstances improve. This may result in an ongoing reliance on pharmacotherapy. The findings from social psychology studies suggest that people may be inclined to overemphasize the role of personality traits in explaining behavior, while ignoring the influence of situational factors (Nisbett & Wilson, 1977). In other words, medication may provide temporary relief for behavioral problems associated with certain personality traits, but does not necessarily address the underlying issues that may be causing those traits to manifest in the first place, which might be predominantly psychological or situational. It is important to consider the role of situational factors and address them as necessary, in addition to any medical interventions that may be prescribed. In this context, nidotherapy, an approach that focuses on modifying the individual's environment to address the underlying factors contributing to personality disorders, could offer a complementary perspective, seemingly addressing aspects beyond the reach of pharmacological interventions (Tyrer, 2019). It has been suggested that numbing emotions like sadness, anger, and fear could potentially lead to social and psychological issues, as the person may not feel motivated to address underlying problems that may be causing distress (Cuijpers et al., 2013; Lebowitz & Ahn, 2015; Moncrieff, 2018).

In his insightful analysis, Dan J. Stein emphasizes that a critical approach, informed by the philosophy of Hegel, reveals that emotional reactions can be understood as culture-bound expressions of distress that reflect the unique concerns and values of a given historical and geographical context. Therefore, such expressions of distress should not be automatically medicalized. Instead, a more nuanced understanding of the social and cultural factors shaping these emotional reactions is necessary in order to develop appropriate and effective interventions (Stein, 2012).

8.4 Philosophical Issues Related to the Use of Medication for Personality Enhancement

When considering the use of medication for personality disorders, there are several complex dilemmas that need to be addressed, which add further nuances to the matter.

8.4.1 Pharmacological Calvinism versus Psychotropic Utopianism

The debate between using psychotropic medication, relevant to our discussion of personality disorders, has been called succinctly the debate between pharmacological Calvinism and psychotropic utopianism (or psychotropic hedonism) (Parens, 2013). Pharmacological Calvinism is the belief that psychiatric medications should only be used as a last resort for severe mental illness and that patients should rely on their own resources, such as therapy or support groups, to manage their conditions. The term "Calvinism" refers to the religious doctrine that emphasizes predestination and the idea that some people are destined for salvation while others are not. In the context of psychiatry, pharmacological Calvinism suggests that some people are simply not meant to be helped by medication and should instead focus on non-pharmacological treatments. On the other hand, psychotropic utopianism is the belief that psychiatric medications can be used to enhance mental and emotional states beyond what is considered "normal" or "healthy." Proponents of psychotropic utopianism argue that medications can be used to improve mood, increase productivity, and even enhance creativity or spirituality. This perspective sees psychiatric medications as a means of achieving a "better" state of being, rather than simply treating a disorder (Stein, 2008).

The notion of medicating temperament raises an ethical dilemma. Temperament, as described by Lee Anna Clark (2005), has a significant influence on both personality and psychopathology. Negative affectivity, a temperament that is frequently observed in neuroticism, borderline personality disorder, and major depressive disorder, is an example of this connection. However, major depressive disorder is not considered to be separate from temperamental predispositions. Consequently, a pressing ethical question arises: Why is it acceptable to manipulate, by way of psychopharmacology, symptoms of major depression that stem from temperamental factors, and not borderline personality disorder? This debate, of course, rests on the assumption that such an intervention is available and safe. On the other hand, viewing temperament, like negative emotionality, as a pharmacological target raises inherent ambivalence regarding intervention. A key aspect of this complexity is that vulnerability factors, such as temperament, are profoundly influenced by the context in which they are situated. Consider the analogy of fair skin – although it's a known risk factor for melanoma, it isn't inherently a pathological condition. In contrast, sickle cell anemia, a genetic trait, can act as a protective factor against malaria, although it can also manifest as a serious illness. The context, therefore, plays a pivotal role in determining whether a specific trait is advantageous or detrimental. Crucially, the precise balance of risk and benefit in any given context can be highly uncertain on an individual level, given the multifaceted nature of human experiences. This raises important ethical questions about whether it is appropriate to intervene and potentially modify aspects of an individual's temperament. Such traits are often deeply intertwined with a person's identity, and altering them could have far-reaching consequences, both in terms of risk and benefit.

8.4.2 Personality Traits Exist Along a Continuum, and There Is No Clear Distinction Between Normal and Abnormal Personality

In the context of medication, the blurry (or debatable) lines between normal and abnormal personality pose a challenge when determining whether medication is necessary. The concept of a continuum highlights the complexity of personality and the diversity of individuals' experiences. Personality is not a static construct, but rather a dynamic and ever-changing aspect of human existence that is influenced by a wide range of factors. When considering whether to medicate a personality, either as treatment or enhancement, it is crucial to acknowledge the potential conflicts between theoretical ideals and real-world practices. It is no secret that the pharmaceutical industry has significant commercial interests at play, which may influence the overdiagnosis of conditions and an overreliance on medication for treatment. Unfortunately, this can result in a rapid influx of medication for many conditions with limited proof of effectiveness and loosening of criteria for many diagnoses. This phenomenon has been dubbed "overmedicalization" by some academic authorities who were involved in forming the diagnostic criteria themselves. In fact, some of these authorities have even publicly mourned the misuse of their work in the name of profit-driven overmedicalization (Frances, 2014). In light of this, it is essential to adopt a nuanced approach to potential use of medication for treatment/enhancement, one that carefully considers the patient's unique needs, in order to avoid any overreliance on medication as a "quick fix" solution.

8.4.3 The Use of Medication to Alter Personality Traits May Challenge an Individual's Sense of Self and Raise Questions about Authenticity and Genuineness

The concept of the self and its relation to personality is a complex topic that extends beyond the scope of this book chapter. However, it is important to consider briefly this relationship when discussing the influence of psychopharmacology on the self. Various concepts, such as self-consciousness, self-concept, self-esteem, identity, and personhood, fall under this topic (Zachar, 2015). The contemporary phenomenological paradigm suggests that the self is embodied, meaning that our consciousness and identity are closely tied to our physical body and experiences. The body is not just a biological machine, but a crucial component of our identity and self-understanding. As such, medication, which can directly alter neurochemistry, always acts on our sense of self, whether we are treating schizophrenia, major depression, or a personality disorder. It is posited that there are several layers of the self, including the pre-reflective self and the narrative-social self (Gallagher & Zahavi, 2012). These layers are not separate but rather constituents of the same self. Personality is made up of characteristics that may not be constantly experienced or displayed by the self, but that have developed into a stable pattern over time and can be exposed under the right circumstances (Svenaeus, 2013). Considering medication's potential impact on different layers of the self is important. For instance, medication used to treat personality disorders may affect the pre-reflective self, which is closely linked to our physical body and experiences. This could alter how individuals with personality disorders experience their own identity and sense of self, potentially affecting their relationship to their own body and physical sensations. Additionally, medication can impact the narrative-social self, which is shaped by cultural and social factors. Altering underlying neurochemistry that contributes to personality disorders may have downstream effects on an individual's relationships, social interactions, and cultural identity. Medication-induced changes in impulsivity or emotional reactivity could change how individuals engage with others and how they are perceived by their social group. Overall, the potential impact of medication on the different layers of the self underscores the importance of considering authenticity and genuineness when discussing the influence of psychopharmacology on the self. For example, if an individual takes medication to enhance their sociability or confidence, does this change their fundamental identity? And is such a change desirable?

According to Carl Elliot, psychopharmaceuticals may threaten a person's authenticity by causing them to lose touch with who they really are. He argues that even if such drugs give someone a better personality, it still isn't their true personality, which goes against an ethics of authenticity (Elliott, 1998). Furthermore, Elliot highlights the social pressures and expectations that lead people to use these drugs to fit in and conform to societal norms, rather than questioning them. Psychopharmaceuticals can help individuals adapt to the patterns and standards required for a "normal" and successful life without questioning the norms themselves (Schermer, 2015).

When individuals experience conditions like depression or schizophrenia, it's commonly seen as an external influence acting upon them, which they may seek to alleviate through treatment (Chung, 2007; Taylor & Fink, 2006). However, with personality disorders, it's frequently perceived as an inherent aspect of their identity. This distinction has profound implications for the ethics of treatment and enhancement. For instance, consider a scenario where an individual with a personality disorder views their condition as an integral part of who they are and resists any form of intervention. Debating the intervention with medication echoes notions about psychiatric disorders and social control (Aftab & Ryznar, 2021). This is one instance where the concept of authenticity is raised, with which a person might assert, "This is who I am, and I don't want to be made into something else." It evokes imagery reminiscent of "A Clockwork Orange," where external forces are used to alter a person's core identity, raising significant ethical questions about the right to autonomy and the boundaries of medical intervention. Conversely, there are cases where individuals with personality disorders might perceive themselves as fundamentally flawed or dysfunctional, desiring change and improvement. Here, the ethical landscape shifts, as they actively seek a different identity, raising questions about the balance between personal agency and societal norms, and whether medication can facilitate this transformation.

One persuasive view has been argued by DeGrazia (2005). He asserts that as long as the choice to use these drugs is autonomous, they can be used to help shape and create one's personality in line with who they truly want to be. DeGrazia argues that pharmaceuticals are simply technological tools to aid in the self-creation process, something humans have always done. The key to authenticity, according to DeGrazia, is honesty toward oneself and others about who one really is (Schermer, 2015). Therefore, if an individual chooses to use mood enhancers to alter a certain aspect of themselves, as long as it is done autonomously and honestly, it can contribute to their authentic self-creation (Levy, 2011).

8.4.4 The Impact of Medication on the Person's Autonomy

The impact of psychopharmaceuticals on a person's autonomy and decision-making abilities is a topic of debate and subject to changing opinions. The US Council on Bioethics, for instance, cautioned against using propranolol as a memory dampener for emotionally charged memories, as it may be considered a form of personality enhancement. They further warned that the use of propranolol could impair decision quality by reducing the physiological arousal that normally guides certain acts (Kass, 2003). Empirical data have since shown that propranolol does affect moral judgment (Sylvia et al., 2013). It is worth noting that propranolol is a medication with wide-ranging applications, from cardiology to the treatment of post-traumatic stress disorder in psychiatry.

As mentioned in the previous discussion, personality traits can be manipulated through external factors such as medication. This raises questions about the extent to which individuals are free to make choices about their personality and the impact of medication on their autonomy. The concept of character, as it was understood historically, was based on moral theories that highlighted virtues and vices. This historical context is relevant to the current discussion on using medication to treat personality disorders. Charland (2004, 2006) argues that some personality disorders should be viewed as moral, rather than medical, conditions. This implies that having a particular type of personality disorder could be equated to being a morally deficient person. If we choose to treat such conditions with medication, we may inadvertently be using medication to shape societal and moral norms.

This leads to the question whether the use of medication for personality enhancement could lead to a society that values conformity over diversity. People may feel compelled to take medication to conform to societal norms, even if they do not have a mental disorder. On the other hand, we could ask if it is always bad. Some conformity is necessary if a society is to function, and absolute diversity in morality is untenable. In this light even Charland said that successful treatment of cluster B personality disorders would lead to their moral improvement. There have been compelling discussions in the bioethical literature suggesting that reinforcing specific social constructs aligns with the goal of psychopharmacological enhancement in reducing social deviance. The risk is that such approaches often overlook the significance of resilience and overemphasize technology, resulting in the dehumanization of individuals (Stein, 2012).

8.5 Conclusion

It is important to note that medication is not a cure for personality disorders, but rather a tool to manage symptoms and improve the patient's overall well-being. As with any treatment, medication should be carefully considered and individualized for each patient, taking into account their specific symptoms, their severity, medical history, and social factors. Many philosophical and ethical conundrums should be addressed in order to help the patient navigate and understand the role of medication. The use of psychotropics for treatment of personality disorders/personality enhancement requires a judicious weighing of the relevant bioethical concerns and risk/benefit ratio.

References

Aftab, A., & Ryznar, E. (2021). Conceptual and historical evolution of psychiatric nosology. *International Review of Psychiatry*, *33*(5), 486–499.

Bortolotti, L. (2020). Doctors without 'disorders'. *Aristotelian Society Supplementary Volume*, *94*, 163–184.

Cameron, A. Y., Benz, M., & Reed, K. P. (2021). The role of guilt and shame in psychosocial functioning in a sample of women with borderline personality disorder. *The Journal of Nervous and Mental Disease*, *209*(1), 13–16.

Cartwright, C., Gibson, K., Read, J., Cowan, O., & Dehar, T. (2016). Long-term antidepressant use: patient perspectives of benefits and adverse effects. *Patient Preference and Adherence*, *10*, 1401–1407.

Charland, L. C. (2004). Personality disorders. In J. Radden (ed.), *The philosophy of psychiatry: A companion*, pp. 64–77. Oxford University Press.

Charland, L. C. (2006). Moral nature of the DSM-IV Cluster B personality disorders. *Journal of Personality Disorders*, *20*(2), 116–125.

Chung, M. C. (2007). Conceptions of schizophrenia. In M. C. Chung, K. W. M. Fulford, & G. Graham (eds.), *Reconceiving schizophrenia*, pp. 29–62. Oxford University Press.

Clark, L. A. (2005). Temperament as a unifying basis for personality and psychopathology. *Journal of Abnormal Psychology*, *114*(4), 505.

Cuijpers, P., Hollon, S. D., van Straten, A., Bockting, C., Berking, M., & Andersson, G. (2013). Does cognitive behaviour therapy have an enduring effect that is superior to

keeping patients on continuation pharmacotherapy? A meta-analysis. *BMJ Open*, *3* (4), e002542.
d'Huart, D., Seker, S., Bürgin, D., . . . Schmeck, K. (2023). The stability of personality disorders and personality disorder criteria: A systematic review and meta-analysis. *Clinical Psychology Review*, *102*, 102284.
DeGrazia, D. (2005). Enhancement technologies and human identity. *The Journal of Medicine and Philosophy*, *30*(3), 261–283.
Elliott, C. (1998). The tyranny of happiness: Ethics and cosmetic psychopharmacology. In E. Parens (ed.), *Enhancing human traits: Ethical and social implications*, pp. 177–188. Georgetown University Press.
Frances, A. (2014). *Saving normal*. Mariner Books.
Gallagher, S., & Zahavi, D. (2012). *The phenomenological mind*, 2nd ed. Routledge.
Hengartner, M. P., & Plöderl, M. (2021). Prophylactic effects or withdrawal reactions? An analysis of time-to-event data from antidepressant relapse prevention trials submitted to the FDA. *Therapeutic Advances in Psychopharmacology*, *11*, 20451253211032052.
Kass, L. (2003). *Beyond therapy: Biotechnology and the pursuit of happiness*. HarperCollins.
Kramer, P. D. (1994). *Listening to Prozac*. Fourth Estate London.
Kramer, P. D. (2016). *Ordinarily well: The case for antidepressants*. Farrar, Straus and Giroux.
Lebowitz, M. S. (2019). The implications of genetic and other biological explanations for thinking about mental disorders. *Hastings Center Report*, *49*, S82–S87.
Lebowitz, M. S., & Ahn, W. (2015). Emphasizing malleability in the biology of depression: Durable effects on perceived agency and prognostic pessimism. *Behaviour Research and Therapy*, *71*, 125–130.
Levy, N. (2011). Enhancing authenticity. *Journal of Applied Philosophy*, *28*(3), 308–318.
Moncrieff, J. (2018). Against the stream: antidepressants are not antidepressants – An alternative approach to drug action and implications for the use of antidepressants. *Psychiatric Bulletin*, *42*(1), 42–44.
Munetz, M. R., & Schulz, S. C. (1986). Minimization and overreaction to tardive dyskinesia. *Schizophrenia Bulletin*, *12*(2), 168–172.
Neacsiu, A. D., Bohus, M., & Linehan, M. M. (2014). Dialectical behavior therapy: An intervention for emotion dysregulation. *Handbook of Emotion Regulation*, *2*, 491–507.
Nisbett, R. E., & Wilson, T. D. (1977). Telling more than we can know: Verbal reports on mental processes. *Psychological Review*, *84*(3), 231–259.
Nosè, M., Cipriani, A., Biancosino, B., Grassi, L., & Barbui, C. (2006). Efficacy of pharmacotherapy against core traits of borderline personality disorder: Meta-analysis of randomized controlled trials. *International Clinical Psychopharmacology*, 21(6), 345–353.
Parens, E. (2013). On good and bad forms of medicalization. *Bioethics*, *27*(1), 28–35.
Pozzi, M., Ferrentino, R. I., Scrinzi, G., . . . Bravaccio, C. (2022). Weight and body mass index increase in children and adolescents exposed to antipsychotic drugs in non-interventional settings: A meta-analysis and meta-regression. *European Child & Adolescent Psychiatry*, *31*, 21–37.

Schermer, M. (2015). Ethics of pharmacological mood enhancement. In J. Clausen & N. Levy (eds.), *Handbook of neuroethics*, pp. 1177–1190. Springer.

Skodol, A. E., Gunderson, J. G., McGlashan, T. H., . . . Morey, L. C. (2002). Functional impairment in patients with schizotypal, borderline, avoidant, or obsessive-compulsive personality disorder. *American Journal of Psychiatry, 159*(2), 276–283.

Stein, D. J. (2008). *Philosophy of psychopharmacology.* Cambridge University Press.

Stein, D. J. (2012). Psychopharmacological enhancement: A conceptual framework. *Philosophy, Ethics, and Humanities in Medicine, 7*(1), 5.

Stone, M. B., Yaseen, Z. S., Miller, B. J., Richardville, K., Kalaria, S. N., & Kirsch, I. (2022). Response to acute monotherapy for major depressive disorder in randomized, placebo controlled trials submitted to the US Food and Drug Administration: Individual participant data analysis. *BMJ, 378*, e067606.

Svenaeus, F. (2013). Psychopharmacology and the Self. In K. W. M. Fulford, M. Davies, R. G. T. Gipps, G. Graham, J. Z. Sadler, G. Stanghellini, & T. Thornton (eds.), *The Oxford handbook of philosophy and psychiatry*, pp. 1171–1184. Oxford University Press.

Sylvia, T., Guy, K., Sarah, M., Julian, S., Neil, L., Miles, H., & Cowen, P. J. (2013). Beta adrenergic blockade reduces utilitarian judgement. *Biological Psychology, 92*(2), 323–328.

Taylor, M. A., & Fink, M. (2006). *Melancholia: The diagnosis, pathophysiology and treatment of depressive illness*. Cambridge University Press.

Tyrer, P. (2019). Nidotherapy: A cost-effective systematic environmental intervention. *World Psychiatry, 18*(2), 144–145.

World Health Organization. (2019). The ICD-11 classification of mental and behavioral disorders. https://icd.who.int/

Yang, M., Tyrer, H., Johnson, T., & Tyrer, P. (2022). Personality change in the Nottingham Study of Neurotic Disorder: 30-Year cohort study. *Australian & New Zealand Journal of Psychiatry, 56*(3), 260–269.

Zachar, P. (2011). The clinical nature of personality disorders: Answering the neo-Szaszian critique. *Philosophy, Psychiatry, & Psychology, 18*(3), 191–202.

Zachar, P. (2015). Personality disorder. Philosophical problems. In T. Schramme & S. Edwards (eds.), *Handbook of the philosophy of medicine*, pp. 1005–1024. Springer.

9 When Do Personality Traits Become Pathological?

An Epistemological and Evolutionary View

Simone Cheli and Martin Brüne

9.1 Personality Traits as Evolved Behavioral Dispositions

The term "personality" is probably one of the most contentious and ill-defined psychological constructs. Since early attempts to define basic elements of human individuality in either ancient West (e.g., the 30 characters of Theophrastus or the four temperaments of Galen) or East (e.g., the five states in the Huangdi Neijing or the three qualities in the Bhagavad Gita), two main goals have been to make predictions about behaviors and to anticipate maladaptive or even pathological trajectories. That said, the complexity of human life is such that after several millennia we still do not fully understand when and how a personality trait can manifest itself as pathological. In this chapter we do not claim to solve this long debate. Instead, we seek to suggest how an evolutionary perspective can help understand how people make sense of their experience. By doing so, we think that several fertile hypotheses may arise about the link between healthy traits and pathological manifestations in the form of personality disorders (PDs) or, broadly speaking, personality pathology.

Indeed, the range of application of evolutionary theory has expanded enormously over the last century. Charles Darwin (1859, 1871) introduced the idea that evolution refers to the change in heritable characteristics of biological populations over time. An enormous amount of evidence has confirmed that the resulting variation is due to random changes in the genetic makeup of populations (i.e., genetic drift) and two main processes, namely natural and sexual selection, both of which shape an individual's reproductive success within that population. All traits (personality traits included) are shaped by these evolutionary forces, but being so shaped does not imply that they are all adaptive. For example, the human belly button has no apparent evolved function, but is nevertheless a by-product of all mammalian amniotes. Moreover, a trait selected in past environments (e.g., possessing a dentition of 32 teeth, which is typical for apes) may be disadvantageous in current environments (e.g., the wisdom teeth may cause health problems due to the increasing use of cooked or processed foods). In addition, sexual selection may directly oppose natural selection: Darwin admitted that the sight of a peacock's tail made him sick, because the flashy tail of the male peacock may attract females, but at the same time impairs escape from predators. It is thus important to keep in mind that evolution is not an intentional process, and therefore adaptation is an ongoing pattern resulting from diverse and intertwined processes.

The early work of Darwin and other scholars on the application of evolution theory to human behavior has led to the development of two intertwined fields. On one hand, the rise of evolutionary psychology has applied general rules and principles of evolution to psychological mechanisms (Buss, 1995), including maladaptive variants that are commonly referred to as "psychopathology" (Brüne, 2016a; Fabrega, 2002). For example, it has been suggested that Cluster B PDs such as borderline and narcissistic personality disorders could reflect an exaggerated form of risk-taking and competitive strategies (Brüne, 2016a; Del Giudice, 2018).

Several attempts have been made to apply evolutionary theory to the study of culture and human socialization practices (Boyd & Richerson, 1988; Dunbar, 2009). Even though social structures may have had an impact on the evolution of the human brain, little is known about how evolutionary principles may explain the role of culture in the development of specific human traits such as personality.

More recently, the rise of dimensional approaches to personality and its pathology have seemingly favored a nuanced and integrated understanding of all these factors: what is defined as personality disorder might be better explored as an inflexible or excessive manifestation of a set of traits distributed in the general population (Bach & Tracy, 2022; Morey et al., 2007; Widiger & Crego, 2019).

Indeed, many researchers consider "personality" to be a set of strategies based on both temperamental and cultural components (Trofimova et al., 2018). Meta-analytic studies indicate how early childhood temperament is related to the development of later personality traits, but childhood and young adulthood seem to be associated with the highest level of change with respect to personality (Bleidorn et al., 2022; Wright & Jackson, 2022). Moreover, temperament and personality traits seem to be strongly predicted by genetic factors with an estimated explained variance ranging between 25 percent and 50 percent and this would imply a similar account of environmental factors across the lifespan (Hopwood et al. 2011; van Wijk et al., 2019): that is, if half of the variance is due to genetic factors, environmental factors contribute the same amount of variance to the development of a trait.

These findings are consistent with neurodevelopmental studies suggesting how adult personality – and its pathological manifestations – would represent the result of diverse interacting factors along general dimensions such as internalizing and externalizing spectra and across specific developmental phases (Cicchetti & Cohen, 2006; McAdams et al., 2021). For example, internalizing and externalizing spectra – emerging during childhood – may equally manifest as a personality pathology in terms of impaired self and/or interpersonal functioning by reducing the ability to understand one's own and other's mental states (Sharp & Wall, 2018). Similarly, several studies on healthy traits such as the Five Factor Model (FFM) and their pathological counterparts (i.e., Alternative Model of Personality Disorders, AMPD) indicate a continuum of experiences ranging from adaptive states and strategies to rigid and inflexible ones corresponding to a personality pathology (Skodol et al., 2015; Widiger & Crego, 2019; Widiger & McCabe, 2020).

From the point of view of evolution theory, these intertwined and multifaceted components could be framed through a general set of evolutionary principles. We will introduce three of them in this chapter.

1. Personality traits can be defined as evolved behavioral and relational dispositions that are shaped by biopsychosocial constraints and provide an individual with a relatively flexible pattern of responses to a broad array of potential challenges from the social and the physical environments.

Indeed, one of the most intriguing assumptions of theoretical biology is based on the autonomy and circular causality of any biological entity (Varela, 1979; von Uexküll, 1926). In short, this means that we experience what we are somehow *designed* to experience. This idea has been traditionally expressed by von Uexküll's assumption that all living beings are embedded in their *Umwelt* (lit. German for "environment"), that is, in their phenomenal world, distinctive from the surrounding world as experienced by others (*Umgebung*). Living beings can be considered autopoietic machines who perpetuate themselves through the very processes that constitute themselves (Maturana & Varela, 1980). Indeed, autopoiesis (from Greek αὐτο- (auto-) "self," and ποίησις (poiesis) "creation") refers to a system capable of producing and maintaining itself by creating its own components. This construct of theoretical biology can better explain the rules of natural and sexual selection. In fact, the theory of biological evolution entails that natural and sexual selection operates on randomly occurring variation (e.g., by mutation) to favor those phenotypes that fit best with current environmental conditions (positive selection) or to eliminate unfavorable phenotypes from the gene pool (negative selection). Conversely, a missed adaptation can be considered as a sort of inertia of autopoietic processes: by trying to maintain its components, a biological entity is closed to change.

The complexity of traits that define a personality probabilistically predicts the kinds of pathological manifestations a person may struggle with. For example, an early externalizing pattern may later expose a person to risk-taking strategies (e.g., dangerous behaviors aimed to attract possible mates), which – when facing recurrent distress – may become rigid or excessive. By perpetuating their core adaptative strategies (i.e., externalizing ones), the person may even be diagnosed with a Cluster B PD such as narcissistic personality disorder or, according to the AMPD, to pathological antagonistic traits.

At the same time, the culturally driven components of traits represent another set of autopoietic processes. The anthropological definition of culture as based on the functional analysis of "the relation between a cultural performance and a human need" (Malinowski, 1960, p. 39) is consistent with the evolutionary idea that "a cultural repertoire is analogous to genotype" (Boyd & Richerson, 1988, p. 36). Culture and genes would have co-evolved over human history; the one influenced the other according to the rules and principles of natural and sexual selection (Richerson & Boyd, 2004; Tomlinson, 2018). According to this culturally relativistic position (Poortinga & van Hemert, 2001), personality traits result from this co-evolution affecting both healthy and pathological manifestations.

Expressed differently, the emerging personality pathology may be better understood as a missing adaptation with respect to a specific pattern of co-evolution. For example, in East Asian countries socially valued perfectionism may be more positively associated with pride after success than in Western countries, and emotion regulation strategies during interpersonal stressful situations seem to be more beneficial for the former than the latter ones (Liddell & Williams, 2019; Stoeber et al., 2013). These findings would be consistent with cultural differences in respect to strategies such as social distancing and emotional avoidance. In this respect a diagnosis of obsessive-compulsive personality disorder – which through the AMPD can be defined in terms of high level of negative affectivity and detachment – would be the joint result of a specific social context, culturally evolved strategies, and an individual endophenotype (i.e., a set of biomarkers that indicate genetic vulnerability independent of clinical state). A clinical example might drive this point home. Clara (fictional name) was a Taiwanese 25-year-old female with a mother with antagonistic traits and a father with detached traits. During her late adolescence in Taiwan, she was diagnosed with borderline personality disorder because of her difficulties regulating emotion in interpersonal contexts as confirmed by relatives and educators. Once she moved to Italy, she experienced severe social and emotional detachment. Friends and acquaintances described her as emotionally cold and socially distant and she described herself in terms of high anxiousness and depressiveness. During the assessment (in Italy) she presented a high level of socially prescribed perfectionism and self-criticism that she has always tried to regulate her emotions with automatic strategies of avoidance. In Taiwan her regulatory strategies were considered maladaptive due to being perceived as impulsive; in Italy they were considered maladaptive due to being perceived as detached.

Regardless of the cultural context in which she lived, Clara exhibited interpersonal distress caused by her painful inner critics and a sense of having to adhere to high social standards. Her difficulty in regulating interpersonal distress using avoidant strategies led her to impulsively run away when she was in contexts perceived as "colder and more controlling" such as Taiwan, and to hide and mask her inner experience in contexts perceived as "warmer and more intrusive" such as in Italy.

9.2 Evolutionary Strategies as Meaning-Making Processes

In the Dao De Jing it is written that "naming that can assign fixed reference to things is not really naming" (Ames & Hall, 2003, p. 145; lit. "the name that can be named is not the enduring name"). One interpretation of this phrase is that life is constantly changing due to human attempts to label and make sense of events. This broad philosophical stance can be applied to any attempt to understand how personality traits develop, including their potential to manifest in pathological ways. The idea of a co-evolution between genetics and culture implies that the complexity of human traits arises from both the biological uniqueness of any individual and the interdependence and connectedness with other members of our species (Cheli, 2018; Maturana & Varela, 1980). Indeed, another form of co-evolution that is constantly operating in humans is the one between individual conspecifics and groups. For example, Clara's story is seemingly defined by a dynamic between her individual strategies in making sense of the world and how – in turn – the surrounding environment interacted with her and constrained her experience. Indeed, several authors have described how both individual and collective attempts to outline and test a theory of the world and of knowledge itself could be better understood through the principles of evolutionary theory (Piaget, 1950; Riedl, 1984; von Glasersfeld, 1985). The more viable theory of the world would be the one that is capable of adjust to the ecological and epistemological constraints it arises within. Consistent with this approach, psychopathology can be framed as a failure in meaning-making in regard to one's own and others' experiences: severe PDs are characterized by a fragmentation of self-to-self and self-to-other patterns (Lysaker et al., 2020).

From this broad perspective we can suggest a second principle:

2. *Evolutionary strategies are epistemological processes that operate at different levels, from single organisms to groups of individuals, in a given ecological niche.*

For example, a personality trait such as Clara's perfectionism is a recursive mechanism aimed at managing her internal and external experience, and to predict and navigate events. As Ronald Laing (1960) said, any symptom – even the severest one – is an attempt to make sense of one's self and a world that otherwise would fall apart. Moreover, the previous definition (2) would imply that an evolutionary strategy works at different levels of adaptation, including same level, top-down, and bottom-up. First, an imbalance of a trait with respect to other related traits can expose an individual to maladaptive experiences. Luria (1968) highlighted in his famous essay on a mnemonist how even a vast memory can represent a source of psychological pain and missing adaptation. Luria describes the tragic story of a man capable of remembering entire articles in a few moments, but incapable of forgetting myriads of details that dominated his life and his experience of himself. Second, a single facet belonging to a trait may influence this very trait and foster or impede adaptation, and vice versa (i.e., a bottom-up pattern). For example, recent advances in the understanding of pathological narcissism suggest how vulnerable and grandiose states would fluctuate and interact over time rather than being exclusively dispositional (Edershile & Wright, 2021; Jauk et al., 2022). This fluctuation – mediated by the need for entitlement and fear of shame in interpersonal relationships – could be considered a failure in valuing the evolutionary advantage of collaboration and reciprocity. Another clinical case may support this contention. John (fictional name) was a 37-year-old male diagnosed with narcissistic personality disorder who reported high levels of antagonism and negative affectivity. He presented a prominent vulnerable phenotype of pathological narcissism that was associated – at the time of diagnosis – with a severe major depression. During his childhood and adolescence, his father had a severe chronic illness and he experienced any attempt to pursue his own needs and wishes as a shameful disinterest in his father's suffering. Gradually, he crystallized a dichotomous belief that pursuing one's own needs was conflicted with being connected with others. He entered therapy due to an interpersonal problem with a former girlfriend, feeling a shameful sense of despair after his girlfriend had left him and the more he tried to contact her, the more she rejected him. Consequently, his shame and covert anger increased and he tried to regulate it by avoiding his own feelings. Unfortunately, this strategy reduced his ability to mentalize his own and other's experience and regulate negative emotions such as shame and anger.

9.3 The Search for a Unifying Theory of Personality Pathology

Despite a long-lasting lack of evolutionary studies on personality and its disorders, recent advances suggest the application of the LHT to this issue (see Box 9.1). Life History Theory is based on Behavioral Ecology, an evolutionary

Box 9.1 Life History Theory

Life History Theory (LHT) is an evolutionary concept derived from Behavioral Ecology. It explains how and why organisms differ in the ways they allocate resources to somatic growth and reproduction. A basic premise of LHT is that limitations in the availability of resources (e.g., food, mates) cause organisms to balance the amount of energy they invest in growth or reproductive activity against one another. Such trade-offs lead to differences in Life History Strategies (LHS) between species, which pertain to growth rate, age and body size at sexual maturation, number and size of offspring, mortality rate, maximum lifespan, and vulnerability to disease (Stearns, 1992). These differences were originally referred to as "r/K selection" (MacArthur & Wilson, 1967), whereby "r" (for growth rate) selected species grow small bodies, mature and reproduce early (and often only once in their lifetimes), have large numbers of offspring, provide little care for offspring, have relatively short lifespans, and are prone to disease, due to constraints on their immune system (among mammals, r-selection is typical for small rodents). By contrast, K-selected species ("K" stands for capacity) grow large bodies, reproduce multiple times over an extended period of time, have small numbers of offspring, invest substantially in offspring survival, have long individual lifespans, and are more immune competent compared to r-selected species (Stearns, 1992). K-selected LHS are typical for large mammals such as whales, elephants, and primates (including humans).

Evolutionary psychologists have suggested that differences in LHS are not only observable between species, but also within species. Specifically, it has been proposed that ecological (environmental) conditions (interacting with genetic factors) determine whether an individual adopts a relatively fast or slow LHS within a species-typical range. These environmental conditions include estimations about current and future resource availability, which are often based on experiences made during early developmental stages (Ellis et al., 2009). Early adversity, for instance, may drive an individual organism toward the adoption of a faster LHS, that is, earlier biological maturation, less investment in body maintenance, and limited parental care in offspring (Ellis et al., 2011a).

Even though it is debated as to what degree these biological rules also explain individual differences in human growth patterns and behavior, the evidence seems quite convincing with regard to psychological traits, and less so for somatic growth and maintenance. Indeed, individual differences in terms of cooperation, risk-taking, interpersonal aggression, and mating

Box 9.1 (cont.)

behavior, as well as executive functioning, inhibitory control, and personality traits seem, in part, to depend on early developmental conditions (Del Giudice, 2014). This view is compatible with findings based on attachment theory. In fact, individuals who grow up in stable, emotionally reliable and predictable familial environmental conditions tend to pursue slower LHS. That is, they tend to mature late, delay reproduction, are generally risk averse, and form stable long-term intimate relationships. Stable conditions in early stages of development are also associated with more cooperative, empathetic behavior, low levels of interpersonal aggression, and superior inhibitory control. As regards personality traits, stability early in life is associated with higher levels of conscientiousness and agreeableness. The opposite seems to be observable in individuals who are exposed to harsh parenting, violence, or poverty. They mature earlier, engage earlier in sexual activity, and are more risk-prone with less inhibitory control (Belsky et al., 1991; Ellis et al., 2011a). A relatively "faster" LHS is also associated with higher scores on extraversion, openness to experience and neuroticism (Del Giudice, 2014).

Whether the concept of LHT can also be applied to psychopathological condition, including personality disorders, is still debated. There is evidence to suggest that borderline personality disorder (Brüne, 2016; Baptista et al., 2023) and antisocial personality disorder (Troisi, 2005) can be likened to the idea of a "fast" LHS, but it seems more difficult to identify personality disorders on the "slower" end of the continuum of LHS. Moreover, some personality disorders are perhaps best described as a mix of fast and slow LHS aspects, as could be the case in schizotypy (Cheli, 2023). In any event, one point of critique from biologists is that the evidence for a differential timing of maturation in personality disorders, as predicted by LHT, is limited to date.

framework aimed to explain the general features of the cycle of life and – more broadly – how natural and sexual selection have designed an organism to achieve reproductive success (Roff, 1992; Stearns, 2000). In doing so, LHT tries to integrate knowledge about factors that are both internal and external to the organism. One of the central tenets of LHT is that an organism cannot invest resources in reproduction and body maintenance at the same time. In other words, there is a trade-off between the two. Accordingly, a number of traits (e.g., size at birth, death rate, growth pattern, age and size at maturity, longevity, etc.) can be explored to determine the general strategy of the organism. For example, we can easily compare a mouse and an elephant in terms of two different fast versus slow strategies (an evolutionary trade-off is a situation in which evolution cannot advance one part of a biological system without distressing another part of it). They present extremely different metabolic, immunological, behavioral, and mating patterns that are consistent with their unique life histories (Mortola, 2023).

Life History Theory has attracted evolutionary psychologists and the number of LHT publications in psychology is about equal to the publications in biology (Nettle & Frankenhuis, 2019). The apparent similarities between LHT's framework and goals and received frameworks in psychology for understanding how a personality evolves over time, the neurodevelopmental role of specific spectra or dimensions, may have favored the application of LHT in psychology.

In the specific field of personality, several authors have discussed a possible application of LHT to, for example, the three clusters of PDs (see Brüne, 2016a): Cluster A (such as schizoid and schizotypal) would be characterized by low-risk strategies and hypervigilance and a specific neurophysiological profile similar to schizophrenia; Cluster B would reflect a high-risk strategy with both hypovigilance (i.e., antisocial PD) and hypervigilance (i.e., borderline PD) toward potential sources of social threat; Cluster C (such as avoidant) would represent a set of diverse strategies based on profiles related to anxiety and depression.

Other authors have tried to more broadly apply LHT to personality and psychopathology. Del Giudice (2018) has proposed three widely used strategies: fast, slow, and defensive. The fast strategy includes psychopathological conditions such as conduct disorder, schizophrenia, and possibly Cluster B PDs that would be based on risk-taking, promiscuous, and antisocial behaviors. The slow strategy (mostly Cluster C) would aim to minimize risk and maintain long-lasting mating strategies. The defensive strategy would refer to general anxiety disorder, obsessive compulsive disorder and other disorders and be motivated by a recurrent harm-reduction model.

Similarly, LHT has been applied to the study of personality pathology using a dimensional approach. Models such as the FFM or the AMPD have fostered the research in the field (Simpson et al., 2010). For example, the degree of severity of personality pathology would be related to the level of parental support and a general K-factor (see Box 9.1) would be an important component of human development being negatively associated with traits such as psychoticism and neuroticism (Figueredo et al., 2005; van der Linden et al., 2012).

Despite the intriguing and fertile link between LHT and evolutionary psychopathology, criticism has also been raised (e.g., the lack of biological factors such growth rate, body size at sexual maturation as specific to psychological traits). The applications of LHT to evolutionary psychopathology and biology have led to two different research programs that are seemingly not sharing the same theoretical and methodological model (Nettle & Frankenhuis, 2020). The main differences would be in the focus of psychologists on behaviors without collecting evidence on biological data, and a limited attention to the life history trade-offs which underlie proposed strategies (Sear, 2020). For example, limited data about body size, sex maturation, and so on are available to confirm the differences between dysregulated and overcontrolled personality traits.

Despite the original formulation of LHT being applied to between-species comparisons because *Homo sapiens* is predominantly characterized by a slow strategy (long parental dependency, slow maturation, low number of offspring, etc.), there is significant variation among humans with regard to the factors usually considered in LHT (Brüne, 2016a; Ellis et al. 2011b). This variation is possibly related to the social complexity of our species and the rise of the so-called social brain and its distinctive functions (e.g., metacognition, mentalizing, social cognition), as well as a wide variety of attachment patterns. Indeed, these variables are suggested to be strictly related to the human phylogenetic history and the specificity of human psychopathology: the enormous process of encephalization in our species is explained in respect to the increased complexity of our social life, and this neurobiological and social complexity would be related to human-specific forms of psychopathology such as schizophrenia (Burns, 2007; Dunbar, 2009; Brüne, 2023). Moreover, these variables would explain the presence of numerous ecological niches favoring diversified evolutionary strategies. Although Westerners and East Asians belong to the same species, the two cultural contexts can favor, for example (see above), even opposite strategies in respect to perfectionism.

We believe that an important line of research in LHT should aim to outline and test multitrait models: a person's personality would be better defined by a set of traits interacting one with another, rather than by a single trait. Therefore, the limited evidence available about the application of LHT in humans would be explained by the use of models suggesting how a psychopathology and a person's life experience would be defined by unique and clear-cut strategy (either fast or slow). If we assume a multitrait approach (i.e., a single personality would be described by both fast and slow strategies), we might foster the LHT research program.

For example, schizotypy is usually associated with a fast strategy, even if a core feature is the presence of social and emotional detachment (i.e., features related to a slow strategy). Consistently, it has been hypothesized that schizotypal traits would represent a joint risk-minimizing and uniqueness-maximizing strategy based on a trajectory linking a basic organization of personality – high openness to experience and introversion – and a resulting maladaptive structure shaped by high psychoticism and detachment (Cheli, 2023; Cheli & Brüne, 2023). The assumption is that genetic–culture co-evolution and the specific niche a person was born in would define a basic organization that may vary

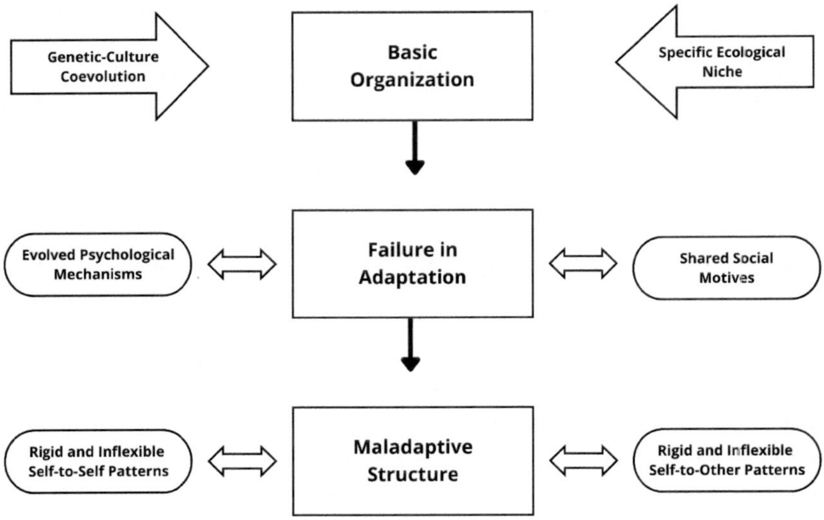

Figure 9.1 A tentative evolutionary model of personality pathology.
© Simone Cheli.

over time and evolve differently, that is in diverse structures (for a definition of organization and structure in biology see Maturana & Varela, 1984). In the case of schizotypal traits several early and developmental experiences may impair the person's ability to socialize their own openness and introversion, finally leading to a rigid and inflexible set of strategies based on odd and detached experiences, and this vulnerability would be explained by the phylogenetic (schizophrenia has seemingly emerged with our species and new brain) and ontogenetic (specific neurophysiological aberrations are consistent with specific psychosocial deficits) studies on the rise of social brain and its pivotal functions such as metacognition (Brüne, 2022; Cheli, 2023).

We can try to extend and generalize this model tested on schizotypal traits to other forms of personality pathology (see Figure 9.1). That is, we can hypothesize a general framework that can be applied to diverse complexes of intertwined traits. This model represents a tentative suggestion for further research, rather than a conclusive formulation.

Evolutionarily speaking, a personality pathology is an extreme of normal variation of strategies that may be pursued in a rigid, inflexible or excessive way. In order to value human complexity and support a research program that is anchored on evidence, we suggest focusing on a trajectory leading from a basic organization (not necessarily pathological even if characterized by specific vulnerabilities) to a final structure (pathological manifestations included).

This trajectory will correspond to a life history shaped by successive trade-offs in response to biopsychosocial constraints and emerging behavioral and epistemological patterns (see (1) and (2)). Consequently, our third principle is:

3. *Personality pathology is a trajectory leading from a basic organization to a maladaptive structure through recursive failures in adapting.*

It is important to underline how a pathological structure of personality results from *both* rigid, inflexible and excessive patterns *and* a mismatch between the individual and the environment. Saul (fictional name), for example, has always experienced paranoid ideation and antagonistic traits, but entered therapy and was diagnosed with paranoid personality disorder only in a specific phase of his life (see Cheli et al., 2021). He has always worked in borderline or even criminal environments where certain traits were adaptive. Once he married again and was preparing to retire from his job the pathology arose: the paranoid attitude that was previously advantageous was used in new contexts (e.g., paranoid jealousy with wife), where it became maladaptive.

Similarly, the emergence of severe disorders such as personality pathology between late adolescence and early adulthood has always been associated with a developmental vulnerability (Galván, 2017; Harrop & Trower, 2001; Sharp & Wall, 2018). Once musculoskeletal, hormonal, and immunological development is nearly complete, the late adolescent is confronted with beginning development of those higher functions distinctive to our species. That is, areas and functions related to the social brain are in the middle of their development, and the surrounding environment is becoming more and more demanding. The prefrontal cortex (an area directly involved in metacognitive processes such as mentalizing one's own and other's mental states) develops up to the age of 25. In the meantime, the reward system is forcing the late adolescent to hypervalue positive experiences and consider negative and even neutral experiences as repulsive. In short, a limited capacity to predict and navigate social complexity is associated with a pervasive impulsivity.

The emergence of a personality pathology may be understood by deepening and revising the standard diathesis–stress model with an evolutionary lens. Because PD is an enduring pattern, it does not manifest simply because the person faces a stressor. Moreover, the perdurance in our species of certain traits is explained by their association with specific advantages (through a direct natural or sexual advantage, a sustainable cost, a trade-off, etc.). The basic structure that defines the morphological constraints of the evolving personality is shaped by several internal and external factors, or broadly speaking evolutionary forces. In this regard, a mismatch between the genetic–cultural repertoire and the ongoing psychosocial demands can trigger and maintain a personality disorder. At the same time, the person can exhibit adaptive behaviors and even traits in specific areas of their lives, consistent with a multitrait approach to LHT. Overcontrolled traits are, for example, associated with altruistic behaviors and can favor an enduring adaptation in certain contexts even if to the point of causing a painful burden and even – through the so-called neurotic paradox – emotional isolation (Lynch et al., 2015).

Several genetic factors have been related to specific traits or spectra. For example, the externalizing spectrum – that is, related to later pathological features such as antagonistic and disinhibited traits – is associated with a set of genetic markers and psychosocial vulnerabilities in regard to behavioral disinhibition and disruptive behaviors (Baselmans et al., 2021; Young et al., 2009). Similar genetic liabilities interact – since birth or even gestation – with the surrounding culture of the broad environment and the specific ecological niche the person was born in. Strong evidence supports the role of general factors such as sociocultural heritage or specific factors such as attachment in psychopathology. For example, living in either collective or individualistic societies predicts how persons would define their own identity (Becker et al., 2012), whereas being exposed to abusive family contexts predicts higher levels of self-criticism in adulthood (Lassri et al., 2013). These complexes of intersecting stressors and vulnerabilities expose the person to diversified psychosocial demands. In trying to adapt to these demands, individuals develop specific evolved mechanisms and motives that are co-construed (in one sense or another) with the social environment in which they live. Indeed, if the organization is defined by a morphological pattern, the structure is progressively modeled by interpersonal interactions consistent with the phylogeny and ontogeny of the human social brain.

A pervasive personality pathology defined by high negative affectivity, antagonism and disinhibition (borderline personality disorder through a categorical perspective) would reflect, from this ecological perspective, a LHS aimed at immediate exploitation of resources, both interpersonal and material, based on predictions shaped by early developmental experiences (Brüne, 2016b). This trajectory may be associated with a genetic vulnerability possibly fueled by abusive family relationships (Bradley et al., 2011) and mating strategies that may be favored by sexual selection but not necessarily natural selection (Brüne et al., 2017). By growing up and possibly facing recurrent stressors the person would automatically exhibit – in pursuing basic human motives such as security and bonding – their prominent strategies that, in turn, might become more and more rigid and inflexible. The complexity of experiences and human relationships may finally lead to self-to-self and self-to-others patterns that are diagnosed as borderline personality disorder.

This broad evolutionary perspective may help understanding of the variety of experiences and traits that are associated with a categorical disorder such as borderline personality disorder and the apparent paradoxes such as the lack of evidence supporting earlier somatic maturation such as age at menarche (in contrast with LHT's assumptions) or the presence of evidence of internalizing (rather than exclusively externalizing) patterns such as depressive symptoms, self-criticism, and perfectionism (Chen et al., 2019; Sansone et al., 2011).

9.4 Conclusions

From an evolutionary point of view, a personality pathology is an extreme of normal variation of strategies that may be pursued in a rigid, inflexible, or excessive way. In this chapter we present personality traits as evolutionary strategies that are shaped by our biopsychosocial constraints and define our behavioral possibilities. At the same time, these strategies can be considered epistemological processes that operate at different levels, from an organism to a species, or even an ecological niche.

By discussing LHT in terms of a multitrait approach to evolutionary psychopathology, we suggest to consider personality pathology as a trajectory leading from a basic organization to a maladaptive structure through recursive failures in adapting. On the one hand, the organization would be morphologically determined by genetic–culture co-evolution and specific ecological niche. On the other hand, the final pathological structure is characterized by rigid, inflexible, and excessive self-to-self and self-to-other relationships that arise from both recursive stressors and a mismatch between the person's mechanisms and motives and the demands from the surrounding environment. Further research is needed to collect evidence about specific multitrait patterns and their pathological manifestations.

References

Ames, R., & Hall, D. (2003). *Dao De Jing: A philosophical translation*. Ballantine Books.

Bach, B., & Tracy, M. (2022). Clinical utility of the alternative model of personality disorders: A 10th year anniversary review. *Personality Disorders: Theory, Research, and Treatment*, *13*(4), 369–379. https://doi.org/10.1037/per0000527

Baptista, A., Chambon, V., Hoertel, N., Olfson, M., Blanco, C., Cohen, D., & Jacquet, P. O. (2023). Associations between early life adversity, reproduction-oriented life strategy, and borderline personality disorder. *JAMA Psychiatry*, *80*(6), 558–566. https://doi.org/10.1001/jamapsychiatry.2023.0694

Baselmans, B., Hammerschlag, A. R., Noordijk, S., Ip, H., van der Zee, M., de Geus, E., Abdellaoui, A., Treur, J. L., & van't Ent, D. (2021). The genetic and neural substrates of externalizing behavior. *Biological Psychiatry Global Open Science*, *2*(4), 389–399. https://doi.org/10.1016/j.bpsgos.2021.09.007

Becker, M., Vignoles, V. L., Owe, E., Brown, R., Smith, P. B., Easterbrook, M., Herman, G., de Sauvage, I., Bourguignon, D., Torres, A., Camino, L., Lemos, F. C. S., Ferreira, M. C., Koller, S. H., González, R., Carrasco, D., Cadena, M. P., Lay, S., Wang, Q., … Yamakoğlu, N. (2012). Culture and the distinctiveness motive: Constructing identity in individualistic and collectivistic contexts. *Journal of Personality and Social Psychology*, *102*(4), 833–855. https://doi.org/10.1037/a0026853

Belsky, J., Steinberg, L., & Draper, P. (1991). Childhood experience, interpersonal development, and reproductive strategy: An evolutionary theory of socialization. *Child development*, *62*(4), 647–670. https://doi.org/10.1111/j.1467-8624.1991.tb01558.x

Bleidorn, W., Schwaba, T., Zheng, A., Hopwood, C. J., Sosa, S. S., Roberts, B. W., & Briley, D. A. (2022). Personality stability and change: A meta-analysis of longitudinal studies. *Psychological Bulletin*, *148*(7–8), 588–619. https://doi.org/10.1037/bul0000365

Boyd, R., & Richerson, P. J. (1988). *Culture and the evolutionary process*. Chicago University Press.

Bradley, B., Westen, D., Mercer, K. B., Binder, E. B., Jovanovic, T., Crain, D., Wingo, A., & Heim, C. (2011). Association between childhood maltreatment and adult emotional dysregulation in a low-income, urban, African American sample: Moderation by oxytocin receptor gene. *Development and Psychopathology*, *23*(2), 439–452. https://doi.org/10.1017/S0954579411000162

Brüne, M. (2016a). *Textbook of evolutionary psychiatry and psychosomatic medicine: The origins of psychopathology* (2nd ed.). Oxford University Press.

Brüne, M. (2016b). Borderline personality disorder: Why 'fast and furious'? *Evolution, Medicine, and Public Health*, *2016*(1), 52–66. https://doi.org/10.1093/emph/eow002

Brüne, M. (2022). Evolution perspectives on schizophrenia spectrum disorders. In R. Abed, & P. St John-Smith (eds.), *Evolutionary psychiatry. Current perspectives on evolution and mental health* (pp. 153–168). Cambridge University Press.

Brüne, M. (2023). Evolutionary inquiries into the origin and nature of mental disorders. Editorial. *JAMA Psychiatry*, *80*(6), 537–538. https://doi.org/10.1001/jamapsychiatry.2023.0662

Brüne, M., Jiaqing, O., Schojai, M., Decker, C., & Edel, M.-A. (2017). Mating strategies and experience of early adversity in female patients with borderline personality disorder: Insights from life history theory. *Personality and Individual Differences*, *113*, 147–154. https://doi.org/10.1016/j.paid.2017.03.024

Burns, J. (2007). *The descent of madness: Evolutionary origins of psychosis and the social brain*. Routledge/Taylor & Francis Group.

Buss, D. M. (1995). Evolutionary psychology: A new paradigm for psychological science. *Psychological Inquiry*, *6*(1), 1–30. https://doi.org/10.1207/s15327965pli0601_1

Cheli, S. (2018) On the eigenform and viability of human complex systems: A view to epistemologically ground current psychotherapy. *Systems Research and Behavioral Science*, *35*, 505–519. https://doi.org/10.1002/sres.2559

Cheli, S. (2023). An evolutionary look at oddity and schizotypy: How the rise of social brain informs clinical practice. *New Ideas in Psychology*, *68*, 100993. https://doi.org/10.1016/j.newideapsych.2022.100993

Cheli, S., & Brüne, M. (2023). Evolutionary aspects of schizotypy. In S. Cheli & P. H. Lysaker (eds.), *A dimensional approach to schizotypy: Conceptualization and treatment* (pp. 19–35). Springer.

Cheli, S., Cavalletti, V., Popolo, R., & Dimaggio, G. (2021). A case study on a severe paranoid personality disorder client treated with metacognitive interpersonal therapy. *Journal of Clinical Psychology*, *77*(8), 1807–1820. https://doi.org/10.1002/jclp.23201

Chen, C., Hewitt, P. L., Flett, G. L., & Roxborough, H. M. (2019). Multidimensional perfectionism and borderline personality organization in emerging adults: A two-wave longitudinal study. *Personality and Individual Differences*, *146*, 143–148. https://doi.org/10.1016/j.paid.2019.04.011

Cicchetti, D., & Cohen, D. J. (eds.). (2006). *Developmental psychopathology: Risk, disorder, and adaptation* (Vol. 3, 2nd ed.). Wiley.

Darwin, C. (1859). *On the origin of species by means of natural selection, or the preservation of favoured races in the struggle for life*. John Murray.

Darwin, C. (1871). *The descent of man, and selection in relation to sex*. John Murray.

Del Giudice, M. (2014). An evolutionary life history framework for psychopathology. *Psychological Inquiry*, *25*(3-4), 261–300. https://doi.org/10.1080/1047840X.2014.884918

Del Giudice, M. (2018). *Evolutionary psychopathology. A unified approach*. Oxford University Press.

Dunbar, R. I. (2009). The social brain hypothesis and its implications for social evolution. *Annals of Human Biology*, *36*(5), 562–572. https://doi.org/10.1080/03014460902960289

Edershile, E. A., & Wright, A. G. C. (2021). Fluctuations in grandiose and vulnerable narcissistic states: A momentary perspective. *Journal of Personality and Social Psychology*, *120*(5), 1386–1414. https://doi.org/10.1037/pspp0000370

Ellis, B. J., Figueredo, A. J., Brumbach, B. H., & Schlomer, G. L. (2009). Fundamental Dimensions of environmental risk: The impact of harsh versus unpredictable environments on the evolution and development of life history strategies. *Human Nature*, *20*(2), 204–268. https://doi.org/10.1007/s12110-009-9063-7

Ellis, B. J., Boyce, W. T., Belsky, J., Bakermans-Kranenburg, M. J., & van Ijzendoorn, M. H. (2011a). Differential susceptibility to the environment: an evolutionary–neurodevelopmental theory. *Development and Psychopathology*, *23*(1), 7–28. https://doi.org/10.1017/S0954579410000611

Ellis, B. J., Shirtcliff, E. A., Boyce, W. T., Deardorff, J., & Essex, M. J. (2011b). Quality of early family relationships and the timing and tempo of puberty: Effects depend on biological sensitivity to context. *Development and Psychopathology*, *23*(1), 85–99. https://doi.org/10.1017/S0954579410000660

Fabrega, H. (2002). *Origins of psychopathology: The phylogenetic and cultural basis of mental illness*. Rutgers University Press.

Figueredo, A. J., Vásquez, G., Brumbach, B. H., Sefcek, J. A., Kirsner, B. R., & Jacobs, W. J. (2005). The K-factor: Individual differences in life history strategy. *Personality and Individual Differences*, *39*(8), 1349–1360. https://doi.org/10.1016/j.paid.2005.06.009

Galván, A. (2017). *The neuroscience of adolescence*. Cambridge University Press.

Harrop, C., & Trower, P. (2001). Why does schizophrenia develop at late adolescence? *Clinical Psychology Review*, *21*(2), 241–265. https://doi.org/10.1016/s0272-7358(99)00047-1

Hopwood, C. J., Donnellan, M. B., Blonigen, D. M., Krueger, R. F., McGue, M., Iacono, W. G., & Burt, S. A. (2011). Genetic and environmental influences on personality trait stability and growth during the transition to adulthood: A three-wave longitudinal study. *Journal of Personality and Social Psychology*, *100*(3), 545–556. https://doi.org/10.1037/a0022409

Jauk, E., Ulbrich, L., Jorschick, P., Höfler, M., Kaufman, S. B., & Kanske, P. (2022). The nonlinear association between grandiose and vulnerable narcissism: An individual data meta-analysis. *Journal of Personality, 90*(5), 703–726. https://doi.org/10.1111/jopy.12692

Kaplan, H. S., & Robson, A. J. (2002). The emergence of humans: The coevolution of intelligence and longevity with intergenerational transfers. *Proceedings of the National Academy of Sciences of the United States of America, 99*(15), 10221–10226. https://doi.org/10.1073/pnas.152502899

Laing, R. D. (1960). *The divided self: An existential study in sanity and madness*. Penguin.

Lassri, D., Soffer-Dudek, N., Lerman, S. F., Rudich, Z., & Shahar, G. (2013). Self-criticism confers vulnerability to psychopathology in the face of perceived stress related to missile attacks: Three longitudinal studies. *International Journal of Cognitive Therapy, 6*(3), 221–234. https://doi.org/10.1521/ijct.2013.6.3.221

Liddell, B. J., & Williams, E. N. (2019). Cultural differences in interpersonal emotion regulation. *Frontiers in Psychology, 10*, 999. https://doi.org/10.3389/fpsyg.2019.00999

Luria, A. (1968). *The mind of a mnemonist: A little book about a vast memory*. Harvard University Press.

Lynch, T. R., Hempel, R. J., & Dunkley, C. (2015). Radically open-dialectical behavior therapy for disorders of over-control: Signaling matters. *American Journal of Psychotherapy, 69*(2), 141–162. https://doi.org/10.1176/appi.psychotherapy.2015.69.2.141

Lysaker, P. H., Kukla, M., Leonhardt, B. L., Hamm, J. A., Schnakenberg Martin, A., Zalzala, A. B., Gagen, E. C., & Hasson-Ohayon, I. (2020). Meaning, integration, and the self in serious mental illness: Implications of research in metacognition for psychiatric rehabilitation. *Psychiatric Rehabilitation Journal, 43*(4), 275–283. https://doi.org/10.1037/prj0000436

Malinowski, B. (1960). *A scientific theory of culture and other essays*. Galaxy Book.

Maturana, H., & Varela, F. (1980). *Autopoiesis and cognition: The realization of the living*. Reidel Publishing Company.

Maturana, H., & Varela, F. G. (1984). *El Arbol del Conocimiento*. Editorial Universitari.

McAdams, D. P., Shiner, R. L., & Tackett, J. L. (2021). *Handbook of personality development*. Guildford Press.

MacArthur, R. H., & Wilson, E. O. (1967). *The theory of island biogeography*. Princeton University Press.

Morey, L. C., Hopwood, C. J., Gunderson, J. G., Skodol, A. E., Shea, M. T., Yen, S., Stout, R. L., Zanarini, M. C., Grilo, C. M., Sanislow, C. A., & McGlashan, T. H. (2007). Comparison of alternative models for personality disorders. *Psychological Medicine, 37*(7), 983–994. https://doi.org/10.1017/S0033291706009482

Mortola, J. P. (2023). The mouse-to-elephant metabolic curve: Historical overview. *Comprehensive Physiology, 13*(2), 4513–4558. https://doi.org/10.1002/cphy.c220003

Nettle, D., & Frankenhuis, W. E. (2019). The evolution of life-history theory: A bibliometric analysis of an interdisciplinary research area. *Proceedings of the Royal Society B, 286*(1899), 20190040. https://doi.org/10.1098/rspb.2019.0040

Nettle, D., & Frankenhuis, W. E. (2020). Life-history theory in psychology and evolutionary biology: One research programme or two? *Philosophical Transactions of the Royal Society B, 375*(1803), 20190490. https://doi.org/10.1098/rstb.2019.0490

Piaget, J. (1950). *Introduction à l'épistémologie génétique. Tome III: La pensée biologique, la pensée psychologique et la pensée sociale*. Presses universitaires de France.
Poortinga, Y. H., & Van Hemert, D. A. (2001). Personality and culture demarcating between the common and the unique. *Journal of Personality, 69*(6), 1033–1060. https://doi.org/10.1111/1467-6494.696174
Richerson, P. J., & Boyd, R. (2004). *Not by genes alone: How culture transformed human evolution*. Chicago University Press.
Riedl, R. (1984). *Biology of knowledge: The evolutionary basis of reason*. John Wiley & Sons.
Roff, D. (1992). *The evolution of life histories: Theory and analysis*. Chapman & Hall.
Sansone, R. A., Chu, J. W., & Wiederman, M. W. (2011). Sexual behaviour and borderline personality disorder among female psychiatric inpatients. *International Journal of Psychiatry in Clinical Practice, 15*(1), 69–73. https://doi.org/10.3109/13651501.2010.507871
Sear, R. (2020). Do human 'life history strategies' exist? *Evolution and Human Behavior, 41*(6), 513–526. https://doi.org/10.1016/j.evolhumbehav.2020.09.004
Sharp, C., & Wall, K. (2018). Personality pathology grows up: Adolescence as a sensitive period. *Current Opinion in Psychology, 21*, 111–116. https://doi.org/10.1016/j.copsyc.2017.11.010
Sharp, C., Wright, A. G., Fowler, J. C., Frueh, B. C., Allen, J. G., Oldham, J., & Clark, L. A. (2015). The structure of personality pathology: Both general ('g') and specific ('s') factors? *Journal of Abnormal Psychology, 124*(2), 387–398. https://doi.org/10.1037/abn0000033
Simpson, J. A., Griskevicius, V., & Kim, J. S. (2010). Evolution, life history theory, and personality. In O. P. John & R. W. Robins (eds.), *Handbook of interpersonal psychology: Theory, research, assessment, and therapeutic interventions* (pp. 75–89). Wiley.
Skodol, A. E., Morey, L. C., Bender, D. S., & Oldham, J. M. (2015). The alternative DSM-5 model for personality disorders: A clinical application. *The American Journal of Psychiatry, 172*(7), 606–613. https://doi.org/10.1176/appi.ajp.2015.14101220
Stearns, S.C. (1992). *The evolution of life histories*. Oxford University Press.
Stearns, S. (2000). Life history evolution: Successes, limitations, and prospects. *Naturwissenschaften, 87*, 476–486. https://doi.org/10.1007/s001140050763
Stoeber, J., Kobori, O., & Tanno, Y. (2013). Perfectionism and self-conscious emotions in British and Japanese students: Predicting pride and embarrassment after success and failure. *European Journal of Personality, 27*(1), 59–70. https://doi.org/10.1002/per.1858
Tomlinson, G. (2018). *Culture and the course of human evolution*. Chicago University Press.
Trofimova, I., Robbins, T. W., Sulis, W. H., & Uher, J. (2018). Taxonomies of psychological individual differences: Biological perspectives on millennia-long challenges. *Philosophical transactions of the Royal Society of London. Series B, Biological Sciences, 373*(1744), 20170152. https://doi.org/10.1098/rstb.2017.0152
Troisi, A. (2005). The concept of alternative strategies and its relevance to psychiatry and clinical psychology. *Neuroscience and Biobehavioral Reviews, 29*(1), 159–168. https://doi.org/10.1016/j.neubiorev.2004.06.012
Varela, F. (1979). *Principles of biological autonomy*. North Holland.

van der Linden, D., Figueredo, A. J., de Leeuw, R. N. H., Scholte, R. H. J., & Engels, R. C. M. E. (2012). The general factor of personality (GFP) and parental support: Testing a prediction from life history theory. *Evolution and Human Behavior*, *33*(5), 537–546. https://doi.org/10.1016/j.evolhumbehav.2012.01.007

van Wijk, I. C., Huffmeijer, R., Bosdriesz, J. R., Bakermans-Kranenburg, M. J., Kolijn, L., van IJzendoorn, M. H., Vrijhof, C. I., & van den Bulk, B. G. (2019). Behavioral genetics of temperament and frontal asymmetry in early childhood. *Journal of Experimental Child Psychology*, 179, 348–361. https://doi.org/10.1016/j.jecp.2018.11.015.

von Glasersfeld, E. (1985). Reconstructing the concept of knowledge. *Archives de Psychologie*, *53*(204), 91–101.

von Uexküll, J. (1926). *Theoretical biology*. Harcourt, Brace & Co.

Widiger, T. A., & Crego, C. (2019). The Five Factor Model of personality structure: An update. *World Psychiatry*, *18*(3), 271–272. https://doi.org/10.1002/wps.20658

Widiger, T. A., & McCabe, G. A. (2020). The alternative model of personality disorders (AMPD) from the perspective of the five-factor model. *Psychopathology*, *53*(3–4), 149–156. https://doi.org/10.1159/000507378

Wright, A. J., & Jackson, J. J. (2022). Childhood temperament and adulthood personality differentially predict life outcomes. *Scientific Reports*, *12*(1), 10286. https://doi.org/10.1038/s41598-022-14666-0

Young, S. E., Friedman, N. P., Miyake, A., Willcutt, E. G., Corley, R. P., Haberstick, B. C., & Hewitt, J. K. (2009). Behavioral disinhibition: Liability for externalizing spectrum disorders and its genetic and environmental relation to response inhibition across adolescence. *Journal of Abnormal Psychology*, *118*(1), 117–130. https://doi.org/10.1037/a0014657

Part III

Novel Conceptual Approaches to Personality Disorder

10 What Does Personality Have to Do with Mental Disorder?

A Cybernetic Perspective

Colin G. DeYoung and Robert F. Krueger

10.1 What Does Personality Have to Do with Mental Disorder? A Cybernetic Perspective

We begin with two assertions that are well supported by empirical evidence: (1) There are no such things as "personality disorders" distinct from other mental disorders. (2) Personality traits contribute to risk for all forms of mental disorder. We expect the first of these claims to be controversial, so it is important to be clear that we are not denying the existence of the sort of mental health problems that have typically been diagnosed as personality disorders. What we are denying is that these problems have some special connection to "personality" that other forms of mental disorder do not (Krueger, 2005). After reviewing the context and evidence for these two assertions, we attempt to clarify their implications with reference to a theory of psychopathology as cybernetic dysfunction (DeYoung & Krueger, 2018a, 2018b, 2023). We argue that personality is necessarily involved in all mental disorders, not just what have historically, and inaccurately, been singled out as "personality disorders."

10.2 Context: Mental Disorders are Dimensional Rather than Categorical

Over the last several decades, it has become clear that common mental disorders are not validly considered discrete categorical entities (Haslam et al., 2020). They are more like high blood pressure than infectious disease. For blood pressure, the threshold drawn to separate those with hypertension from those without is clearly somewhat arbitrary, a practical demarcation of a continuous dimension of risk. For most infectious diseases, by contrast, the pathogen is either present or absent, and its presence is the categorical marker of disease. In official nosologies, such as the *Diagnostic and statistical manual of mental disorders* (DSM; American Psychiatric Association, 2013) and the

International classification of diseases (ICD; World Health Organization, 2018), most mental disorders are assumed to be like infectious disease, in that people with the diagnosis are deemed categorically, not just quantitatively, distinct from people without it. Given a great deal of evidence that this assumption is incorrect, a movement has arisen to study mental disorders as dimensional constructs and to devise new dimensional nosologies (Insel et al., 2010; Kotov et al., 2017; Krueger et al., 2012).

These new dimensional approaches additionally address another long-standing problem with the official nosologies, namely that the traditional categories group symptoms together in ways that reflect neither underlying etiology nor typical patterns of co-occurrence. (Throughout, we use "symptom" to refer to outwardly observable behaviors as well as subjective experiences.) Although the categorical diagnoses of DSM and ICD are typically presented as "syndromal" – intending to describe common aggregations of symptoms – extensive empirical investigations of the co-occurrence of symptoms have demonstrated that they often do not (Forbes et al., 2024b). And the categorical personality disorders (PDs) are some of the worst offenders in proposing putatively distinct clusters of symptoms that fail to reflect how symptoms actually covary (Sharp et al., 2015).

Largely because of these failures, but also because the concept of trait dimensions is so familiar in personality research, diagnosis of PDs has recently been transformed in revisions of DSM and ICD. Although DSM-5 retains the 10 categorical personality disorders as the official diagnostic system for PDs, it also includes an alternative diagnostic model of personality disorder (AMPD) in section III, "Emerging measures and models," in which personality disorder is defined in relation to overall self and interpersonal impairment (Criterion A) and a set of 25 "pathological personality traits" grouped into five broader trait dimensions (Criterion B). The 11th revision of the ICD went further by eliminating the categorical diagnostic system entirely and replacing it with a single diagnosis of personality disorder based on self and interpersonal dysfunction, which can then be specified using five symptom dimensions describing "maladaptive traits" (four of which are nearly identical to AMPD dimensions).

In changing to a dimensional system of diagnoses, the PDs are the leading edge of a larger movement. Empirical investigations of the covariation of many different forms of mental illness have led to new mappings of the covariation among symptoms, not just within personality disorders, but across the full range of mental disorders. The most prominent such mapping currently is the Hierarchical Taxonomy of Psychopathology (HiTOP), a new nosology that describes people not by placing them into a specific disorder category but by indicating the intensity of their symptoms in various symptom dimensions organized into six broader spectra (Kotov et al., 2017, 2021). HiTOP attempts to reflect the "consensus of evidence" from quantitative research on patterns of co-occurrence of symptoms, and the evidence it summarizes indicates two things about personality disorders.

First, no one has a "personality disorder" in the way that one might have an infectious disease. Hence, if any personality disorder exists, it must be like having high blood pressure, reflecting a persistently high level of some qualities that other people have to lesser degrees. Second, the symptoms that were used to identify PDs in the traditional categorical nosologies do not form a coherent cluster or clusters but rather reflect nearly all the dimensions of symptoms that are present in other putatively distinct types of mental disorder. They are spread across the HiTOP model, with the five dimensions of the AMPD being essentially equivalent to five of HiTOP's spectra. (The 25 trait dimensions of the AMPD were designed to cover all the symptoms listed as criteria in the 10 traditional categorical diagnoses; Krueger et al., 2012.) Thus, the dimensions of psychopathology represented in HiTOP describe symptoms equally well for people diagnosed with personality disorders or with other disorders. This can also be demonstrated using the traditional PD diagnoses instead of specific symptom measures: a factor-analytic meta-analysis of co-occurrence of diagnoses showed the categorical PDs spread across five HiTOP spectra (although they are most prominently represented in the detachment and antagonism spectra; Ringwald et al., 2022).

10.3 Are Personality Disorders Characterizable by Temporal Stability or Impairments in Self and Interpersonal Functioning?

Even if personality disorders are not categorical entities and they involve symptoms that can also be found in many other diagnostic categories not traditionally deemed to be personality disorders, one might wonder if there are nonetheless some specific classes of PD symptoms that might distinguish them from other disorders. Certainly, clinicians have long had a sense that some people have problems better diagnosed as personality disorders than as what were known – before DSM-5 – as "Axis I" disorders (with personality disorders constituting Axis II). We are not denying that these clinicians may often have been picking up on characteristics that were genuinely different about these individuals, compared to those diagnosed with depression, anxiety, bipolar disorder, and so on, and it is worth exploring both what these might be and why they do not suffice to qualify them as "personality" disorders in any way that clearly distinguishes them from other disorders.

First, it might be the case that PDs could be identified by their developmental course. Both the traditional categorical PD model and the AMPD require that PDs have onsets beginning at latest "in adolescence or early adulthood" and that they are "relatively stable across time." The assumption that PD symptoms are more stable and persistent than those of other disorders was core to the rationale for separating PDs as Axis II in DSM-III and -IV. This assumption has been questioned, however, based on findings that PDs may remit (i.e., have symptom levels drop below the diagnostic threshold) at rates not unlike those of Axis I disorders (Krueger, 2005; Shea & Yen, 2003). PDs appear to be less stable than originally assumed, and many Axis I disorders also emerge in childhood or adolescence and show considerable stability across time (Campbell et al., 2003; Kessler et al., 1994; Krueger, 2005). For both PDs and Axis I disorders, symptoms wax and wane over time, while maintaining relatively high rank-order stability. These findings contributed to the decision to eliminate the axial system in DSM-5, instead simply including the PDs as another chapter in the general section for official diagnoses.

The ICD-11 has again gone further by reducing the stability requirement to persistence for "an extended period of time (e.g., lasting 2 years or more)" (World Health Organization, 2018). And no longer must the onset be in early life – ICD-11 states that early onsets are typical but not required. This change reflects the evidence that the developmental course of illness cannot be used to distinguish personality disorder from other disorders. It is simply not the case that PD symptoms are "maladaptive traits" whereas symptoms of other disorders are not trait-like.

The HiTOP consortium has suggested that any symptom dimension within the HiTOP model can be considered both as a temporary symptom or as a more persistent trait, merely based on whether it is true in general of the person over time (trait) versus being present over a specific time frame (symptom) (DeYoung et al., 2022). This means that symptoms that last sufficiently long become indistinguishable from traits. Because traits are assessed using a general rather than specific time frame or recall period (e.g., by rating what is true "in general" or "typically" for the person), the recall period beyond which a symptom measure becomes undifferentiable from a trait measure is an empirical question, but one that has not yet been well-studied. Given the limitations and biases of human memory, it seems unlikely to be longer than a few months. (How long, conceptually, some pattern of behavior should last to be considered a trait is a separate question; most traits fluctuate over time, but are nonetheless reasonably stable over periods of many years; Bleidorn et al., 2022.) Obviously, some people have episodes of psychopathology that last for only a few months or less and are relatively inconsistent with their general personality traits, but more typically, when people have brief episodes of mental illness, those reflect a temporary increase of an already high (but subclinical) level of the symptom dimension(s) in question (DeYoung et al., 2022; Shea et al., 2004). This suggests that psychopathology described by any dimension of HiTOP can be a "personality disorder" (in the sense of being a maladaptive trait) if it is sufficiently persistent, and this means that "personality" does not single out any particular group of disorders.

Given that the presence of persistent trait-like symptoms is insufficient to distinguish qualitatively different groups of disorders, it is worth considering the more substantive component of the redefinition of PDs in ICD-11 and the AMPD. In both these systems, the core defining features of PD are persistent impairments in self and interpersonal functioning. (Note that the interpersonal emphasis is consistent with the clustering of many of the old categorical PD diagnoses around the detachment and antagonism spectra, precisely the two spectra that explicitly describe interpersonal behavior, or lack thereof; Wright & Ringwald, 2022.) These impairments are elaborated through four more-specific constructs: lack of self-direction, disturbed or incoherent sense of identity, difficulty maintaining intimate relationships, and lack of empathy. Undeniably, these are characteristics that may cause or stem from mental health problems. Further, they are not symptoms that are explicitly attributed to many other disorders in the official nosologies (although there are exceptions; e.g., interpersonal problems are included in the diagnosis of autism). Perhaps, then, the new PD diagnoses provide important coverage of forms of mental disorder that are not well covered elsewhere.

Self and interpersonal impairments may be important forms of psychopathology and thus important to recognize diagnostically, but does that mean they constitute "personality" disorder whereas other forms of impairment do not? Personality is typically defined as encompassing all reasonably persistent patterns of behavior, emotion, cognition, and motivation. Therefore, although persistent self and interpersonal impairments are clearly elements of personality, so are all the other symptom dimensions that can be listed in HiTOP (or similar nosologies), as long as they are sufficiently persistent. To illustrate our point by example, we see no reason why having chronic problems with a lack of empathy should be more worthy of being considered a problem of "personality" than having chronic problems with inattention, impulsivity, anhedonia, or anxiety.

Also worth noting in this context is that, when factor-analyzed with a wide range of other symptoms, the impairments of self have been found to fall within HiTOP's internalizing spectrum (which is labeled "neuroticism" or "negative affectivity" in other contexts) and the interpersonal impairments to fall within the detachment and antagonism spectra (Clark & Ro, 2014). This finding indicates that, although problems with self-direction, identity, intimate relationships, and empathy may be important features of mental illness, they are not independent of the more general covariance structure of psychopathology and can be considered elements within the broader HiTOP spectra (Widiger et al., 2019a). Further, even if they had been shown to constitute separate factors beyond the current spectra (Zimmerman et al., 2015), this would not render the current spectra less personality-like. HiTOP is intended to be expanded based on empirical evidence; it is likely to add another spectrum reflecting many symptoms of the so-called "neurodevelopmental disorders" (e.g., autism), and it can add others as needed (Forbes et al., 2024a). But all spectra will always contain constructs that can be trait-like (and hence part of personality) despite sometimes occurring over much shorter time periods for some people.

10.4 Personality Traits as Risk for Psychopathology

As we have seen, the covariance structure of psychopathology can be considered a structure of traits as well as a structure of temporary symptoms (DeYoung et al., 2022; Widiger et al., 2019b). Having higher levels on these trait/symptom dimensions indicates higher risk for psychopathology. (We think this claim is more defensible than to say that being above some level on these dimensions is necessarily pathological, for reasons that will become clear below.) Not only that, the covariance structure of normal personality variation is very similar to the covariance structure of psychopathology, and various assessments of psychopathology have been shown to be measuring the same underlying latent trait dimensions as assessments of normal personality variation (Griffith et al., 2010; Stepp et al., 2012; Suzuki et al., 2015). This means that most persistent symptoms of psychopathology are extreme or maladaptive variants of normal personality traits.

The major dimensions of covariation among personality traits are typically described by the Big Five (neuroticism, extraversion, conscientiousness, agreeableness, and openness/intellect), and, psychometrically, the first four of these correspond almost perfectly to the symptom dimensions internalizing or negative affect, (low) detachment, (low) disinhibition, and (low) antagonism. (Openness/intellect is more complicated, but psychoticism or thought disorder can be considered a maladaptive variant of the Openness to Experience subfactor of the broader Big Five dimension; DeYoung & Krueger, 2018a.) Because of this correspondence, it is clear that most major dimensions of personality are major dimensions of risk for psychopathology – and not just risk for what have traditionally been labeled "personality disorders" but for psychopathology described by the Axis I disorders as well. Even for the few mental disorders or symptom dimensions that do not fit neatly into the general factor structure of normal personality variation, we know of none that have failed to show significant associations with some normal personality traits. Thus, it is uncontroversial to say that personality traits contribute to risk for all forms of mental disorder.

10.5 The Cybernetic Dysfunction Theory

Drawing on the empirical discoveries described above, as well as a mechanistic theory of personality called Cybernetic Big Five Theory (CB5T; DeYoung, 2015), we have developed a theory of psychopathology as cybernetic dysfunction (DeYoung & Krueger, 2018a, 2018b, 2023). We define psychopathology as "persistent failure to move toward one's goals, due to failure to generate effective new goals, interpretations, or strategies when existing ones prove unsuccessful." Note that such definitional endeavors are inherently philosophical, in the sense that they cannot be resolved purely by empiricism. To collect empirical evidence regarding psychopathology (or any other phenomenon), one must measure it, and to measure it one must define what it is that will be measured. If one does not have an explicit definition, then one is necessarily accepting some implicit definition through one's choice of instrument. A number of philosophical analyses defining "mental disorder" and "psychopathology" have been produced (e.g., Bolton, 2008; Boorse, 1977; Kendell, 1975; Wakefield, 1992), and we have compared our theory to them in previous articles (DeYoung & Krueger, 2018a, 2023). Our purpose here is to review our theory briefly and to explain how it sheds light on the role of personality in mental disorders.

First, some additional definitional considerations: Cybernetics (also known as *control theory*) is the study of goal-directed systems that self-regulate via feedback (Wiener, 1961; Powers, 1973). Cybernetic systems must incorporate at a minimum three elements: (1) one or more controlled variables, physically instantiated within the system, that the system works to bring into a certain range (goals); (2) a sensor of the current state of the variable allowing feedback comparison of the goal state with the current state; and (3) some operator(s) that can act to move the current state toward the goal state. All organisms are cybernetic systems. In keeping with the broad cybernetic conception of goals, in our theory goals are understood to encompass not just explicit, detailed representations of a future state toward which one is committed to working (Elliot & Fryer, 2008), but also any desired state of the world, including broad, vague, and even potentially unconscious desires, values, and basic needs. Goals govern people's behavior and interpretations of events, and the inability to pursue one's goals effectively, coupled with an inability to adapt one's goals or one's habits of thinking, feeling, and acting in such a way as to get back on track in the pursuit of goals, is how we propose to define psychopathology.

Although we won't here rehash comparisons of our definition to other philosophical accounts, we will compare it to the general definition of mental disorder that appears in the DSM, given that the DSM is the main source of most current conceptions of personality disorder. DSM-5 uses the terms "mental disorder" and "psychopathology" interchangeably. We prefer to gloss them differently, with "mental disorder" reserved for official diagnostic entities (DeYoung & Krueger, 2018a). Whereas we take psychopathology to be a matter of objective fact (because, at a given time, there is a fact of the matter regarding any individual's goals and how effectively they are being pursued), the determination of what form and level of psychopathology counts as a mental disorder necessarily involves sociopolitical processes of negotiation among various stakeholders. For present purposes, however, we can ignore this distinction much as the DSM does. The core of the DSM-5 definition (APA, 2013, p. 20) comprises two sentences (which are followed by exclusionary qualifiers not relevant here): "A mental disorder is a syndrome characterized by clinically significant disturbance in an individual's cognition, emotion regulation, or behavior that reflects a dysfunction in the psychological, biological, or developmental processes underlying mental functioning. Mental disorders are usually associated with significant distress or disability in social, occupational, or other important activities." This definition is not philosophically rigorous because many of its key elements, such as "dysfunction" and "clinically significant," are never defined. The DSM is a manual for practice, a pragmatic tool, and it leaves clinicians to decide what is significant and how to define "dysfunction" (which has several different definitions in biology; Wouters, 2003). Further, clinicians rarely have cause to refer to this general definition because the important part of the DSM-5 is the list of official diagnoses in section II, each of which specifies its own criteria, without reference to the general definition. Something particularly interesting about the general definition, from our perspective, is that the word "usually" entails that distress and impairment are neither necessary nor sufficient for the presence of mental disorder as such. In the individual diagnostic categories, most do make distress or impairment necessary, but some do not. None of them make it sufficient. Further, the subsequent text is apologetic about including impairment as a criterion in many diagnoses despite "substantial efforts . . . to separate the concepts of mental disorder and disability (impairment in social, occupational, or other important areas of functioning)" (APA, 2013, p. 21). The text goes on to express a wish for "clear biological markers or clinically useful measurements of severity" that could obviate the need to ask whether people's symptoms are interfering with their personal concerns and outcomes before providing a diagnosis.

Our solution to these difficulties is to move in the opposite direction (DeYoung & Krueger, 2023). Rather than looking for biological signs that would necessarily indicate the presence of disease, independently of the individual's specific concerns and outcomes, we identify the latter as the essence of psychopathology. In our view, all mental processes supervene on biological processes, meaning that biological processes can change without changing mental processes, but mental processes cannot change without change in their underlying biological processes. Both biological and mental or psychological processes are physical, but they are descriptions of the physical world at different levels of resolution and analysis, and *psycho*pathology, *mental* illness, is most cogently defined at the psychological level rather than the biological level. Someone with an unusual pattern of brain function should not be deemed mentally ill unless that pattern prevents them from pursuing their goals effectively. (This means it is possible for someone to have a neurological illness, based on assessment of brain pathology, without yet having a mental illness.) Thus, from our perspective, distress or impairment (understood cybernetically as goal failure) is not only necessary but also sufficient to identify psychopathology, as long as subsequent attempts at adaptation have failed. We believe our definition of psychopathology is largely consistent with common medical and lay perceptions of who is mentally ill, even though it diverges from common essentialist intuitions and emphasis on specific symptoms.

Our approach resolves a core dilemma of the DSM, namely that it relies primarily on checklists of symptoms to diagnose specific mental disorders, while simultaneously recognizing that symptoms alone are not sufficient to diagnose mental disorder. Symptoms are not inherent indicators of disease, but rather clues to the possible presence of disease. No surprise, then, that the DSM admits "it has not been possible to completely separate normal and pathological symptom expressions contained in diagnostic criteria" (APA, 2013, p. 21). Not everyone who experiences a lot of anxiety is mentally ill, nor is everyone who hears voices (Linscott & van Os, 2013; Powers et al., 2017). Despite the DSM's disclaimer, we perceive that its ethos, as well as current cultural attitudes toward mental illness, revolve around the assumption that having certain combinations of symptoms generally entails having a mental disorder. One way to undercut this assumption is to emphasize that the symptom dimensions of psychopathology (which, as just noted, are markers of risk for psychopathology rather than sufficient indicators thereof) are all also personality traits. Just as having an unusual pattern of brain function never, by itself, constitutes mental illness, so having unusual personality traits never reflects mental illness without being accompanied by cybernetic dysfunction. Extreme traits often constitute risks for dysfunction, but a risk is not the thing itself.

10.6 Traits versus Characteristic Adaptations: Personality as the Foundation of All Mental Disorder

Our argument thus far may seem to have led to a paradox. If extreme personality traits, even those that are often considered "symptoms," are never sufficient to identify psychopathology, how is it possible for us to claim that personality is necessarily involved in all mental disorders? We resolve this apparent paradox with reference to a distinction made by CB5T between personality traits and characteristic adaptations, the two exhaustive components of personality. We have mentioned that personality is typically defined as encompassing all reasonably persistent patterns of behavior, emotion, cognition, and motivation. This means that all persistent psychological individual differences are elements of personality, whether they have traditionally been labeled as such or as symptoms of psychopathology, cognitive abilities, attitudes, or anything else. Some personality psychologists equate all such differences with "personality traits," but this has the unfortunate consequence of qualifying things like love of spaghetti as personality traits, if they are persistent (DeYoung, 2017). It is more in keeping with the usage of psychologists and others to reserve the label "personality traits" for certain kinds of psychological individual differences and to describe the rest as "characteristic adaptations."

CB5T defines personality traits as probabilistic descriptions of relatively stable patterns of emotion, motivation, cognition, and behavior, in response to classes of stimuli that have been present in human environments over evolutionary time, and it asserts that they are due to variation in parameters of evolved mechanisms that are present in every intact human brain (such as those governing sensitivity to reward, for extraversion versus detachment, or sensitivity to punishment, for neuroticism versus emotional stability). In contrast, characteristic adaptations are relatively stable goals, interpretations, and strategies, specified in relation to an individual's particular life circumstances. They are not evolutionary adaptations (genetic changes from generation to generation), but rather adaptations learned during a lifetime – persistent, but updateable, contents of memory, which is to say habits of thinking, feeling, and acting (and wanting, perceiving, etc.). To illustrate the distinction, being generally prevention-focused is a trait; checking the stove every time one leaves the house is a characteristic adaptation.

The three categories of characteristic adaptation correspond to the three basic elements of a cybernetic system, with *goals* being the controlled variables, *interpretations* reflecting the model of the current (and past) state of the world against which goals are compared, and *strategies* being the cognitive and behavioral operations that are used to pursue one's goals. Relatively abstract general goals that are presumably innate in all people (such as the desire to gain information or to avoid punishment), but that vary in strength from person to person in a way that qualifies them as personality traits, cannot be accomplished without more specific characteristic adaptations (including nested subgoals) that allow the person to navigate their own particular circumstances. Thus, all actual functioning, from moment to moment, depends on our characteristic adaptations.

Sometimes people encounter situations sufficiently novel that their existing adaptations are insufficient to allow them to maintain effective goal pursuit.

Then one must adapt, figure out something new, and, if that new adaptation is subsequently remembered and persists, it becomes a new characteristic adaptation, part of one's enduring personality. Characteristic adaptations are likely to change more readily and rapidly than personality traits (Henry & Mõttus, 2020), but many are strikingly persistent and make up much of a person's personality.

If psychopathology is an inability to pursue one's goals and to develop new characteristic adaptations that would permit a return to effective goal pursuit, then the failure of characteristic adaptations is the essence of psychopathology. Hence, a personality that is not sufficiently adapted to one's current situation is fundamental to all psychopathology. The complement to this conclusion is that if one's characteristic adaptations are generally working effectively in pursuit of one's goals, and one can develop new ones when they fail, then one is not mentally ill, no matter how peculiar or "symptomatic" one is. Having extreme traits, even those typically considered to be symptoms of psychopathology, is not sufficient to identify mental disorder (as even the DSM grudgingly acknowledges in most cases) because someone may have compensated for those extreme traits with characteristic adaptations that allow them to circumvent or capitalize on their unusual traits. The person who hears voices, for example, may be successfully self-employed as a novelist or a psychic (Powers et al., 2017). (Hearing voices is an interesting example of a trait because it may be tempting to think that it is not present to any degree in many healthy brains – yet consider dreaming or the ability to imagine a conversation with another person. Clearly, the underlying mechanism is an evolved human standard.)

Only one form of mental illness remains a potential challenge for the perspective we've presented here, and that is an episode of mental illness with symptoms strikingly different from the person's normal personality trait profile. For someone who is generally depressive but functional, to slide occasionally into a dysfunctional depressive episode is unsurprising, requiring only a small fluctuation. But what about someone with a generally sunny disposition who goes through a single episode of serious clinical depression, lasting maybe a few months or a year, and then recovers back to their usual happy self? In what way can a temporary episode of psychopathology, in which the person's symptoms are dramatically out of keeping with their usual personality traits, be considered a breakdown of personality? The simple answer is that, although there may have been no personality trait contributing causally as a risk factor in this case, characteristic adaptations were nonetheless involved. For whatever reason, the person's existing goals, interpretations, and strategies were not sufficient to keep them functioning effectively during a period of low mood, and they were not able to develop new adaptations that would allow them to get back on track – hence the need for clinical help. Certainly, such a person might struggle through a depressive episode on their own without ever receiving help, but that would not mean they had avoided an episode of psychopathology (which is not summoned into existence by a formal diagnosis). We would do well, as a society, to move away from seeing mental illness as an essential part of a person's being and to seeing it as something that many people will encounter and recover from during their lives, just like physical illness. Personality can break down, but it can also be repaired.

10.7 Conclusion

All mental disorders involve a breakdown in the functioning of personality, not because they necessarily entail extreme personality traits but rather because they involve the failure of our characteristic adaptations to allow us to pursue our important goals effectively. Thus, in an important sense, all disorders are personality disorders, and the term is useless for discriminating among different forms of disorder. Let us reiterate that the developmental course of psychopathology cannot single out some disorders as "personality disorders." Whether effective characteristic adaptations are never developed in some domain of life, or whether they are developed but then fail to be updated adequately at later stages of development or in novel circumstances, the involvement of personality is clear. Even short-term episodes of mental illness involve a breakdown in personality functioning, as previously effective characteristic adaptations no longer allow people to get what they want and need.

What should people do with our argument in this chapter? Although we think mental health professionals and lay people alike would benefit from adopting our cybernetic perspective on mental illness, we recognize that this is a tall order. A more likely development in the relatively near future is the abandonment of the categorical diagnostic systems of the DSM and ICD, replacing them with a dimensional nosology like HiTOP. If all mental health problems were characterized not by assigning a categorical diagnosis but by evaluating people's standing on the full range of symptom dimensions, then there would be no cause to worry about which problems were disorders of "personality." Where prominent features of disorder involved detachment, antagonism, distrust, lack of empathy, or inability to reason about others' mental states, then one might refer to "interpersonal disorders" (Wright & Ringwald, 2022), but only with the recognition that this is not simply a relabeling of the traditional "personality disorders," which do not exist as natural kinds, nor of the new "personality disorder" of ICD-11 or the AMPD, which does not capture the full range of dysfunction centered around interpersonal issues. In short, even if people struggle with the idea that all mental disorders are personality disorders because they involve failure of characteristic adaptations, we hope they will pay more attention to the fact that mental disorders in general can be described using dimensions of psychological variation that constitute personality traits.

References

American Psychiatric Association. (2013). *Diagnostic and statistical manual of mental disorders* (5th ed.). American Psychiatric Association.

Bleidorn, W., Schwaba, T., Zheng, A., Hopwood, C. J., Sosa, S. S., Roberts, B. W., & Briley, D. A. (2022). Personality stability and change: A meta-analysis of longitudinal studies. *Psychological Bulletin*, *148*(7–8), 588–619.

Bolton, D. (2008). *What is mental disorder? An essay in philosophy, science, and values*. Oxford University Press.

Boorse, C. (1977). Health as a theoretical concept. *Philosophy of Science*, *44*(4), 542–573.

Campbell, L. A., Brown, T. A., & Grisham, J. R. (2003). The relevance of age of onset to the psychopathology of generalized anxiety disorder. *Behavior Therapy*, *34*(1), 31–48.

Clark, L. A., & Ro, E. (2014). Three-pronged assessment and diagnosis of personality disorder and its consequences: Personality functioning, pathological traits, and psychosocial disability. *Personality Disorders: Theory, Research, and Treatment*, *5*(1), 55–69.

DeYoung, C. G. (2015). Cybernetic Big Five Theory. *Journal of Research in Personality*, *56*, 33–58.

DeYoung, C. G. (2017). A cybernetic perspective on integrating personality structure, personality process, and personality development. *European Journal of Personality*, *31*, 538–539.

DeYoung, C. G., Chmielewski, M., Clark, L. A., Condon, D. M., Kotov, R., . . . & the HiTOP Normal Personality Workgroup. (2022). The distinction between symptoms and traits in the Hierarchical Taxonomy of Psychopathology (HiTOP). *Journal of Personality*, *90*, 20–33.

DeYoung, C. G., & Krueger, R. F. (2018a). A cybernetic theory of psychopathology. *Psychological Inquiry*, *29*, 117–138.

DeYoung, C. G., & Krueger, R. F. (2018b). Understanding psychopathology: Cybernetics and psychology on the boundary between order and chaos. *Psychological Inquiry*, *29*, 165–174.

DeYoung, C. G., & Krueger, R. F. (2023). A cybernetic perspective on the nature of psychopathology: Transcending conceptions of mental illness as statistical deviance and brain disease. *Journal of Psychopathology and Clinical Science*, *132* (3), 228–237.

Elliot, A. J., & Fryer, J. W. (2008). The goal construct in psychology. In J. Y. Shah & W. L. Gardner (eds.), *Handbook of motivation science* (pp. 235–250). Guilford.

Forbes, M. K., Ringwald, W. R., Allen, T. A., Cicero, D. C., Clark, L. A., DeYoung, C. G., . . . Wright, A. G. (2024a). Principles and procedures for revising the Hierarchical Taxonomy of Psychopathology. *Journal of Psychopathology and Clinical Science*, *133*(1), 4–19.

Forbes, M. K., Baillie, A. J., Batterham, P., Calear, A., Kotov, R., Krueger, R., . . . Clark, L. (2024b). Reconstructing psychopathology: A data-driven reorganization of the symptoms in DSM-5. *Clinical Psychological Science*. https://doi.org/10.31234/osf.io/7um9a

Griffith, J. W., Zinbarg, R. E., Craske, M. G., Mineka, S., Rose, R. D., Waters, A. M., & Sutton, J. M. (2010). Neuroticism as a common dimension in the internalizing disorders. *Psychological Medicine*, 40, 1125–1136.

Haslam, N., McGrath, M. J., Viechtbauer, W., & Kuppens, P. (2020). Dimensions over categories: A meta-analysis of taxometric research. *Psychological Medicine*, *50*(9), 1418–1432.

Henry, S., & Mõttus, R. (2020). Traits and adaptations: A theoretical examination and new empirical evidence. *European Journal of Personality*, *34*(3), 265–284.

Insel, T., Cuthbert, B., Garvey, M., Heinssen, R., Pine, D. S., Quinn, K., Sanislow, C., & Wang, P. (2010). Research domain criteria (RDoC): Toward a new classification framework for research on mental disorders. *American Journal of Psychiatry*, *167* (7), 748–751.

Kendell, R. E. (1975). The concept of disease and its implications for psychiatry. *The British Journal of Psychiatry*, *127*(4), 305–315.

Kessler, R. C., McGonagle, K. A., Zhao, S., Nelson, C. B., Hughes, M., Eshleman, S., Wittchen, H. U., & Kendler, K. S. (1994). Lifetime and 12-month prevalence of DSM-III-R psychiatric disorders in the United States: Results from the National Comorbidity Survey. *Archives of General Psychiatry*, *51*, 8–19.

Kotov, R., Krueger, R. F., Watson, D., Achenbach, T. M., Althoff, R. R., … Zimmerman, M. (2017). The Hierarchical Taxonomy of Psychopathology (HiTOP): A dimensional alternative to traditional nosologies. *Journal of Abnormal Psychology*, *126*(4), 454–478.

Kotov, R., Krueger, R. F., Watson, D., Cicero, D. C., Conway, C. C., DeYoung, C. G., … & Wright, A. G. (2021). The Hierarchical Taxonomy of Psychopathology (HiTOP): A quantitative nosology based on consensus of evidence. *Annual Review of Clinical Psychology*, *17*, 83–108.

Krueger, R. F. (2005). Continuity of Axes I and II: Toward a unified model of personality, personality disorders, and clinical disorders. *Journal of Personality Disorders*, *19* (3), 233–261.

Krueger, R. F., Derringer, J., Markon, K. E., Watson, D., & Skodol, A. E. (2012). Initial construction of a maladaptive personality trait model and inventory for DSM-5. *Psychological Medicine*, *42*, 1879–1890.

Linscott, R. J., & van Os, J. (2013). An updated and conservative systematic review and meta-analysis of epidemiological evidence on psychotic experiences in children and adults: On the pathway from proneness to persistence to dimensional expression across mental disorders. *Psychological Medicine*, *43*(6), 1133–1149.

Powers, A. R., Kelley, M. S., & Corlett, P. R. (2017). Varieties of voice-hearing: Psychics and the psychosis continuum. *Schizophrenia Bulletin*, *43* 84–98.

Powers, W. T. (1973). *Behaviour: The control of perception*. Aldine.

Ringwald, W. R., Forbes, M. K., & Wright, A. G. (2023). Meta-analysis of structural evidence for the Hierarchical Taxonomy of Psychopathology (HiTOP) model. *Psychological Medicine*, *53*(2), 533–546.

Sharp, C., Wright, A. G., Fowler, J. C., Frueh, B. C., Allen, J. G., Oldham, J., & Clark, L. A. (2015). The structure of personality pathology: Both general ('g') and specific ('s') factors? *Journal of Abnormal Psychology*, *124*(2), 387–398.

Shea, M. T., Stout, R. L., Yen, S., Pagano, M. E., Skodol, A. E., Morey, L. C., . . . & Zanarini, M. C. (2004). Associations in the course of personality disorders and Axis I disorders over time. *Journal of Abnormal Psychology, 113*(4), 499–508.

Shea, M. T., & Yen, S. (2003). Stability as a distinction between Axis I and Axis II disorders. *Journal of Personality Disorders*, 17, 373–386.

Stepp, S. D., Yu, L., Miller, J. D., Hallquist, M. N., Trull, T. J., & Pilkonis, P. A. (2012). Integrating competing dimensional models of personality. *Personality Disorders: Theory, Research, and Treatment*, *3*, 107–126.

Suzuki, T., Samuel, D. B., Pahlen, S., & Krueger, R. F. (2015). DSM-5 Alternative Personality Disorder Model traits as maladaptive extreme variants of the Five-Factor Model: An item–response theory analysis. *Journal of Abnormal Psychology, 124*, 343–354.

Wakefield, J. C. (1992). Disorder as harmful dysfunction: A conceptual critique of *DSM-III-R*'s definition of mental disorder. *Psychological Review, 99*, 232–247.

Widiger, T. A., Bach, B., Chmielewski, M., Clark, L. A., DeYoung, C. G., Hopwood, C. J., . . . & Thomas, K. M. (2019a). Criterion A of the AMPD in HiTOP. *Journal of Personality Assessment*, *101*(4), 345–355.

Widiger, T. A., Sellbom, M., Chmielewski, M., Clark, L. A., DeYoung, C. G., Kotov, R., . . . & Wright, A. G. C. (2019b). Personality in a hierarchical model of psychopathology. *Clinical Psychological Science*, *7*, 77–92.

Wiener, N. (1961). *Cybernetics – Or control and communication in the animal and the machine* (2nd ed.). MIT Press/Wiley.

World Health Organization (2018). *International classification of diseases for mortality and morbidity statistics* (11th revision).

Wouters, A. G. (2003). Four notions of biological function. *Studies in History and Philosophy of Science Part C: Studies in History and Philosophy of Biological and Biomedical Sciences*, *34*, 633–668.

Wright, A. G. C., & Ringwald, W. R. (2022). Personality disorders are dead; long live the interpersonal disorders: Comment on Widiger and Hines (2022). *Personality Disorders: Theory, Research, and Treatment*, *13*(4), 364–368.

Zimmermann, J., Böhnke, J. R., Eschstruth, A., Mathews, A., Wenzel, K., & Leising, D. (2015). The latent structure of personality functioning: Investigating Criterion A from the alternative model for personality disorders in DSM-5. *Journal of Abnormal Psychology*, *124*, 532–548.

11 Self-Illness Ambiguity in Personality Disorders

Is It Me or My Disorder (that Makes Me Do X)?

Roy Dings, Nina S. de Boer, Léon de Bruin, and Gerrit Glas

This chapter provides an explorative analysis of self-illness ambiguity in personality disorders. Self-illness ambiguity is a particular form of *self-ambiguity*. Self-ambiguity occurs when someone is unclear about whether a particular thought, feeling, or behavior is really *theirs* (Dings, 2020). Such cases cover trivial as well as more existential domains of our lives. For instance, did I really think my partner did something wrong when I scolded her, or did I have a short fuse because I was hungry? Do I really want to move to another city, or am I just trying to please my partner? Am I smiling because I am happy, or because I have to smile all day in my job as a waitress (cf. Hochschild, 2012)?

In Section 11.1, we introduce and explain the concept of self-illness ambiguity, and summarize recent research on this topic. In Section 11.2, we draw on research on lived experience to show that self-illness ambiguity does seem common in the context of personality disorders, and suggest that this may be(partially) due to how personality disorders are conceptualized in the *Diagnostic and statistical manual of mental disorders* (DSM). In Section 11.3, we elaborate on this suggestion by turning to the recent development of interpreting personality disorders in terms of maladaptive traits. We demonstrate how trait maladaptivity in personality disorders is both similar and dissimilar to other cases of trait maladaptivity. On the view we propose, personality disorders involve strongly maladaptive traits, and the differences between weak, moderate, and strong cases of maladaptivity help to clarify how personality disorder diagnoses may give rise to a unique form of self-illness ambiguity. Section 11.4 zooms in on this particular form of self-ambiguity that can arise in the context of personality disorders, namely self–self-ambiguity. In Section 11.5, we supplement this analysis by examining various forms of implicit self-relating and their connection to common clinical concepts (e.g., self-regulation) and interventions.

11.1 Self(-Illness) Ambiguity

Self-illness ambiguity is a relatively novel concept, yet it describes a phenomenon that is quite common in psychiatric contexts. Its origins can be traced back to sociologist David Karp's (1992) work on "illness ambiguity." Psychiatrist and philosopher John Sadler (2007) offered the first philosophical analysis of self-illness ambiguity. Although self-ambiguity is ubiquitous, it manifests itself in a peculiar way in psychiatric contexts. For example, if a person diagnosed with depression finds themselves not wanting to go to a party to which they were invited, they might start questioning this lack of desire: "Is it really that *I* do not want to go, or is this the depression acting up, making me feel like I do not want to go?" They might also recall that their therapist warned them of becoming too avoidant. "Is this one of those cases where I am being avoidant of social interaction?" They might also be uncertain about the impact of their antidepressant medication on their actions, thoughts, and feelings. In the words of David Karp (2006): "Is it me or my meds?" In these contexts, we can speak of self-*illness* ambiguity: the difficulty in distinguishing one's self, or "who one is," from a mental disorder or diagnosis (Dings, 2020). In other words, "Is it me or my disorder (that makes me do *x*)?"

Building on the work by Karp and Sadler, recent years have witnessed several studies exploring the dynamics and phenomenology of self-illness ambiguity (e.g., Bortolan, 2022; Jeppsson, 2022); its implications for self-understanding and recovery (Dings & Glas, 2020; Drożdżowicz, 2023); its ethical implications (e.g., Dings & de Haan, 2022); and its clinical implications (e.g., Glas, 2023). In addition, there have been specific investigations into self-illness ambiguity for addiction (McConnell & Golova, 2023), anorexia nervosa (Drożdżowicz, 2023), and bipolar disorder (Carls-Diamante, 2023). It goes beyond the scope of this chapter to provide a complete account of the research into self-illness ambiguity (but see Dings & de Bruin, 2023, for an overview). Instead, this section presents some initial distinctions that can be used to explicate and clarify the concept (cf. Dings, 2020; Dings & Glas, 2020; Glas, 2023).

The first distinction relevant to understanding self-illness ambiguity is between *identity*- and *agency*-related concerns. Identity-related concerns occur when someone has to make sense of the relation between themselves (their identity) and the disorder. For instance, someone may wonder: "How do I relate to my depression diagnosis? Is the depression best conceptualized as a part of who I am, or as something external? Does my diagnosis make me a different person?" Agency-related concerns, in contrast, occur when someone has to make sense of an action, feeling, or thought in relation to themselves and the disorder: "Does this particular action or thought belong to myself or the depression?"[1]

A second distinction relates to dealing with self-illness ambiguity from a *first-person* or a *third-person* perspective. When you receive a diagnosis, you may experience agency- or identity-related concerns yourself, but your partner, friends, or colleagues might also wonder whether, say, a particular choice or statement should be seen as belonging to your "self" or rather, to the illness that you were diagnosed with (cf. Bröer & Besseling, 2017).

A third distinction pertains to the "levels" at which self-illness ambiguity may occur. On a *conceptual level*, one may reflectively wonder about both identity- and agency-related concerns. That is, one may consciously ask oneself "How do I relate to my depression?" or discuss this matter with other people. On a *phenomenological level*, self-illness ambiguity occurs pre-reflectively. For instance, one may have a (bodily) sense that "this is not me" or "this does not feel like mine." To be clear: although most of our everyday agential experiences involve actions, feelings, or thoughts which are experienced as "internal" (i.e., as originating in oneself) or "external" (i.e., as being an outside force), there may be cases where it is unclear, experientially, whether an action feeling or thought has an origin within or outside of oneself.[2] Those are cases of agential self-ambiguity on a phenomenological level. Once one starts reflecting on those experiences, the phenomenon shifts to the conceptual level. Finally, if one starts to think about what such ambiguous actions or feelings mean for your identity, then we are moving from agency-related to identity-related concerns.

In short, self-illness ambiguity can be identity- or agency-related; can be a first- or a third-person experience, and may occur on a conceptual as well as a phenomenological level. With these basic distinctions in place, we will now explore how self-illness ambiguity may manifest itself in personality disorders.

11.2 Self-Illness Ambiguity in Personality Disorders

At first glance, self-illness ambiguity is relevant for understanding the self-experience of people who receive personality disorder diagnoses because such diagnoses seem to directly concern a person's self.[3] Indeed, people struggling

[1] Of course, identity- and agency-related concerns are often intertwined. For instance, if you consider a lot of your actions or thoughts to be due to your disorder (=agency), this will likely impact how you think about the relation between your self and your disorder (=identity).

[2] This also means that self-ambiguity is not the same as *ambivalence*, where one is "divided" in the sense that one has two incompatible but *internal* motivations (cf. Dings & de Haan, 2022).

[3] For present purposes, we use "self" and "person" interchangeably, referring to the complex and multidimensional individual who receives a personality disorder diagnosis (for a more fine-grained analysis, see Glas, 2006).

with a personality disorder explicitly state that they often do not trust their own experiences, lack a clear sense of self, and have many ambiguous and conflicting thoughts, feelings, and actions (Gillard et al., 2015). We see identity-related concerns reflected in first-person testimonials of people who have received a personality disorder diagnosis. For instance, in a first-person testimonial of someone with a borderline personality disorder diagnosis, Gary H. (2018) writes: "[T]his is the story of a non-person, of a walking diagnosis, of a set of 'symptoms'" (p. 70). Later in the paragraph, however, Gary H. describes himself as "[s]omeone who knows deep down that I am a person, that I am a human being. (. . .) A person who is figuring out who this someone actually is. I am ME" (p. 70). Furthermore, in a recent study by Lamph et al. (2022) on the impact of a personality disorder diagnosis on people's sense of identity, participants stated that "[the label] implies there is something wrong with the very core of who I am" (p. 40), but also that "I'm not just [a personality disorder] – there's more to me" (p. 38).

Receiving a personality disorder diagnosis may also give rise to agency-related concerns of self-illness ambiguity, because the diagnosis can force a person to re-evaluate the relation between themselves and their traits and dispositions. Marcia (2006) illustrates this process of re-evaluation: "The histrionic person may insist that their emotional storms are simply 'being honest.' The obsessive-compulsive individual can prize 'being cautious, thoughtful, and consistent.' The schizoid personality can take refuge in valuing 'solitude, creativity, and introspectiveness'" (pp. 587–588). Importantly, self (-illness) ambiguity occurs when a person is uncertain about how to evaluate this relation between self and traits. Self-illness ambiguity as a concept acknowledges the insufficiency of *dichotomous* views on the self-illness relation. It goes against the idea that a (personality) disorder is *either* ego-syntonic (i.e., in line with one's self-concept) *or* ego-dystonic (i.e., not in line with one's self-concept); *either* alienating *or* not; or that an action, feeling, motivation, or disposition is felt as *either* internal *or* external (cf. Dings, 2020). The point of self-illness ambiguity is that the relation (between self and illness in the case of identity-related concerns, or between self, illness, and the action in the case of agency-related concerns) may be unclear, both conceptually and phenomenologically. As such, self(-illness) ambiguity should be seen as a supplement (rather than a replacement) of existing views on such relations, allowing for more valid and fine-grained analyses of human (self-)understanding an (self-) experience.

In light of self-illness ambiguity in personality disorders, it is worthwhile to note that the DSM, from its third edition onward, holds that "[a] common misconception is that a classification of mental disorders classifies individuals, when actually what are being classified are disorders that individuals have" (American Psychiatric Association, 1980, p. 6). Diagnoses are not meant to classify people, but to classify *disorders*. This also goes for personality disorder diagnoses: according to the DSM, personality disorders are conditions that people have, not something with which they should be identified. In other words, the DSM relies on a somewhat confusing *conceptual* distinction between the person and their (psychopathological) personality.[4] Needless to say, this distinction is difficult to maintain: the descriptions of personality disorder criteria are about tendencies, feelings, and behaviors that most people would consider as belonging to who one is as a person. For instance, borderline personality disorder supposedly involves an "unstable self-image" (American Psychiatric Association, 2013, p. 766) and "[i]nstability in goals, aspirations, values, or career plans" (American Psychiatric Association, 2013, p. 766). Relatedly, obsessive-compulsive personality disorder is thought to involve a "[s]ense of self derived predominantly from work or productivity" (American Psychiatric Association, 2013, p. 768), "constricted experience and expression of strong emotions" (American Psychiatric Association, 2013, p. 768), and "rigid and unreasonably high and inflexible internal standards of behavior" (American Psychiatric Association, 2013, p. 768). All these criteria are easily interpreted as pertaining to a person.

In sum, personality disorder diagnoses may invoke self-illness ambiguity, but the experience may differ from that related to other mental disorder diagnoses. That is, because personality disorder characteristics seem more closely related to one's self than to an acquired disorder, it is difficult to separate the two. Indeed, this is what makes diagnosing personality disorders so complicated: their characteristics are so closely related to someone's (sense of) self that receiving a personality disorder diagnosis could easily be interpreted as labeling a person's self as pathological. In the next section, we will explore the specifics of self-illness ambiguity in personality disorders in more detail by focusing on trait maladaptivity.

11.3 Personality Disorder, Trait Maladaptivity, and Self-Illness Ambiguity

There have been various recent proposals for dimensional models of personality disorders, such as the alternative model of personality disorder (AMPD) in chapter III of DSM-5 (for an overview, see Krueger & Hobbs, 2020) and the hierarchical taxonomy of psychopathology (HiTOP; Kotov et al., 2017). What these models converge on is that they conceptualize personality

[4] It is worth flagging that in the DSM-5 this conceptual distinction seems to break down to a large extent, as the alternative model of personality disorder holds that "[d]isturbances in self and interpersonal functioning constitute the core of personality psychopathology" (American Psychiatric Association, 2013, p. 762).

disorders in terms of maladaptive personality traits. For instance, the AMPD holds that personality disorders should be diagnosed based on the presence of "[m]oderate or greater impairment in personality (self/interpersonal) functioning" (American Psychiatric Association. 2013, p. 761) (Criterion A) and "[o]ne or more pathological personality *traits*" (American Psychiatric Association. 2013, p. 761, emphasis added)[5] (Criterion B), including negative affectivity, detachment, antagonism, disinhibition, and psychoticism. Importantly, the AMPD states that the difference between maladaptive and adaptive traits is *gradual*: "personality disorders represent maladaptive variants of personality traits that merge imperceptibly into normality and into one another" (American Psychiatric Association, 2013, p. 646). So, personality disorders are conceptualized based on the presence of personality traits that fall on a spectrum from normal to abnormal, with personality disorders falling on the strongly abnormal-maladaptive end of the spectrum.

This shift toward dimensionality and the emphasis on (maladaptivity of) traits have received ample attention (see e.g., Clark & Watson, 2022, for a recent discussion). In this chapter, we will focus on what it implies for self-illness ambiguity in personality disorders. For this purpose, we should first zoom in on what it means for traits to be (mal)adaptive, and how to make statements about the relative maladaptivity of traits. Adaptivity presupposes a relation between an agent (or an agent's traits more specifically) and their social, cultural, and material context. A trait is considered adaptive if it "fits," that is, if it meets social and cultural expectations or norms and does not hinder a person's agency. However, traits may also be "maladaptive" when they fit poorly with sociocultural expectations or norms and hinder a person's agency.

The (mal)adaptivity of traits has been extensively debated (see e.g., DeYoung, 2010, 2015), but for present purposes, we will highlight three aspects of traits that we can use to compare their relative maladaptiveness. First, trait maladaptivity has a *temporal* aspect: a trait can be maladaptive only incidentally, for instance when it is maladaptive in a specific context in which an agent seldomly finds themselves. Conversely, traits may be maladaptive in a more chronic sense, for instance when the trait is incompatible with a very common social norm. Let us take an introverted academic as an example (introversion will be discussed in more detail later in the section). If this person spends most of their time working behind their desk and interacting with other introverted people, their introversion may be only incidentally maladaptive (when they have to present at conferences, for instance). However, if they

[5] We are aware that these criteria are contested, because they do not make space for the potential of flourishing while having a personality disorder diagnosis (see Chapman & Carel, 2022, who explore a similar claim for autism).

decide to switch careers and go into marketing, then their introversion may be more chronically maladaptive, given that socializing is a strong social norm in this work context.

A second aspect of maladaptivity is the *severity of the consequences* of not engaging in trait management. The – often social – consequences of (not) managing traits depend on both the traits in question and on the sociocultural context, as two traits (or the same trait in different cultures) may be maladaptive in different ways. Some traits, such as introversion, may be merely frowned upon (i.e., weakly maladaptive), whereas others, such as paranoid ideation, may have more severe social consequences (i.e., strongly maladaptive). A third aspect is a person's *attitude* toward their maladaptive trait. This attitude includes a metacognitive, affective, and a behavioral element. For instance, one's attitude can be more positive or more negative. One can feel comfortable or dissatisfied with a trait, and one can identify with a trait or distance oneself from it. As we will see, one's attitude towards a maladaptive trait (and in particular whether and to what extent one identifies with it) plays an important role in the dynamics of self(-illness) ambiguity.

These three aspects of trait maladaptivity can help distinguish among traits that are weakly, moderately, and strongly maladaptive. Below we will elaborate on each, show their similarities and differences, and discuss their relation to self-(illness) ambiguity. On the proposed view, personality disorders involve strongly maladaptive traits, and the differences between weak, moderate, and strong cases of maladaptivity help to clarify how personality disorder diagnoses may give rise to a unique form of self-illness ambiguity (which we will elaborate on in Section 11.4). Thus, we aim to show how traits in personality disorders are both similar to non-pathological traits (in line with the dimensional approach) and dissimilar.

11.3.1 Weak Trait Maladaptivity: Introversion Versus Extraversion

Weakly maladaptive traits constitute the non-pathological end of the spectrum of maladaptiveness. We know from research in social psychology that many people engage in impression management and often display behavior that in some sense is "not really them" (Goffman, 1959). One common form of impression management in Western society is that introverted people sometimes feel the need to act in a more extraverted way (Fleeson & Wilt, 2010). That is, Western society favors extraverted behavior, meaning that being an introvert is taken to be undesirable or maladaptive (and is often experienced as such, cf. Cain, 2012). We can explain why introverted behavior is *weakly* maladaptive by looking at the three aspects discussed above. First, regarding temporality, most introverts only incidentally suppress their traits or alter their behavior, for instance when they have to operate in new social situations.

Second, regarding the severity of the consequences, the consequences of not suppressing introverted behavior are not that severe. They may affect one's social life but do not typically have harmful consequences for an individual or their surroundings. Finally, the attitude that people have towards these acts of temporarily "acting differently" is fairly carefree and unconcerned: they know or feel that they "are" introverted and that they are only acting differently (i.e., inhibiting their introverted tendencies) for the sake of a particular social circumstance (e.g., they think that doing so will make it easier for them to get a promotion at work). Thus, engaging in impression management is transparent and unambiguous: an introverted person is typically aware of acting more extraverted for the sake of some social goal.

How is weak trait adaptivity related to self-ambiguity? Even in the case of the introvert, there may be situations where self-ambiguity arises. For instance, when introverted people act in a more extraverted manner, they sometimes report feeling more authentic (compared to acting introverted, which would be seemingly more in line with their actual traits, cf. Fleeson & Wilt, 2010). We can easily imagine that this leads to tensions or ambiguity in one's self-understanding: "Am I a person who is more introverted or extraverted?" Self-ambiguity also may arise when it is unclear whether a particular state one is in is due to one's traits or due to situational influences. Following Nisbett and Wilson's (1977) famous study on the unconscious alteration of judgment, it is generally agreed upon that for most people, most of the time, who they are and what they do is the result of some interplay between situational factors and their personality. We can again easily imagine that people may be uncertain whether it is them who decides to act more extrovertedly, or whether it has a social determinant such as peer pressure (Dings & de Bruin, 2022). So, even in cases of weak trait maladaptivity, self-ambiguity may arise.

11.3.2 Moderate Trait Maladaptivity: Camouflaging

Moving up the spectrum of trait maladaptivity, we use an example of a phenomenon highlighted by the neurodiversity movement: autistic camouflaging (or camouflaging, for short).[6] Camouflaging refers to a set of strategies that people with autism report engaging in for the sake of fitting in and meeting social expectations (Hull et al., 2017). (For a recent overview of camouflaging research see Cook et al., 2021.) Camouflaging entails two types of behavior. First, it concerns *masking*, that is, the inhibition of autistic traits and behaviors. For instance, someone may suppress their urge to engage in self-soothing or

[6] This example differs from the other two in that it is not strictly about personality traits. Indeed, we do not want to suggest that autism is a form of personality disorder. Nevertheless, we think it serves as a good illustration of the broader phenomenon in which people may actively adapt their behavior in light of social norms.

"stimming" behaviors, such as making sounds or shaking one's body. Second, it concerns *compensating*, that is, the display of behavior that autistic individuals would not display were it not for the social norms that prescribe those behaviors, such as making eye contact during conversation. Trait maladaptivity in the case of camouflaging seems more severe than in the previous case. First, in contrast to the introverted person who incidentally acts extraverted, people with autism report feeling the need to camouflage more frequently. They have to suppress the way that they would prefer to act in most social, neurotypical settings. Second, the consequences seem more severe, in the sense that not engaging in camouflaging in neurotypical environments may result in stigmatization or exclusion. This combination of chronicity and severity may help explain the impact of camouflaging on mental health more generally: having to consistently camouflage has various short- and long-term consequences including exhaustion ("autistic burnout"; Cook et al., 2021; Hull et al., 2017). The attitude aspect of maladaptivity is important here as well. Many people with autism value their camouflaging activities negatively: they would rather not perform them. They identify with their "own" traits and behavioral tendencies and report that acts of camouflaging sometimes challenge their self-perception (Bargiela et al., 2016; Hull et al. 2017). In this respect, Hull et al. (2017) stress that camouflaging is extremely effortful for autistic individuals and more challenging to their identity in comparison to the impression management that neurotypical individuals engage in (p. 2520).

How is moderate trait maladaptivity related to self-ambiguity? Although a fully fledged analysis of self-ambiguity in people with autism goes beyond the scope of this chapter, it seems clear that camouflaging (as a more chronic and high-stakes form of impression management) leads to experiences of self-ambiguity. For example, a participant in the study by Hull et al. (2017) remarks: "Sometimes, when I have had to do a lot of camouflaging in a high-stress environment, I feel as though I've lost track of who I really am, and that my actual self is floating somewhere above me like a balloon (Female, 22)" (p. 2529).

11.3.3 Strong Trait Maladaptivity: Personality Disorder

Let us now turn to the maladaptivity of traits in personality disorders, which seems to be situated on the severe end of the spectrum. Regarding temporality, the maladaptive traits in personality disorders do not pertain to incidental cases of maladaptivity, but to traits that are maladaptive all of the time or in a significant amount of (social) contexts. Regarding the severity of consequences, the very idea of a personality *disorder* suggests that maladaptivity pertains to a trait being *pathological*. That is, the trait is not just being frowned upon, or hindering social advancements, but directly contributes to "dysfunctional" behavior and makes it difficult for the individual to participate in society and adhere to societal norms. The consequences are thus severe. Finally, what is typical (and distinct) for trait maladaptivity in personality disorders is the *attitude* of the person who receives the personality disorder diagnosis toward their presumedly maladaptive trait. In the "everyday case" of the introvert who acts in an extraverted manner, but also in the case of autistic camouflaging, people still *identify with* their maladaptive trait. Camouflaging behavior, for instance, is deemed an unfortunate yet necessary requirement to fit in with society, but there is typically no identification with this camouflaging behavior itself.[7] In contrast, a person diagnosed with a personality disorder may sometimes *reject* their personality traits. Examples include impulsivity, inability to tolerate feelings of being alone and/or extreme dependence on significant others. Persons with these traits may try to find ways to manage or cope with them and even try to not (or no longer) identify with them.

Where introverts and autistic people typically identify with "what comes naturally to them" (and only rely on, e.g., impression management for social reasons), people with a personality disorder diagnosis may distance themselves from "what comes naturally," given that "what comes naturally" to them is considered pathological or has proven to be maladaptive. Instead, they may identify with the metacognitive, affective, and behavioral coping mechanisms that they rely on to thwart that which comes natural to them (Lester et al., 2020).[8]

To illustrate, a participant with a personality disorder diagnosis in the study by Gillard et al. (2015) remarks that, as a coping mechanism, "[I have to] talk to myself and say 'this is part of your illness, it'll pass in a minute,' what thoughts are there that shouldn't be there or that aren't doing me any good so I have to, like, sit down, identify it, face it and then take steps to counteract it" (p. 9). This is a difficult and exhausting process, as another participant adds that "[s]ome of these feelings are . . . so deeply ingrained in me that however much I try (. . .) I'm not sure that I can turn everything round because your history's your history, however much you try" (Gillard et al., 2015). In a similar vein, Ng et al. (2019) note that a crucial element in recovering from borderline personality disorder is to "not be blindsided" by emotions (p. 5), to gain the skill of recognizing and "tolerating" one's "negative affectivity." Finally, a participant in the study by Castillo et al. (2013) remarked that, in the process of recovering from a personality disorder, she stopped disliking *herself* and instead disliked

[7] Although this might happen in some cases of self-ambiguity, as we have discussed above (see also Dings & de Bruin, 2022).

[8] In fact, this is in line with what occurs in dialectical behavior therapy, one of the most well-known forms of psychotherapy for borderline personality disorder: this therapy begins with attempts to let patients de-identify with their most disturbing personality traits.

her *behavior* (p. 271). These quotes illustrate that people with a personality disorder diagnosis may come to actively reject certain maladaptive traits.

To be clear, we do not wish to claim that such a rejection occurs in all individuals with a personality disorder diagnosis. Those that *do* reject certain traits may be motivated by self-recrimination. Yet, some people diagnosed with a personality disorder may occasionally "use" a trait associated with their diagnosis (Hart et al., 2018). For instance, the (typically maladaptive) trait of antagonism may prove useful in certain contexts, such as when a person intimidates someone else into giving them a special treatment.

This brief analysis of various forms of maladaptivity has shown that, much like non-pathological phenomena such as impression management, people with personality disorder diagnoses may modulate their traits in various ways. Similar to camouflaging in autism, this trait management may be quite chronic and require a lot of time and effort. Yet personality disorders seem distinct in the sense that they, or at least some of them and for some individuals, involve a distancing or disidentification with the maladaptive trait.[9] In the next section, we discuss the ramifications this distancing and/or disidentification has for self-understanding, and suggest that it may lead to a particular form of self-illness ambiguity, namely, *self–self-ambiguity.*

Before doing so, three further remarks are in place. First, we do not know the *prevalence* of self–self-ambiguity in personality disorders, for it has not been explicitly (and empirically) investigated. Nonetheless, our examples will show that it at least occurs for some individuals with some personality disorder diagnoses. Second, research has shown that establishing a more coherent and healthy sense of self is an important factor in the recovery of people with a personality disorder diagnosis (e.g., Katsakou et al., 2012; Lester et al., 2020; Shepherd et al., 2016).[10] This process typically involves accepting a diagnosis, coming to terms with it, and incorporating it into one's self-narrative or identity. Self–self-ambiguity is "located" within that process: it highlights the ambiguity at stake in the process of accepting a diagnosis, coming to terms with maladaptive traits, and establishing a sense of self. Third, we wish to reiterate a point made in Section 11.2, namely that the concept of self–self-ambiguity is meant to capture something that is left out by dichotomous approaches. In fact, the (albeit scarce) literature on whether personality disorders are ego-syntonic or ego-dystonic seems to illustrate precisely the need for such a concept, as this literature shows that there is evidence

[9] Antisocial and narcissistic personality disorders are candidate cases in which such distancing or disidentification with people's maladaptive traits might be lacking. In addition, we may think of schizotypical, schizoid, and paranoid personality disorders.

[10] A relevant point here concerns the attitude many people with personality disorder diagnoses have toward recovery. For many other mental health conditions, a key goal in recovery is to regain a balanced sense of self. Yet, people with personality disorder diagnoses often note that they never had a balanced sense of self in the first place, so there is no self to "regain." They cannot *recover* a sense of self but have to *discover* it (e.g., Gillard et al., 2015).

for *both* ego-syntonic elements *and* ego-dystonic elements of personality disorder traits (see e.g., Hart et al., 2018; Sleep et al., 2019). For instance, traits typically associated with personality disorders were reported to both have functional benefits but were also more likely to evoke self-recrimination.

11.4 Self-Illness Ambiguity in Personality Disorder: "Self–Self-Ambiguity"

The unique form of self-illness ambiguity that arises in the context of personality disorder diagnoses could be called "self–self-ambiguity." To understand why this somewhat paradoxical term nevertheless aptly describes the phenomenon in question, we have to zoom in on the various strategies that people may engage in to compensate for the maladaptive nature of a trait. Impression management, as we saw, is fairly common and entails an incidental inhibition of a certain tendency or the presentation of a tendency that does not come naturally. Camouflaging entails a more elaborate set of strategies that similarly serve to suppress or enhance certain traits. In both cases, however, it seems apparent to the person engaging in these strategies that their sense of self and their performed behavior are clearly separable. They *know* or *feel* that this is compensatory behavior, merely for the sake of adhering to social norms, among others.

In the case of personality disorders, when a person would come to *reject* a trait, a different strategy seems required. The trait can no longer serve as a reference point on which to build a *coping strategy*, nor can one only temporarily suppress it. Instead, someone with a personality disorder diagnosis who rejects their maladaptive trait may feel the need to establish a "new way of being," that is, to become a person who has, or at least acts in accordance with, non-pathological (adaptive) traits. That is, their "default self," consisting of what comes naturally to them and what has been the basis for their self-understanding up until that point, has to be "managed" because it is apparently pathological (or strongly maladaptive) (Dings & Glas, 2020).

If someone increasingly feels that their default self is flawed in some way, then they might develop a *subsidiary (or "as if") self.*[11] Such a subsidiary self has a strong metacognitive character in that it aims to "monitor" the default self in the hope of detecting its deviant or pathological elements and substituting these with other, non-deviant or non-pathological elements. In substituting these elements, one is essentially *pretending* to *be* different (which is why we may also label the subsidiary self as an "as if" self). Over time, this may

[11] The term "as-if" does not refer here to the so-called as-if personality in the psychoanalytic literature. The psychoanalytic concept refers to a pathological self that masks a deeper, other kind of personality problem (narcissistic, borderline, and/or antisocial). The as-if personality we aim at refers to emerging new habits and core convictions about oneself and the world that are the result of some (therapeutic) process.

inevitably lead to *self–self-ambiguity*, where the person struggles to determine whether a particular action is part of their default or subsidiary self. In other words, one may struggle to disentangle the pretense, subsidiary ("as if") self from one's default self.

This phenomenon is illustrated in Sørensen et al.'s (2019) study on the lived experience of people with an avoidant personality disorder diagnosis. People with avoidant personality disorder struggle with excessive social anxiety and severe feelings of inadequacy and/or inferiority, and adopt avoidance of social situations as a (maladaptive) coping strategy. Thus, according to the AMPD, avoidant personality disorder involves pathological traits like negative affectivity (specifically: anxiousness) and detachment (specifically: withdrawal, anhedonia, or intimacy avoidance) (cf. Skodol et al., 2015). Furthermore, people with this diagnosis are often aware of the discrepancy between themselves as more isolated individuals and others who are inherently social. This may lead to insecurity because "*others* are being themselves" (Sørensen et al., 2019 p. 11, italics added). If persons with an avoidant personality disorder compare themselves to other people and simultaneously tries to suppress their avoidant tendencies in social contexts, this may lead to a "multiplication of selves." That is, a subsidiary self could be created that, in contrast to their default self, is more social and fitting to societal conventions. As a result, in situations where both selves might plausibly be involved, this person may struggle to navigate between and ultimately, also, distinguish their subsidiary from their default self. Sørensen et al. (2019) illustrate this as: "Some participants did express that they had quite clear opinions when they were on their own. However, they reported that they usually kept such opinions to themselves to avoid uncomfortable discussions or having to defend their views. The participants often felt that they lost their sense of knowing their own experiences when anticipating others' judgments" (p. 11). Furthermore,

> Some participants described a sense that their agency had become blurred, as though they had lost touch with their own will after years of adapting to that of others. Some said they sometimes felt they had lost control over their bodies or that they did not know themselves. They expressed feeling confused when thinking about who they are. Some questioned the entire concept of identity, asking whether other people usually had a clear sense of themselves: "I feel like me as a person is not present. I feel like I do not know myself anymore . . . I do not feel like I know who I am. That is kind of what I would like to know" (Amanda). (Sørensen et al., 2019)

In an attempt to disambiguate "who they are," the participants in this study resorted to a meticulous analysis of their own thoughts, feelings, and actions, illustrating the metacognitive character of their subsidiary self. However, this turned out to be a non-viable strategy as "they found no certain answers to confirm or disconfirm their interpretations" (Sørensen et al., 2019). They struggled with the fact that they could not rely on a clear phenomenology of what was "theirs" and what was not. Indeed, Sørensen et al. (2019) note that:

> [A] disturbing sense of emptiness in place of their feelings seemed an unwanted consequence of the participants' intention of avoiding thinking or feeling. In particular, positive feelings, such as enjoyment and love, were described as somehow distant, or even lost, within themselves: "I think that it is real fun or should be, but I do not feel anything" (Eva). Some participants searched within to regain connection with their emotions, questioning whether they felt anything at all. (p. 11)

These examples depict (arguably) pathological traits such as anxiousness, withdrawal, and anhedonia, and illustrate how these may be "managed" by developing a subsidiary self with a strong metacognitive, reflective character. To fully grasp the complexity of self–self-ambiguity in personality disorders, we should also explicate more implicit, non-reflective ways of self-relating. We turn to those in the next section, where we also explore self–self-ambiguity from a clinical perspective, through the lens of self-referentiality and self-regulation.

11.5 Self-Illness Ambiguity in Personality Disorder: Self-Relatedness and Self-Referentiality

In the previous section, we argued that personality disorders may be associated with developing a subsidiary (metacognitive or "as if") self. We suggested that people with a personal disorder diagnosis could be more or less aware of what they want to avoid or correct while developing this subsidiary self. The clinician, however, will also take into account *implicit* forms of self-relating (where ambiguity may arise as well). The current section examines these implicit forms of self-relating using the concept of *self-referentiality*. We will show that there are various layers of self-relating, and that self(–self)-ambiguity may occur within each of these layers.

We have developed the concept of self-referentiality in earlier work and have applied it to self-management (Dings & Glas, 2020; Glas, 2017), self-knowledge in psychotherapy (Strijbos & Glas, 2018), the understanding of psychopathology (Glas, 2019), and self-illness ambiguity in psychiatric illness (Glas, 2023). Self-referentiality builds on the idea that who one is as a person also comes to expression in how one relates to oneself. Selfhood can be defined in terms of identifiable features such as character traits, habits, and core convictions about oneself and others; however, selfhood can also be seen as an expression of how one relates to these traits, habits, and convictions, that is, one's *self-relatedness*. A fictitious person, called Jim, can be described as sincere, but also as somewhat rigid and hot-tempered. Who Jim is does not only become apparent in these character traits but also in how Jim relates to them. Is he aware of his character flaws? Does he thoughtfully deal with them or does he ignore how his rigidity and temper affect his relations with others? In short, identity is not only the sum of one's traits but also a manifestation of how one relates to oneself. Yet, we are often unaware of how we relate to ourselves in our behavior, inclinations, and interactions. This implicit self-relatedness is nonetheless *meaningful*. When the meaning of our self-related behavior, inclinations, and interactions remains implicit or non-conscious to us, we call it "self-referential." In other words, self-referentiality refers to the *implicit (non-conscious) self-signification* in one's behaviors, inclinations, and interactions (for more information about this, see Glas, 2019, 2023). Self-referentiality also applies to personality traits: how people deal with their (maladaptive) personality traits shows who they are or intend to be. We will illustrate the self-referentiality of maladaptive personality traits using avoidant personality disorder as an example (see also Strijbos & Glas, 2018). To do so, we introduce a fictitious person, Anne, who is diagnosed with avoidant personality disorder.

Anne shows signs of insecurity, introversion, and fear in social situations. As a child and adolescent, Anne is unaware of these traits but tends to avoid social situations. This avoidance is self-referential, for it implicitly says something about her fear of being exposed to social situations. In her early twenties, her habit of avoiding becomes a problem. Social expectations have made her aware that she is an avoidant person, and that there is a conflict between what she is expected to do (engage in social situations) and inclines to avoid. Here, we see an example of self-relatedness: Anne is relating to her tendency to avoid and experiences a conflict. Her awareness of this conflict may cause her to see herself as weak and unable to live a normal social life. Anne may leave it at this: she may be aware of the conflict, without showing any attempt to do something about it. This implicit "avoidance" of doing something about her internal conflict is again self-referential: it shows that Anne implicitly adopts an avoidant stance toward her inner conflict. There may, of course, be reasons for this "secondary" avoidance, but in clinical cases, they are often not so clear – at least not for the person themself. For instance, Anne may feel embarrassed about her avoidant tendencies and may withdraw from any engagement with her conflict because it seems unsolvable. This withdrawal may lead to a state of forgetfulness or even plain denial, at least for a while. This state is, again, self-referential: it signifies something about who Anne is.

In her late twenties, Anne's avoidance of dealing with her inner conflict may become explicit, for instance, due to remarks by a loved one or a missed opportunity to make new friends. This may cause Anne to interpret herself in a new way, for instance as a person who is failing because of her enduring tendency to avoid social situations despite the obvious disadvantages. However, after a couple of years of therapy, Anne has learned to cope with certain social situations and to accept some of her shortcomings. By training her social skills and via psychoeducation, Anne has learned to relate differently to her maladaptive traits. Changes in her relations with relatives and friends have helped her to construe and maintain a holding environment that exerts a healthy influence on how she relates to herself. Insight-oriented and experiential forms of psychotherapy have targeted how Anne implicitly relates to her maladaptive traits, leading to a fuller understanding and correction of her self-relating. Finally, acceptance and commitment therapy (ACT) has made her focus on who she has become as a person with a life-long prevalence of certain personality traits.[12] Initially, all of this is part of an explicit process in which Anne learns to relate differently to herself. She learns to overcome some of her avoidant tendencies and to accept some of the remaining social problems she experiences. After a while, her coping may become so habitual that she is no longer aware of it. Anne has become more self-confident and this becomes manifest in situations that she previously tended to avoid. Anne has internalized a new attitude toward some of her maladaptive traits. The glow of self-confidence in her behavior is the self-referential expression that her identity has changed. During the process, Anne has become aware of how she regulates the emotions and behaviors that come along with her personality traits. Such self-regulation encompasses much more than learning to adapt to her problems: it requires adapting to the demands of her context, self-image and desires, and the expectations of herself and others. This awareness and the self-interpretations that follow from her self-regulation add new layers to her already existing self-image, layers that are gradually internalized and become part of a more differentiated and layered self-concept.

11.6 Conclusion

In this chapter, we have argued that receiving a personality disorder diagnosis can lead to self-illness ambiguity. We explored this phenomenon in three ways. First, we examined how the increasingly common construal of personality disorders in terms of maladaptive personality traits shows how personality disorders are both similar as well as different from "non-pathological" cases of trait maladaptivity (e.g., introverts acting more extrovertedly). Second, we showed how trait management in personality disorders may result in self–self-ambiguity, where a person may be uncertain whether an action or tendency should be seen as part of their default or rather their subsidiary ("as if") self. Third, we explored how people with a personality disorder diagnosis may implicitly relate to their maladaptive personality traits and how ambiguity could arise here too. We hope that our analysis serves as a starting point to further elucidate the relationship between personality disorders and selfhood.

[12] Note that these interventions do not need to be reflectively understood to be helpful: they may exert a healthy influence on Anne's self-relating even if it occurs outside of her awareness.

References

American Psychiatric Association. (1980). *Diagnostic and statistical manual of mental disorders (DSM-III)*. American Psychiatric Publishing.

American Psychiatric Association. (2013). *Diagnostic and statistical manual of mental disorders (DSM-5)*. American Psychiatric Publishing.

Bargiela, S., Steward, R., & Mandy, W. (2016). The experiences of late-diagnosed women with autism spectrum conditions: An investigation of the female autism phenotype. *Journal of Autism and Developmental Disorders*, *46*(10), 3281–3294. https://doi.org/10.1007/s10803-016-2872-8.

Bortolan, A. (2022). Selves hijacked: Affects and personhood in 'self-illness ambiguity'. *Philosophical Explorations*, *25*(3), 343–362. https://doi.org/10.1080/13869795.2022.2093393.

Bröer, C., & Besseling, B. (2017). Sadness or depression: Making sense of low mood and the medicalization of everyday life. *Social Science & Medicine*, *183*, 28–36. https://doi.org/10.1016/j.socscimed.2017.04.025.

Cain, S. (2012). *Quiet: The power of introverts in a world that can't stop talking*. Crown Publishers.

Carls-Diamante, S. (2023). Know thyself: Bipolar disorder and self-concept. *Philosophical Explorations*, *26*(1), 110–126. https://doi.org/10.1080/13869795.2022.2147982.

Castillo, H., Ramon, S., & Morant, N. (2013). A recovery journey for people with personality disorder. *International Journal of Social Psychiatry*, *59*(3), 264–273. https://doi.org/10.1177/0020764013481891.

Chapman, R., & Carel, H. (2022). Neurodiversity, epistemic injustice, and the good human life. *Journal of Social Philosophy*, *53*(4), 614–631. https://doi.org/10.1111/josp.12456.

Clark, L. A., & Watson, D. (2022). The trait model of the DSM-5 alternative model of personality disorder (AMPD): A structural review. *Personality Disorders: Theory, Research, and Treatment*, *13*(4), 328–336. https://doi.org/10.1037/per0000568.

Cook, J., Hull, L., Crane, L., & Mandy, W. (2021). Camouflaging in autism: A systematic review. *Clinical Psychology Review*, *89*, 102080. https://doi.org/10.1016/j.cpr.2021.102080.

DeYoung, C. G. (2010). Toward a theory of the Big Five. *Psychological Inquiry*, *21*(1), 26–33. https://doi.org/10.1080/10478401003648674.

DeYoung, C. G. (2015). Cybernetic Big Five Theory. *Journal of Research in Personality*, *56*, 33–58. https://doi.org/10.1016/j.jrp.2014.07.004.

Dings, R. (2020). Not being oneself? Self-ambiguity in the context of mental disorder. PhD thesis, Radboud Universiteit, Nijmegen.

Dings, R., & de Bruin, L. C. (2022) What's special about 'not feeling like oneself'? A deflationary account of self(-illness) ambiguity. *Philosophical Explorations 25*(3), 269–289. https://doi.org/10.1080/13869795.2022.2051592.

Dings, R., & de Bruin, L. C. (2023). Editorial: Self-illness ambiguity and narrative identity. *Philosophical Explorations*, *26*(2), 147–154. https://doi.org/10.1080/13869795.2023.2203709.

Dings, R., & de Haan, S. (2022). The role of self-illness ambiguity and self-medication ambiguity in clinical decision-making. *The American Journal of Bioethics*, *22*(6), 58–60. https://doi.org/10.1080/15265161.2022.2063436.

Dings R., & Glas, G. (2020). Self-management in psychiatry as reducing self-illness ambiguity. *Philosophy, Psychiatry and Psychology*, *27*(4), 333–347. https://doi.org/10.1353/ppp.2020.0043.

Drożdżowicz, A. (2023). Self-illness ambiguity and anorexia nervosa. *Philosophical Explorations*, *26*(1), 127–145. https://doi.org/10.1080/13869795.2023.2168033.

Fleeson, W., & Wilt, J. (2010). The relevance of Big Five trait content in behavior to subjective authenticity: Do high levels of within-person behavioral variability undermine or enable authenticity achievement? *Journal of Personality*, *78*(4), 1353–1382. https://doi.org/10.1111/j.1467-6494.2010.00653.x.

Gary H. (2018). A diagnosis of "Borderline Personality Disorder" Who am I? Who could I have been? Who can I become? *Psychosis*, *10*(1), 70–75. https://doi.org/10.1080/17522439.2018.1431691.

Gillard, S., Turner, K., & Neffgen, M. (2015). Understanding recovery in the context of lived experience of personality disorders: A collaborative, qualitative research study. *BMC Psychiatry*, *15*(1), 183. https://doi.org/10.1186/s12888-015-0572-0.

Glas, G. (2006). Person, personality, self, and identity: A philosophically informed conceptual analysis. *Journal of Personality Disorders*, *20*(2), 126–138. https://doi.org/10.1521/pedi.2006.20.2.126.

Glas, G. (2017). Dimensions of the self in emotion and psychopathology: Consequences for self-management in anxiety and depression. *Philosophy, Psychiatry, & Psychology*, *24*(2), 143–155. https://doi.org/10.1353/ppp.2017.0019.

Glas, G. (2019). *Person-centered care in psychiatry: Self-relational, contextual, and normative perspectives*. Routledge.

Glas, G. (2023). Dimensions of self-illness ambiguity – A clinical and conceptual approach. *Philosophical Explorations*, *26*(2), 165–178. https://doi.org/10.1080/13869795.2023.2199013.

Goffman, E. (1959). *The presentation of self in everyday life*. Anchor.

Hart, W., Tortoriello, G. K., & Richardson, K. (2018). Are personality disorder traits ego-syntonic or ego-dystonic? Revisiting the issue by considering functionality. *Journal of Research in Personality*, *76*, 124–128. https://doi.org/10.1016/j.jrp.2018.08.001.

Hochschild, A. R. (2012). *The managed heart: Commercialization of human feeling*. University of California Press.

Hull, L., Petrides, K. V., Allison, C., Smith, P., Baron-Cohen, S., Lai, M.-C., & Mandy, W. (2017). "Putting on my best normal": Social camouflaging in adults with autism spectrum conditions. *Journal of Autism and Developmental Disorders*, *47*(8), 2519–2534. https://doi.org/10.1007/s10803-017-3166-5.

Jeppsson, S. M. I. (2022). Solving the self-illness ambiguity: The case for construction over discovery. *Philosophical Explorations*, *25*(3), 294–313. https://doi.org/10.1080/13869795.2022.2051589.

Karp, D. A. (1992). Illness ambiguity and the search for meaning: A case study of a self-help group for affective disorders. *Journal of Contemporary Ethnography*, *21*(2), 139–170.

Karp, D. A. (2006). *Is it me or my meds? Living with antidepressants*. Harvard University Press.

Katsakou, C., Marougka, S., Barnicot, K., Savill, M., White, H., Lockwood, K., & Priebe, S. (2012). Recovery in borderline personality disorder (BPD): A qualitative study of service users' perspectives. *PLoS One*, *7*(5), e36517. https://doi.org/10.1371/journal.pone.0036517.

Kotov, R., Waszczuk, M. A., Krueger, R. F., Forbes, M. K., Watson, D., Clark, L. A., Achenbach, T. M., Althoff, R. R., Ivanova, M. Y., Michael Bagby, R., Brown, T. A., Carpenter, W. T., Caspi, A., Moffitt, T. E., Eaton, N. R., Forbush, K. T., Goldberg, D., Hasin, D., Hyman, S. E., . . . Zimmerman, M. (2017). The Hierarchical Taxonomy of Psychopathology (HiTOP): A dimensional alternative to traditional nosologies. *Journal of Abnormal Psychology*, *126*(4), 454–477. https://doi.org/10.1037/abn0000258.

Krueger, R. F., & Hobbs, K. A. (2020). An overview of the DSM-5 alternative model of personality disorders. *Psychopathology*, *53*(3–4), 126–132. https://doi.org/10.1159/000508538.

Lamph, G., Dorothy, J., Jeynes, T., Coak, A., Jassat, R., Elliott, A., McKeown, M., & Thornton, T. (2022). A qualitative study of the label of personality disorder from the perspectives of people with lived experience and occupational experience. *Mental Health Review Journal*, *27*(1), 31–47. https://doi.org/10.1108/MHRJ-05-2020-0035.

Lester, R., Prescott, L., McCormack, M., Sampson, M., & North West Boroughs Healthcare, NHS Foundation Trust. (2020). Service users' experiences of receiving a diagnosis of borderline personality disorder: A systematic review. *Personality and Mental Health*, *14*(3), 263–283. https://doi.org/10.1002/pmh.1478.

Marcia, J. E. (2006). Ego identity and personality disorders. *Journal of Personality Disorders*, *20*(6), 577–596. https://doi.org/10.1521/pedi.2006.20.6.577.

McConnell, D., & Golova, A. (2023). Narrative, addiction, and three aspects of self-ambiguity. *Philosophical Explorations*, *26*(1), 66–85. https://doi.org/10.1080/13869795.2022.2115532.

Ng, F. Y. Y., Townsend, M. L., Miller, C. E., Jewell, M., & Grenyer, B. F. S. (2019). The lived experience of recovery in borderline personality disorder: A qualitative study. *Borderline Personality Disorder and Emotion Dysregulation*, *6*(1), 10. https://doi.org/10.1186/s40479-019-0107-2.

Nisbett, R. E., & Wilson, T. D. (1977). Telling more than we can know: Verbal reports on mental processes. *Psychological Review*, *84*(3), 231–259.

Sadler, J. Z. (2007). The psychiatric significance of the personal self. *Psychiatry*, *70*(2), 113–129. https://doi.org/10.1521/psyc.2007.70.2.113.

Shepherd, A., Sanders, C., Doyle, M., & Shaw, J. (2016). Personal recovery in personality disorder: Systematic review and meta-synthesis of qualitative methods studies. *International Journal of Social Psychiatry*, *62*(1), 41–50. https://doi.org/10.1177/0020764015589133.

Skodol, A. E., Morey, L. C., Bender, D. S., & Oldham, J. M. (2015). The alternative DSM-5 model for personality disorders: A clinical application. *American Journal of Psychiatry*, *172*(7), 606–613. https://doi.org/10.1176/appi.ajp.2015.14101220.

Sleep, C. E., Lamkin, J., Lynam, D. R., Campbell, W. K., & Miller, J.D. (2019). Personality disorder traits: Testing insight regarding presence of traits, impairment, and desire for change. *Personality Disorders: Theory, Research, and Treatment*, *10* (2), 123–131. https://doi.org/10.1037/per0000305.

Sørensen, K. D., Råbu, M., Wilberg, T., & Berthelsen, E. (2019). Struggling to be a person: Lived experience of avoidant personality disorder. *Journal of Clinical Psychology*, *75*(4), 664–680. https://doi.org/10.1002/jclp.22740.

Strijbos, D., & Glas, G. (2018). Self-knowledge in personality disorder: Self-referentiality as a stepping stone for psychotherapeutic understanding. *Journal of Personality Disorders*, *32*(3), 295–310. https://doi.org/10.1521/pedi.2018.32.3.295.

12 On Personality Dimensions and Disorders

Is a Trait-Based Approach Really the Answer?

Simon Boag

12.1 Introduction

The inadequacies of the categorical approach to personality disorders are widely recognized, and there is growing consensus among researchers and clinicians concerning the advantages of a dimensional approach for understanding personality pathology (Hopwood et al., 2018; Morey et al., 2015; Trull & Durret, 2005; Tyrer et al., 2019; Watson & Clark, 2020; Widiger & Crego, 2019; Widiger et al., 2018). Unlike the categorical approach, which assigns individuals to discrete diagnostic categories, the dimensional approach emphasizes the continuous nature between normal and pathological personality. Although there are various dimensional models available (see Trull & Durret, 2005), personality pathology is generally taken here to represent maladaptive variants of personality traits found within the general population. Personality traits seem particularly well-suited here given the wealth of empirical evidence from studies in both general and clinical populations (Watson & Clark, 2020; Widiger et al., 2019). Moreover, the trait approach is also seen to allow for a more nuanced and comprehensive assessment of personality pathology that captures variations in severity and co-occurrence of symptoms, while promising greater diagnostic accuracy and guidance for treatment planning (Hopwood et al., 2018; Krueger et al., 2014; Widiger et al., 2018).

The shift towards a trait based approach to personality pathology is reflected in the recent 11th revision of the International Classification of Diseases and Related Health Problems (ICD-11) and the fifth edition of the American Psychiatric Association's (APA) *Diagnostic and statistical manual of mental disorders* (DSM-5; American Psychiatric Association, 2013), both of which introduced dimensional approaches to disordered personality functioning. With respect to the latter, DSM-5 retains the former categorical approach found in previous DSM editions, while also advancing an Alternative Model of Personality Disorders (AMPD) with two components: the Criterion A level of personality functioning (i.e. impairments or deficits in the sense of self and interpersonal relatedness) and the Criterion B five-domain maladaptive trait model. The theoretical basis for both systems is often attributed to personality trait approach exemplified by the Five-Factor Model (FFM; McCrae & Costa, 1995, 2008, 2021). The FFM is widely regarded as the leading personality trait model and is seen as providing a particularly well-suited conceptualization of normal personality that can be extended to personality pathology (Widiger, 2005; Widiger & Costa, 2012; Widiger & McCabe, 2020). The Five Factor Theory (FFT) underlying the model proposes that five traits (neuroticism, extraversion, openness to experience, agreeableness, conscientiousness) are universal, endogenous tendencies or dispositions (McCrae & Costa, 1997, 1999, 2008, 2021). DSM-5 acknowledges five 'maladaptive variants' of these domains (p. 773) in the form of negative affectivity, detachment, psychoticism, antagonism, and disinhibition within the AMPD trait model (APA, 2013). Extending upon this, Widiger and McCabe (2020) claim that both Criterion A self–other deficits and the Criterion B traits can be understood as maladaptive variants of the FFM: 'To the extent that the Big Five includes every maladaptive trait term, it naturally follows that the FFM, aligned with the Big Five, accounts for virtually every maladaptive personality trait' (p. 150).

Nevertheless, although many endorse extending the FFM framework for understanding disordered personality, some question the suitability of these traits due to both conceptual and methodological issues (e.g. Livesley & Jang, 2005; Livesley, 2021; Wright, 2011). Shedler et al. (2010), for example, raise doubts about whether traits identified in the general population apply similarly to clinical samples, writing '[w]e endorse the value of dimensionalizing well-recognized clinical constructs (e.g., severity), but do not agree with the use of non-clinical concepts drawn from academic personality psychology' (p. 1027). On the other hand, critics further argue that trait approaches are generally too limited (e.g. Rauthmann, 2024), as well as obscuring the role of situational variables for explaining behaviour through aggregating scale responses and averaging across situations (Cervone, 2004, 2005, 2023; Cervone & Little, 2019; Mischel, 2004; Nowak et al., 2005).

There are also long-standing conceptual concerns regarding trait theory in general. For example, although trait scores may capture individual differences across subjects, they cannot point to within-person attributes that underlie such variation (Borsboom et al., 2003; Cervone, 2004, 2005; Lamiell, 2013). Furthermore, some trait researchers recognize that trait information provides descriptive summaries rather than explanation (e.g., Goldberg, 1990). These summaries are nevertheless then mistakenly treated by some as inherent attributes within individuals and fallaciously used to explain individual behaviour (Boag, 2011, 2015; Cervone, 1999, 2004, 2005). If these latter arguments prove valid, then serious doubts emerge regarding whether trait-based approaches can provide a coherent theoretical framework for comprehending personality pathology.

This chapter evaluates the theoretical soundness of the FFM trait approach for comprehending personality pathology. To achieve this, the chapter first examines the conceptual standing of traits in relation to the generally under-appreciated conceptual distinction between nonrelational properties and relations. A discussion of the theoretical problems of reification and circular explanation is then used as a basis for critically evaluating both the concept of traits and their application to understanding personality pathology. Although traits might help discern individual differences in the population, they are logically precluded from explaining personality pathology. An alternative approach for comprehending personality pathology is then put forward that integrates motivational, cognitive, and affective processes, while satisfying logical requirements determined by philosophical enquiry. Finally, this chapter discusses the need for greater conceptual research for understanding personality pathology and psychology generally.

12.2 What are Personality Traits?

Although providing a one-size-fits-all account of traits is difficult, trait theorists generally view these as 'temperament-like variables' (McCrae & Costa, 1995, 2008, 2021), emphasizing the significance of innate, enduring, and context-independent factors in shaping individuals and their behaviour (e.g., Eysenck, 1997; McCrae & Costa, 1995, 2008, 2021). The precise number of traits varies from anywhere between three, five, seven, and 16 (see Cattell, 1957; Cloninger et al., 1993; Eysenck, 1997; Goldberg, 1990; McCrae & Costa, 1995, 2008, 2021), and identifying traits has been generally guided by the lexical approach to personality, emerging with Galton, and traceable through figures such as Thurstone and Cattell (Goldberg, 1990). With the lexical approach, extensive sets of adjectives are analysed via factor analysis to construct hierarchical models, which identify higher-level broad factors from clusters of lower-level traits and specific acts (Eysenck, 1997; Goldberg, 1990; McCrae & Costa, 2008).

Understanding the precise nature of traits is critical for valid assessment, because valid assessment necessitates demonstrating that the attribute causally influences fluctuations in test scores (Borsboom et al., 2004). This requires both that (i) the attribute in question exists, and (ii) that differences in the attribute are causally reflected in differences in scores upon the assessment outcomes (Borsboom et al., 2004; Michell, 1999, 2004, 2005). As Borsboom et al. (2004) write:

If something does not exist, then one cannot measure it. If it exists but does not causally produce variations in the outcomes of the measurement procedure, then one is either measuring nothing at all or something different altogether. Thus a test is valid for measuring an attribute if and only if (a) the attribute exists and (b) variations in the attribute causally produce variations in the outcomes of the measurement procedure. (p. 1061)

Implicated within these criteria is the necessity for variations in test performance to reflect changes in the attribute, which requires an account of process – a theory of response behaviour – to address how the attribute comes to be reflected in test performance (Borsboom et al., 2004). Accordingly, if we assert that individuals possess disordered personalities and that personality tests are purportedly evaluating maladaptive traits, it becomes essential to ascertain precisely what these tests are measuring and how traits are reflected in test scores.

12.3 Traits within the Five Factor Model and Theory

One immediate issue here, however, concerns the nature of the FFT traits and the evidence for them. We learn from McCrae and Costa (1999) that '[t]raits . . . are directly accessible neither to public observation nor to private introspection. Instead, they are deeper psychological entities that can only be *inferred* from behaviour and experience' (p. 143, italics in original). In this respect, McCrae and Costa consistently argue that traits are not biological attributes, writing instead that 'traits are . . . real psychological structures' (McCrae, 2004, p. 4; cf. McCrae & Costa, 1995, 1999, 2021). As they note: 'ours is a psychological theory of personality. We do not equate basic dispositions with biological constructs, nor have we offered a psychobiological theory of personality' (McCrae & Costa, 1995, p. 239). Nevertheless, it is not precisely clear what kind of psychological entities traits might actually be. Traits do not seem to correspond to typical psychological states like desires and beliefs, the latter instead perceived as outcomes of traits rather than the traits themselves ('characteristic adaptations'; McCrae & Costa, 1995; McCrae, 2004). Thus, at first blush, the specific nature of traits is unclear.

Despite their indefinite character, traits are nonetheless considered genuine attributes of individuals and relevant to explaining what people do (e.g. Costa & McCrae, 2009; McCrae & Costa, 1995, 2008). In this sense, traits are latent variables that play an explicit explanatory role in the form of intra-individual dispositional 'temperament-like variables' (McCrae & Costa, 1995, 2008, 2021). The Five Factor Theory (FFT) here explicitly proposes that these traits are the 'underlying causes of behaviour' (McCrae & Costa, 1995, p. 236; cf. McCrae & Costa, 2008), with McCrae and Costa (1995) writing: 'the causal argument is in principle clear: traits as underlying tendencies cause and thus explain (in general and in part) the consistent patterns of thoughts, feelings, and actions that one sees' (p. 236). These traits serve as distal causes rather than proximal ones, however, with McCrae and Costa (2021) recently writing that '[t]raits are not seen as direct causes of behavior; instead, they lead to the development of concrete and contextualized adaptations which in turn interact with the demands and opportunities of the environment to shape action and experience' (p. 7). Considering that traits are theorized to be attributes causally reflected both in behaviour and personality test scores (e.g. Costa & McCrae, 1995, 2008, 2021), we need to specifically know then how to characterize the FFM/FFT traits. Therefore, determining the suitability of traits for understanding personality pathology necessitates a closer examination of how traits are conceptualized.

12.4 Realism, Relations, and Reification

If traits are not observable by either oneself or others, and can only ever be inferred from behaviour and experience (McCrae & Costa, 1995, 1999), then further empirical research is unlikely to provide definitive insights into the exact nature of traits. Nevertheless, conceptual analysis can serve as a method for addressing the coherency of claims made about traits. Conceptual research has a long history in science generally (Machado & Silva, 2007) and can be used to extricate the logically sound features of theories and reject incoherent aspects to help clarify what we are specifically talking about. Conceptual analysis, in fact, precedes empirical testing of theory because a clear theory is essential for meaningful empirical evaluation (Michell, 2000; Petocz & Newbery, 2010; Petocz & Mackay, 2013). Indeed, attempting to empirically assess logically flawed theories would be futile, as such theories could never accurately represent reality. As Petocz and Newbery (2010) write, '[i]f the logical tests are failed, if our conceptual analysis reveals confusions, ambiguities, contradictions, implicit assumptions, and so forth, then we know without going any further (i.e., without taking the next step into any specific observational analysis) that the situation as envisaged is either *not yet clear enough* or *could not possibly be the case*' (p. 130, italics in original).

There are various possible forms of conceptual research (see Banicki, 2012), and the approach applied here can be described as a realist one,[1] in part due to it clarifying the important, but often poorly appreciated, distinction between *qualities* (or nonrelational properties) and *relations*. With respect to this distinction, Mackie (1962) writes that 'a quality is an intrinsic feature of a thing, it

[1] There are also various types of realisms, and the one employed here has its basis in the philosophy of John Anderson (see Anderson, 1962; Baker, 1986). This is not the place to provide a detailed exposition and defence of this position, but the interested reader is referred to both Mackay and Petocz (2010) and Petocz and Mackay (2013).

belongs to the thing itself, whereas a relation holds between two or more things' (p. 266). Relations are real features of situations (existing in the same spatio-temporal universe as the things standing within relations) and come in various forms (e.g. spatial relations, temporal relations, logical relations). What these all have in common is that they involve at least two or more *terms* standing with respect to one another (where the terms are whatever stands in relation to other things).[2] These terms must be logically independent from one another, so in the relation *a*R*b*, the terms *a* and *b* must be logically independent situations with their own nonrelational properties. Maze (1983) here writes:

> Anything that can stand ... in any relation at all, must have at least some intrinsic properties. If that were not the case . . . then we could not understand what it was that was said to have those relationships. A relation can only hold between two or more terms, and a part of what is involved in seeing those terms as related is being able to see them as distinct, that is, as each having its own intrinsic properties, so that we can say what the terms *are* that are related. This means that each term of the relation must be able in principle to be described without the need to include any reference to its relation to the other. (p. 24, italics in original; cf. Maze, 1954; Michell, 1988)

Failing to recognize the distinction between nonrelational properties and relations can lead to several conceptual errors. One such error is that of reification. Reification is commonly conceived of in terms of confusing the 'abstract' with the 'concrete', which can be taken to involve mistaking relations with nonrelational properties or entities (Bell et al., 2000; Passmore, 1935). To illustrate this error, consider the concept of 'individual differences' as found in personality research. 'Difference' is a relation between two terms that somehow differ from one another (e.g. person A differs from person B). Taken as such, 'difference' is a relation that cannot be reduced to either person A or B alone, even if both people necessarily have features that they differ from one another on. However, 'individual differences' are commonly confused with attributes of individuals in personality psychology. As Lamiell (2013) writes, 'in the hands of mainstream personality investigators, the dimensions of individual differences ... have been regarded as entities existing, in varying amounts, within individuals, rather than as mathematical constructions intended to facilitate discussions of between-person variations within populations' (p. 67). As such, reification here involves the mistake of attributing a nonrelational quality of 'difference' to individuals rather than recognizing its relational character (Bell et al., 2000).[3]

[2] The term 'term' here only refers to what stands within the relation and does not refer to a linguistic entity specifically (unless talking about certain linguistic relations).

[3] Confusing what something does with what it is also constitutes an example of reification, as 'doing' is also a relation (*S* does *x*). For example, 'strength' refers to what a set of muscles can *do*, and so to mistakenly treat 'strength' as a property of the muscle would also be to engage in reification (Passmore, 1935).

A related problem arises when description is mistaken for explanation. Broadly speaking, description involves classification (taxonomy), whereas explanation addresses the causal factors responsible for bringing the observed phenomenon into being (Boag, 2011, 2018). Description is logically independent of explanation because it is possible to describe something without providing an explanation for it. For example, one can describe someone as a narcissist or compare levels of narcissism between people without having any insight into the causal factors that explain those traits. Confusing description with explanation is problematic because it leads to *circular explanation* (Boag, 2011). Circular explanation occurs when the explanation of some effect (the *explanans*) is equivalent to the effect that it is said to explain (the *explanandum*), such that the explanation for some occurrence is the occurrence itself (i.e. when saying A causes B and A is equivalent to B; Bell et al., 2000; Boag, 2011, 2017). Circular explanation can easily occur when a label initially describing someone or some set of behaviours is then used to explain that same occurrence. For instance, one might use 'extraversion' as a descriptive label for outgoing and sociable behaviour. However, using 'extraversion' then as an explanation of that same outgoing and sociable behaviour provides an instance of circular explanation because the explanans and explanandum are not logically distinct from one another. This problem of circular explanation has been raised at various times in the history of modern psychology (Maze, 1954; Skinner, 1953) and described as 'verbal-magic': 'giving a name to a certain kind of event and then using the name as if it accounted for the *occurrence* of that kind of event' (Maze, 1954, p. 226; italics in original). Because something cannot be both a description and explanation of the same phenomenon, avoiding circular explanation involves appreciating that causes and effects must be logically distinct from one another.

12.5 Evaluating the Trait Account

Although we have little specific guidance as to what traits specifically consist of, we know that traits are conceptualized as dispositions or tendencies that play a causal role in behaviour (McCrae & Costa, 2021). A such, we can logically assess conceptual claims in relation to traits as dispositions. Here Hampshire (1953) notes that a disposition 'is a statement which summarizes what tends to happen or is liable on the whole to happen' (p. 5), and a 'tendency' can be similarly taken to be a summary of what someone is likely to do. As such, a 'disposition' or 'tendency' is generally a disposition or tendency to *do something*, which can be taken to mean that both tendencies and dispositions are relational concepts (e.g. '*S* tends to do *x*'; '*S* is disposed to do *y*'). As relations, dispositions or tendencies cannot be reduced to a feature of persons responsible for what they do because the person is simply one term in the doing relation (i.e. the relation '*S* does *x*' cannot be reduced simply to *S*). Moreover, neither dispositions nor tendencies offer insight into the causes that lead to these 'tending' or 'disposing' relations (see also Cervone, 2004, 2005).

The trait theorist might be tempted here to appeal to 'dispositional properties' in the same way that we might describe a physical object as fragile. By analogy, for instance, we might attempt to explain why a person becomes upset easily in terms of their being 'psychologically fragile'. The topic of dispositional properties is, itself, complex (e.g. single versus multiple; passive versus active dispositions – see Mackie, 1977), but a dispositional statement is essentially a relational one, meaning nothing more than an 'if . . . then . . . ' contingency (Maze, 1983). Taken as such, psychological fragility as a dispositional concept would be a description of a relation between an individual and some other situation, meaning simply that if the person comes into contact with a certain situation (e.g. criticism), then they become more easily upset compared to other people. However, as a relation between the individual and such situations, the disposition cannot be reduced to nonrelational properties of the person. Of course, there will be causal factors that explain any such disposition: an individual might, for example, become easily upset due to beliefs and associated fears concerning rejection. However, those causal factors should not be confused with the disposition itself because causes and effects must be logically independent of one another. Additionally, if the disposition to become upset can be explained by reference to such cognitive and affective factors on the part of the person, then the term 'psychological fragility' adds nothing to the explanation of getting upset (even if the concept may allow prediction of how the person is likely to react under certain circumstances).

Consequently, dispositions and tendencies cannot be characteristics of persons that explain what people do because they are not conceptually distinct from what they are meant to explain. Additionally, conceptualizing traits in terms of dispositions and 'tendencies' provides no real idea of what it is that is relevant to explaining behaviour or test performance. Attempting then to explain behaviour *x* by reference to a 'tendency to do *x*' cannot help but be circular, as the 'tendency' is not logically independent of the effect *x*. Accordingly, if traits are understood as either 'tendencies' or 'dispositions' then they are incapable of standing as independent causal factors of those same behaviours.

Nevertheless, Terracciano and McCrae (2012) attempt to defend the causal role of traits by analogy with explaining the flocking behaviour of birds via the concept of a 'flocking instinct':

> Presumably some species flock because they have evolved a mechanism, or suite of mechanisms, that allow each bird to respond to its environment in ways that give rise to

flocking behaviour. Loosely, we can call this set of mechanisms a *flocking instinct*, present in some species but not others. Surely it is meaningful to say that the innate flocking instinct is *a cause* of flocking behaviour, because when it is absent, flocking does not occur. (p. 449, italics in original)

On this view, we essentially have a situation where we observe some behaviour (in this instance, flocking), and based on that same observation postulate an instinct to explain that behaviour (a flocking instinct that explains flocking behaviour). However, a major problem with this strategy has been long recognized, as seen in criticisms of the early twentieth-century instinct theorist McDougall (1923). McDougall proposed that instincts could be identified by observing behavioural goals, so that we could explain someone's sociability and outgoingness in terms of their gregarious instinct, whereas a combative instinct could explain a pugnacious person's actions. Holt, commenting on McDougall's instinct theory, was aware of the pitfalls of such an explanatory strategy:

... man is impelled to action, it is said, by his instincts. If he goes with his fellows, it is 'herd instinct' which activates him; if he walks alone, it is the 'anti-social instinct'; if he fights, it is the 'pugnacity instinct'; if he defers to another it is the instinct of 'self-abasement'; if he twiddles his thumbs, it is the thumb-twiddling instinct; if he does not twiddle his thumbs, it is the thumb-not-twiddling instinct. Thus, everything is explained with the facility of magic – word magic. (Holt in Yankelovich, 1973, p. 413)

The specific problem here is that without independent evidence of these instincts, we have as many instincts as there are recognizable acts of behaviour, and the 'evidence' for the instinct is always available (Maze, 1983). As such, if traits are identified solely from what people do (or say that they do), and subsequently used to explain the same behaviour that they are inferred from, then traits are essentially the thumb-twiddling instincts of the twenty-first century (cf. Boag, 2015).

12.6 Can Traits Be Placeholders?

McCrae and Costa (2008), however, propose that traits may nevertheless stand as legitimate explanatory placeholders. In this respect, they believe that traits are causes in the same sense that we might say that a car breaks down because it is 'unreliable'. Being 'unreliable', they say, is not simply a description of what the car does but can also serve as a causal explanation of a car's breaking down because it points to other problems:

... unreliability can be seen under the hood, if one knows where to look. It is seen in the poor design, in the shoddy workmanship, in the flimsy materials used to construct the car. Any good mechanic could point these out, even without knowing the performance history of that model. Unreliability is an elliptical explanation, pointing to unspecified features that provide a more mechanistic explanation, but it is no less an explanation for being abstract. (p. 289)

Presumably, there could be numerous sources of any such unreliability, such that one car might be unreliable because of a faulty battery, and another because of a problem with the fuel line. However, even if we were to accept trait unreliability as a placeholder, we can then potentially explain the situation with respect to a variety of possible causes, *without any need of invoking 'trait unreliability'*. Presumably, then, once we have identified the specific causal influences responsible for unreliable performance (and presumably, if the analogy holds, these may be various), 'trait unreliability' becomes causally redundant. One would expect that advances in knowledge would eventually make 'explanatory' traits irrelevant to personality psychology (Boag, 2015).

12.7 What Does This All Mean for the Trait Approach?

The above analysis reveals that traits as dispositions are, at best, descriptive summaries of what a person is likely to do under different circumstances. As dispositions, traits are relational concepts logically linked to what they seek to explain and so logically precluded from explaining what people do. Furthermore, as there is no independent evidence for traits apart from the behaviour that traits are said to explain, we simply have again 'an instance of word-magic, an instance of the fallacy of reification, inventing entities in an *ad hoc* fashion to do explanatory jobs. Such entities have no qualitative nature of their own; their sole existence lies in observed relations of certain kinds' (McMullen, 1982, p. 224). Consequently, trait theory cannot provide a coherent substantive theory of personality and so, by extension, maladaptive traits cannot help us to comprehend personality pathology. In fact, the same logical issues are already evident with respect to maladaptive traits because facets such as emotional lability, suspiciousness, and grandiosity in the Personality Inventory for DSM-5 (PID-5; Hopwood et al., 2013) are all essentially descriptions of what instead requires explanation. Thus, although the latent trait approach to personality may hold descriptive value, it should not become a distraction away from developing substantive theory of personality pathology (cf. Shedler et al., 2010).

As noted earlier, however, not all trait accounts necessarily fall into the trap of reification or conflate description with explanation (e.g. Goldberg, 1990; Saucier et al., 2000). Furthermore, the arguments presented above do not negate the potential descriptive utility of dimensional trait approaches. The value of dimensional approaches, for example, may be evident when considering examples like intellectual disability. As Hyman (2010) writes, '[t]his dimensional representation [of intellectual disability] is entirely appropriate given the continuous distribution of IQ in the population', and despite diverse causes underlying such disability, 'IQ remains a clinically useful and predictive clinical dimension in that an IQ of 70 or below has been convincingly correlated with significant impairment' (p. 165).[4] However, there is no logical requirement that any observed act has a single corresponding underlying cause (cf. Lamiell, 2013). Thus, reducing complex phenomena such as sociability and outgoing behaviour to a single factor such as 'extraversion' simply grossly under-estimates the complexity of the human situation (Asendorpf, 2016; Nilsson, 2014). It is also worth pointing out that tenets of trait theory are also not empirically supported. For instance, the claim that traits are stable, and that personality is inherently resistant to change, is contradicted by the available evidence (cf. Bleidorn et al., 2021; Krueger et al., 2014).

12.8 Personality and Causal Explanation

If the aim instead is to use theory to comprehend personality, normal or otherwise, then any adequate theory of personality needs to move beyond description and address causal mechanisms (Asendorpf, 2016). Achieving this essentially entails two inter-related considerations. One such consideration relates to identifying the relevant components and processes of persons for developing a theoretically sound integrative account of human behaviour. In this respect, given that the concept of personality 'disorder' implies some sense of personality *order* (Leising et al., 2009), the starting point for making sense of personality requires addressing the component parts of persons and their interactions that contribute to what people do. Addressing this requires a metapsychological position whereby a theory of personality provides a general theory of human behaviour (cf. Petocz & Mackay, 2013). Such a metapsychology will necessarily address motivational, cognitive, and affective processes and explain how these processes interact with both one another and contexts in the production of behaviour (see Boag, 2017).

Developing such a coherent metapsychology requires further philosophical enquiry because any theoretical position entails metaphysical postulates that constrain what is logically possible and therefore theoretically permissible (Hibberd, 2014). For example, any consideration of personality pathology necessarily entails broader theoretical and philosophical assumptions including the relationship between mind and body. Accordingly, developing scientific theory is inherently philosophical because we need to also address the broader metaphysical conditions that any coherent theory of personality must conform

[4] Be this as it may, 'intelligence' (intellectual ability), like 'traits' lends itself easily to reification and circular explanation because such terms are commonly defined relationally (i.e., *S* is able to do *x*; Howe, 1990; Passmore, 1935).

to. Although providing a comprehensive account of these metaphysical conditions is beyond the scope of this chapter (for a more detailed discussion, refer to Hibberd, 2014), one example relevant to claims about personality and explanation concerns the nature of causality. On the position proposed here, causality can only be deterministic whereby all events arise out of causes and go on to cause other events (Anderson, 1962; McMullen, 1996)[5]. Such determinism is more than a simple cause–effect chain, however, because causality involves a network whereby causes and effects operate within a *causal field* in which both causes and effects operate ('a background against which the causing goes on' – Mackie, 1974, p. 63).

If this metaphysical position is accepted, then any theory of personality is thus constrained philosophically because explaining human behaviour necessarily requires eschewing conceptions entailing either teleological or self-directed accounts of human behaviour (Boag, 2017; Maze, 1983). This then means that any theory of personality claiming that persons act freely or in a self-directed manner can be rejected as such claims are simply incoherent. This view of causality further constrains how we understand motivational processes. Rather than striving towards goals, motivation needs to be instead conceptualized in terms of causal antecedents that push or drive the person into action and determine the direction of any such activity (Maze, 1983). This, in turn, points to the importance of motivation for explaining human action. For example, within a desire–belief model of human action, cognition alone is insufficient for explaining what people do because cognition is policy-neutral: the one and the same belief might be either acted or not acted upon depending upon one's motivational policy (what one 'desires'; Maze, 1983). Thus, the concept of motivation takes on special significance for explaining what people do (Mackay & Petocz, 2010).

Given the importance of motivation for explaining behaviour, any theory that neglects the concept is consequently incapable of sufficiently addressing personality. For example, dynamic personality theories view personality as a dynamic organization of within-person (intra-individual) characteristics interacting with situations across time (e.g., Cervone, 2004, 2005, 2023; Cervone & Little, 2019; Mischel, 2004; Vallacher et al., 2002). These perspectives offer the advantage of addressing psychological mechanisms underlying individual differences, making these accounts potential candidates for providing a coherent alternative to the trait position. Nevertheless, these dynamic

[5] There are, of course, various approaches to the topics of causality and explanation including interventionist–counterfactual models (e.g., Woodward, 2003) and probabilistic models (e.g., Dawid, 2000). Such approaches are partly premised on the practical difficulties associated with identifying causal relationships, and although space does not permit going into detailed argument here, it can nevertheless be pointed out that such approaches are not logically incompatible with the metaphysical account of determinism as understood here.

theories tend to emphasise cognition at the expense of motivation. For example, Cervone's (2004) Knowledge-and-Appraisal Personality Architecture (KAPA) model places the emphasis on the distinction between knowledge and appraisal for explaining how people respond and act. When interacting with situations, knowledge informs appraisal, which is then in turn reciprocally influenced by situations (Cervone, 2004, 2005). However, there is no explicit role for motivation in Cervone's account (see Boag, 2018), and so the KAPA model is currently incomplete because it provides no account of motivational policy. Although this is not a fatal flaw for the theory – this gap may potentially be filled – an explicit and coherent account of motivation must be provided if the theory is to provide a coherent explanation for what people do.

One theoretical perspective that in principle addresses the logical requirements for a coherent explanation of human action can be found in Freudian metapsychology, albeit divested of certain problematic postulates.[6] Freud's metapsychology, broadly speaking, was an attempt at developing a general theory that integrates motivation, cognition, and affects for understanding both normal and pathological human activity. Maze (1983) here writes, 'Freud's metapsychology, though, unfinished, was the one great systematic attempt in modern psychology to outline a deterministic, physiologically based theory of motivation and extend it to embrace all of human behaviour, bodily and mental' (pp. 142–143). An important component of Freud's theory of motivation is his 'drive' concept (Freud, 1915), whereby psychobiological systems underly human action and determine any person's motivational policy.[7] These action systems are substantiated in neurophysical 'biological engines', while their operations are guided by cognitive and affective states (Maze, 1983). Although these drives initially operate according to inbuilt action programmes (*consummatory actions*), these programmes are highly plastic and modifiable, becoming elaborated through learning experiences and motor development, and potentially distorted due to conflict between the drives. Freudian metapsychology here thus integrates motivational, cognitive, and affective processes, while addressing biological processes without reducing the mind to brain.

One advantage of this metapsychological position is that Freud (1915) acknowledges that drives need to be identified by their somatic sources to prevent postulating drives ad hoc and ad libitum. In this respect, Freud

[6] Freud's metapsychology can be construed variously, and the position promoted here should not be confused with the narrow Freudian one involving some type of mental *economy* (entailing a system of psychical energy). For further discussion see Boag (2017).

[7] Freud used the German word *Trieb*, which was translated by Freud's editor Strachey as 'instinct'. This translation is problematic because the English 'instinct' commonly refers to unmodifiable or stereotyped species-specific behaviour patterns (Laplanche & Pontalis, 1973). Although there is no single English equivalent for *Trieb*, the word 'drive' provides a fair approximation (see Boag, 2017; Maze, 1983).

recognizes that any attempt at specifying drives based on behaviour alone remains only more or less arbitrary:

> What instincts should we suppose there are, and how many? There is obviously a wide opportunity here for arbitrary choice. No objection can be made to anyone's employing the concept of an instinct of play or of destruction or of gregariousness, when the subject-matter demands it and the limitations of psychological analysis allow of it. Nevertheless, we should not neglect to ask ourselves whether instinctual motives like these, which are so highly specialised on the one hand, do not admit of further dissection in accordance with the *sources* of the instinct, so that only primal instincts – those which cannot be further dissected – can lay claim to importance. (Freud, 1915, pp. 123–124, italics in original)

Freud thus recognizes that if behaviour is the only evidence for postulating drives, then we have a problem because we could propose as many drives (or instincts) as there are things that people do.[8] However, identifying drives in terms of their somatic sources means that the number and specification of drives is ultimately resolved empirically: drives are empirically identifiable biological (neural) structures that stand logically distinct from the behaviours that they generate. Consequently, such drives stand as potential explanatory candidates because they are logically independent of the behaviours that they are said to cause (see Boag, 2017; Maze, 1983).

None of this is to pretend that identifying such drives is straightforward, and one needs to go further than simply postulating some brain centre or circuitry for any given drive. Instead, the further requirement is demonstrating that any postulated centre or circuity is causally relevant to the production of behaviour for any specific drive. This is an empirical challenge, however, rather than a logical one, and Panksepp and colleagues seem to have gone some way to addressing this (e.g. Panksepp & Biven, 2012). For example, Panksepp has identified distinct neural circuits responsible for generating and regulating different basic emotions and corresponding behavioural responses via animal studies manipulating brain regions and observing resulting changes in behaviour. Although there may still be limitations here surrounding inference, this research nevertheless shows that postulating drives based on somatic sources is not speculative reductionism as there are empirical avenues for substantiating which basic drives actually exist.

The evidence of such affective–motivational (action) systems that anchor mind and personality within the body provides a physiological–motivational basis for understanding both rational and irrational actions in conjunction with

[8] Freud (1915) further recognizes that several drives may contribute to any behavioural act and that a drive may find substitutive aims (e.g. as may occur with emotional eating). Consequently, identifying the 'true' goal of any activity requires some intuitive interpretation of what someone is really doing, and thus does not provide an objective basis for identifying drives (see also Maze, 1983).

both cognition and the environment (Panksepp & Biven, 2012). With respect to personality theory, as biological creatures, our minds are necessarily embodied and integrated with motivational, affective, and cognitive states, and so personality pathology can accordingly be theoretically grounded in terms of drives or action systems and the experiences that shape their response modalities (e.g. traumatization).

12.9 Conclusion

Zachar and Krueger (2013) write: There are very few, if any, constructs in psychiatry that are more conceptually encumbered than that of personality disorder. How so? Because personality disorder inherits not only all the problems associated with the concept of "personality," but also all the problems associated with the concept "psychiatric disorder" (p. 889). As discussed above, personality traits as 'dispositions' are, at best, descriptive summaries of what a person is likely to do under different circumstances. At worst, however, such summaries become reified into within-subject attributes and then fallaciously used to explain individual behaviour. Consequently, although some propose that trait approaches provide a basis for conceptualizing disordered personality (e.g. Widiger, 2005), the latent trait approach is conceptually problematic and so not up to the task of providing a coherent theoretical foundation for understanding either personality generally or personality pathology more specifically. Whether alternative accounts succeed where trait accounts fail requires further conceptual and theoretical research, and one potential alternative candidate is a metapsychological position integrating motivational, cognitive, and affective processes, while informed and constrained by philosophical enquiry.

Reification can be avoided by using conceptual analysis to clarify the distinction between entities, properties, and relations, which points to an essential role for philosophical scrutiny when developing scientific theory. Although psychological science tends to perceive itself as emancipated from its philosophical foundations, the neglect of conceptual and theoretical research contributes to the proliferation of vague and ambiguous concepts as found within the trait approach (cf. Banicki, 2012). The history of psychology further demonstrates that reification and circular explanation are not recently arisen problems, but instead persistent ones (cf. faculty psychology; Passmore, 1935). None of this is to say that dimensional approaches are without value, but substituting empirical and statistical success for coherent theory leads to apparent short-term gains at the expense of long-term theoretical dead ends. Thus, the future success of scientific psychology for addressing personality pathology requires rigorous and critical attention to its theoretical foundations.

Acknowledgement: I would like to thank the Editors of this volume for their very thoughtful and constructive feedback and suggestions.

References

American Psychiatric Association. (2013). *Diagnostic and statistical manual of mental disorders* (DSM-5) (5th ed.). American Psychiatric Association.

Anderson, J. (1962). *Studies in empirical philosophy.* Angus & Robertson.

Asendorpf, J. B. (2016). Causal unity of broader traits is an illusion. *European Journal of Personality, 30*, 304–340.

Baker, A. J. (1986). *Australian realism*. Cambridge University Press.

Banicki, K. (2012). Connective conceptual analysis and psychology. *Theory & Psychology, 22*, 310–323.

Bell, P., Staines, P., & Michell, J. (2000). *Logical psych*. University of New South Wales Press.

Bleidorn, W., Hopwood, C. J., Back, M. D., Denissen, J. J., Hennecke, M., Hill, P. L., . . . & Zimmermann, J. (2021). Personality trait stability and change. *Personality Science, 2*, 1–20.

Boag, S. (2011). Explanation in personality research: 'Verbal magic' and the Five-Factor Model. *Philosophical Psychology, 24*, 223–243.

Boag, S. (2015). Personality assessment, 'construct validity', and the significance of theory. *Personality & Individual Differences, 84*, 36–44.

Boag, S. (2017). *Metapsychology and the foundations of psychoanalysis: Attachment, neuropsychoanalysis and integration*. Routledge.

Boag, S. (2018). Personality dynamics, motivation, and the logic of explanation. *Review of General Psychology, 22*, 427–436.

Borsboom, D., Mellenbergh, G. J., & van Heerden, J. (2003). The theoretical status of latent variables. *Psychological Review, 110*, 203–219.

Borsboom, D., Mellenbergh, G. J., & van Heerden, J. (2004). The concept of validity. *Psychological Review, 111*, 1061–1071.

Cattell, R. B. (1957). *Personality and motivation: Structure and measurement.* World Book Company.

Cervone, D. (1999). Bottom-up explanation in personality psychology: The case of cross-situational coherence. In D. Cervone & Yuichi Shoda (eds.), *The coherence of personality: Social-cognitive bases of consistency, variability, and organization* (pp. 303–341). Guilford Press.

Cervone, D. (2004). The architecture of personality. *Psychological Review, 111*, 183–204.

Cervone, D. (2005). Personality architecture: Within-person structures and processes. *Annual Review of Psychology, 56*, 423–452.

Cervone, D. (2023). Theory and application in personality science: The case of social-cognitive theory. *Psychology & Developing Societies, 35*, 220–250.

Cervone, D., & Little, B. R. (2019). Personality architecture and dynamics: The new agenda and what's new about it. *Personality & Individual Differences, 136*, 12–23.

Clark, L. A. (2007). Assessment and diagnosis of personality disorder: Perennial issues and emerging reconceptualization. *Annual Review of Psychology, 58*, 227–257.

Cloninger, C. R., Svrakic, D. M., & Przybeck, T. R. (1993). A psychobiological model of temperament and character. *Archives of General Psychiatry, 50*, 975–990.

Costa, P. T., & McCrae, R. R. (2009). The five-factor model and the NEO inventories. In J. N. Butcher (ed.), *Oxford handbook of personality assessment* (pp. 299–322). Oxford University Press.

Dawid, A. P. (2000). Causal inference without counterfactuals. *Journal of the American Statistical Association, 95*, 407–424.

Eysenck, H. J. (1997). Personality and experimental psychology: The unification of psychology and the possibility of a paradigm. *Journal of Personality and Social Psychology, 73*, 1224–1237.

Freud, S. (1915). *Instincts and their vicissitudes. Standard edition* (Vol. 14). Hogarth.

Goldberg, L. R. (1990). An alternate 'description of personality': The Big-Five Factor structure. *Journal of Personality and Social Psychology, 59*, 1216–1229.

Hampshire, S. (1953). Dispositions. *Analysis, 14*, 5–11.

Hibberd, F. J. (2014). The metaphysical basis of a process psychology. *Journal of Theoretical & Philosophical Psychology, 34*, 161–186.

Hopwood, C. J., Kotov, R., Krueger, R. F., Watson, D., Widiger, T. A., Althoff, R. R., . . . & Zimmermann, J. (2018). The time has come for dimensional personality disorder diagnosis. *Personality & Mental Health, 12*, 82–86.

Hopwood, C. J., Wright, A. G., Krueger, R. F., Schade, N., Markon, K. E., & Morey, L. C. (2013). DSM-5 pathological personality traits and the Personality Assessment Inventory. *Assessment, 20*, 269–285.

Howe, M. J. A. (1990). Does intelligence exist? *The Psychologist, 3*, 490–493.

Hyman, S. E. (2010). The diagnosis of mental disorders: the problem of reification. *Annual Review of Clinical Psychology, 6*, 155–179.

Krueger, R. F., Hopwood, C. J., Wright, A. G., & Markon, K. E. (2014). DSM-5 and the path toward empirically based and clinically useful conceptualization of personality and psychopathology. *Clinical Psychology: Science and Practice, 21*, 245–261.

Lamiell, J. T. (2013). Statisticism in personality psychologists' use of trait constructs: What is it? How was it contracted? Is there a cure? *New Ideas in Psychology, 31*, 65–71.

Laplanche, J., & Pontalis, J.-B. (1973). *The language of psychoanalysis*. Karnac.

Leising, D., Rogers, K., & Ostner, J. (2009). The undisordered personality: Normative assumptions underlying personality disorder diagnoses. *Review of General Psychology, 13*, 230–241.

Livesley, W. J. (2021). Why is an evidence-based classification of personality disorder so elusive? *Personality and Mental Health, 15*, 8–25.

Livesley, W. J., & Jang, K. L. (2005). Differentiating normal, abnormal, and disordered personality. *European Journal of Personality, 19*, 257–268.

Machado, A. & Silva, F. J. (2007). Toward a richer view of the scientific method: The role of conceptual analysis. *American Psychologist, 62*, 671–681.

Mackie, J. L. (1962). The philosophy of John Anderson. *Australasian Journal of Philosophy, 40*, 265–282.

Mackie, J. L. (1974). *The cement of the universe: A study of causation*. Oxford University Press.

Mackie, J. L. (1977). Dispositions, grounds, and causes. *Synthese, 34*, 361–370.

Mackay, N., & Petocz, A. (eds.). (2010). *Realism and psychology: Collected essays*. Brill.

Maze, J. R. (1954). Do intervening variables intervene? *Psychological Review, 61*, 226–234.

Maze, J. R. (1983). *The meaning of behaviour*. Allen & Unwin.

McCrae, R. R. (2004). Human nature and culture: A trait perspective. *Journal of Research in Personality, 38*, 3–14.
McCrae, R. R. & Costa, P. T. Jr. (1995). Trait explanations in personality psychology. *European Journal of Personality, 9*, 231–252.
McCrae, R. R., & Costa, P. T., Jr. (1997). Personality trait structure as a human universal. *American Psychologist, 52*, 509–516.
McCrae, R. R. & Costa, P. T. Jr. (1999). A five-factor theory of personality. In L. A. Pervin & O. P. John (eds.), *Handbook of personality: Theory and research* (pp. 139–153). Guilford Press.
McCrae, R. R., & Costa, P. T., Jr. (2008). Empirical and theoretical status of the five-factor model of personality traits. In G. Boyle, G. Matthews, & D. Daklofske (eds.), *Sage handbook of personality theory and assessment* (pp. 273–294). Sage.
McCrae, R. R., & Costa Jr, P. T. (2021). Understanding persons: From Stern's personalistics to Five-Factor Theory. *Personality & Individual Differences*, *169*, 109816.
McDougall, W. (1923). *An outline of psychology*. Methuen & Co.
McMullen, T. (1982). A critique of humanistic psychology. *Australian Journal of Psychology, 34*, 221–229.
McMullen, T. (1996). Psychology and realism. In C. R. Latimer & J. Michell (eds.), *At once scientific and philosophic: A festschrift for John Philip Sutcliffe* (pp. 59–66). Boombana.
Michell, J. (1988). Maze's direct realism and the character of cognition. *Australian Journal of Psychology, 40*, 227–249.
Michell, J. (1999). *Measurement in psychology*. Cambridge University Press.
Michell, J. (2000). Normal science, pathological science and psychometrics. *Theory and Psychology, 10*, 639–667.
Michell, J. (2004). The place of qualitative research in psychology. *Qualitative Research in Psychology, 1*, 307–319.
Michell, J. (2005). The logic of measurement: A realist overview. *Measurement, 38*, 285–294.
Mischel, W. (2004). Toward an integrative science of the person. *Annual Review of Psychology, 55*, 1–22.
Morey, L. C., Benson, K. T., Busch, A. J., & Skodol, A. E. (2015). Personality disorders in DSM-5: Emerging research on the alternative model. *Current Psychiatry Reports, 17*, 1–9.
Nilsson, A. (2014). Personality psychology as the integrative study of traits and worldviews. *New Ideas in Psychology, 32*, 18–32.
Nowak, A., Vallacher, R. R., & Zochowski, M. (2005). The emergence of personality: Dynamic foundations of individual variation. *Developmental Review, 25*, 351–385.
Panksepp, J., & Biven, L. (2012). *The archaeology of mind: Neuroevolutionary origins of human emotions*. WW Norton & Company.
Passmore, J. A. (1935). The nature of intelligence. *Australasian Journal of Psychology & Philosophy, 13*, 279–289.
Petocz, A., & Mackay, N. (2013). Unifying psychology through situational realism. *Review of General Psychology, 17*, 216–223.
Petocz, A., & Newbery, G. (2010). On conceptual analysis as the primary qualitative approach to statistics education research in psychology. *Statistics Education Research Journal, 9*, 123–145.

Rauthmann, J. F. (2024). Personality is (so much) more than just self-reported Big Five traits. *European Journal of Personality, 38*, 863–866.

Saucier, G., Hampson, S. E., & Goldberg, L. R. (2000). Cross-language studies of lexical personality factors. In S. E. Hampson (Ed.), *Advances in personality psychology* (Vol. I). Psychology Press.

Skinner, B. F. (1953). *Science and behavior.* The Free Press.

Shedler, J., Beck, A., Fonagy, P., Gabbard, G. O., Gunderson, J., Kernberg, O., . . . & Westen, D. (2010). Personality disorders in DSM-5. *American Journal of Psychiatry, 167*, 1026–1028.

Terracciano, A., & McCrae, R. R. (2012). Why do (some) birds flock? Causality and the structure of characteristic adaptations. *European Journal of Personality, 26*, 449–450.

Trull, T. J. & Durrett, C. A. (2005). Categorical and dimensional models of personality disorder. *Annual Review of Clinical Psychology, 1*, 355–380.

Tyrer, P., Mulder, R., Kim, Y. R., & Crawford, M. J. (2019). The development of the ICD-11 classification of personality disorders: An amalgam of science, pragmatism, and politics. *Annual Review of Clinical Psychology, 15*, 481–502.

Vallacher, R. R., Read, S. J., & Nowak, A. (2002). The dynamical perspective in personality and social psychology. *Personality and Social Psychology Review*, 6, 264–273.

Watson, D., & Clark, L. A. (2020). Personality traits as an organizing framework for personality pathology. *Personality & Mental Health, 14*, 51–75.

Widiger, T. A. (2005). Five factor model of personality disorder: Integrating science and practice. *Journal of Research in Personality, 39*, 67–83.

Widiger, T. A., & Costa, P. T. (2012). Integrating normal and abnormal personality structure: The five-factor model. *Journal of Personality, 80*, 1471–1506.

Widiger, T. A., & Crego, C. (2019). The Five Factor Model of personality structure: An update. *World Psychiatry*, 18, 271–272.

Widiger, T. A., & McCabe, G. A. (2020). The alternative model of personality disorders (AMPD) from the perspective of the five-factor model. *Psychopathology, 53*, 149–156.

Widiger, T. A., Sellbom, M., Chmielewski, M., Clark, L. A., DeYoung, C. G., Kotov, R., . . . & Wright, A. G. (2019). Personality in a hierarchical model of psychopathology. *Clinical Psychological Science, 7*, 77–92.

Widiger, T. A., Crego, C., Rojas, S. L., & Oltmanns, J. R. (2018). Basic personality model. *Current Opinion in Psychology, 21*, 18–22.

Woodward, J. (2003). *Making things happen: A theory of causal explanation*. Oxford University Press.

Wright A. G. (2011). Qualitative and quantitative distinctions in personality disorder. *Journal of Personality Assessment, 93*, 370–379.

Yankelovich, D. (1973). The idea of human nature. *Social Research, 40*, 407–428.

Zachar, P., & Krueger, R. F. (2013). Personality disorder and validity: A history of controversy. In K. W. M. Fulford, M. Davies, R. Gipps, G. Graham, J. Z. Sadler, G. Stanghellini, & T. Thornton (eds.), *The Oxford handbook of philosophy & psychiatry* (pp. 889–910). Oxford University Press.

13 A Dual-Aspect Approach to Personality Disorder

Locating the Normal in the Abnormal

Huw Green

13.1 Two Views of Personality Disorder

For the purposes of this chapter, I want to make a distinction between two approaches to thinking about personality disorder. I take it as read that my distinction is just an approximation of existing attitudes in this field, but it is an approximation that I think is helpful and likely gets at something real.

On the one hand there is what I will call the orthodox approach to personality disorder. This comes in a variety of flavors, but some common elements are: that personality disorder represents a diagnosable set of facts about a person that disrupts their social relating in a clinically significant way. That these facts of disrupted relating have something to do with deployment of defense mechanisms, dysregulated affect, distorted perceptions of self and other, or of a high "loading" on some personality trait(s) (such as aggressivity) and a low "loading" on some other personality trait(s) (e.g., "agreeableness"). The orthodox approach to personality disorder posits a disorder that resides in an individual, which has to do with their personality. The disordered behavior and coping styles may be rooted in biological facts. The standard diagnostic criteria for personality disorders, the work of Otto Kernberg (1984, 1992) and of Marsha Linehan (1993) are all good examples of the orthodox approach. I would anticipate that many clinicians would adhere to some version of the orthodox view.

On the other hand are what I will call relational/ameliorative (RA) views of personality disorder. These are somewhat dissenting perspectives, and as such come in a broader variety. RA views of personality disorder have in common an attempt to dissolve the very concept of personality disorder by revealing it to be either socially constructed or fundamentally relational in nature. They tend toward what Hacking (1999) termed a "revolutionary" attitude to the concept. That is, they frame the concept of personality disorder as not inevitable, they suggest the concept is a bad thing, and they imply that we would be better off without it.

A key example of this revolutionary RA approach is the work of Judith Herman (2015). Herman has done much to make salient the role of trauma in the sorts of symptoms that are liable to attract a label of personality disorder. Her work has had a broad cultural influence on psychiatry and psychology. Herman (1992) proposed the diagnostic construct complex post-traumatic stress disorder (cPTSD), which was subsequently adopted by the World Health Organization (WHO)'s International Statistical Classification of Diseases (ICD) in 2018. Although Herman stops short (on my reading) of calling for the abandonment of the term personality disorder, she notes that: "In survivors of childhood abuse, these disturbances in relationship are further amplified. Oscillations in attachment, with formation of intense, unstable relationships, are frequently observed. These disturbances are described most fully in patients with borderline personality disorder, the majority of whom have extensive histories of childhood abuse" (Herman, 1992, p. 385).

Herman's work offers a framework in which the notion of "personality disorder" might be reframed not as an intrapersonal "disorder" but as a cluster of trauma sequelae that are more or less intelligible as such by the community in which the survivor finds themself. A dissolution of the notion of individual personality pathology is implied. The traumatized individual is manifesting the consequences of their social/interpersonal context. If the behaviors and emotions concerned can be understood in terms of the understandable consequences of earlier traumatic experiences then it is hoped that they can also be substantially mitigated by the social/relational context of the trauma survivor.

What Herman doesn't herself say but what I think is strongly implied in her work and in the ethos of the trauma-informed care framework which her work has facilitated is that the focus on trauma is intended to provide redress for a form of epistemic injustice, specifically hermeneutic injustice (Fricker, 2007). Epistemic injustice is a wrong done to someone in their capacity as a knower. Hermeneutic injustice is a particular form of epistemic injustice in which the form of the wrong done is that an individual is deprived of a particular interpretative framework for making sense of their experience. An example Fricker gives of a relevant interpretative framework is the concept of "sexual harassment." When this concept was introduced in the 1970s, women were able to make better sense of a pervasive and upsetting pattern of behavior perpetrated very largely by men.

By drawing attention to the role of trauma and proposing a new diagnostic entity stripped of reference to personality, Herman encourages a wholesale reconceptualization of a familiar symptom set. I think the upshot of her work is supposed to be twofold. She offers an alternative diagnosis and treatment approach. She also encourages a form of political consciousness raising, in the service of furthering hermeneutic justice for trauma survivors. One upshot of the latter intervention is that clinicians and society at large are encouraged to have a different attitude toward women who attract the diagnosis of personality disorder. They are not in possession of disordered personalities, they are manifesting dysregulated emotional responses that are intelligible in the light of a trauma history.

I take it that Herman's position therefore calls for not only a specific approach to treatment, but also makes a sort of moral relational demand on society more generally. It is imperative, in the trauma-informed clinical landscape that Herman helped to foster, for everyone (not only clinicians) to be sensitive to the emotional needs of trauma survivors. It is important to gerrymander diagnostic criteria so that the interpersonal manifestations of trauma are not considered disorders of individual personality.

To contrast the orthodox and RA views of personality disorder like this is to reveal, I think, a dialectic. The orthodox view of personality disorders arises out of a tradition that is analogous to physical medicine. It rules the theoretical roost by virtue of its presence in diagnostic manuals and textbooks. The trauma-informed ameliorative perspective arises as a sort of antithesis to this perspective. Certainly they are often presented as alternative or opposed views.

So one way of characterizing what I am up to in this chapter is to say I am trying to articulate a synthesis between these two approaches. I hope that by offsetting them against each other I can arrive at something closer to a singular articulation of what a personality disorder is, which does justice to both the conventional and RA perspectives. It is a mistake to suppose that one or the other of these attitudes gets it right about personality disorder. Clinical experience suggests that each pole of the dialectic exists for a reason. Different clinicians and advocates, working in different contexts, are exposed to different aspects of the total interpersonal experience of people diagnosed with personality disorders. These different people consequently develop different perspectives on the extent to which individuals with the diagnosis are culpable, understandable, and reasonable. I attempt to illustrate this below.

13.2 The Argument from Clinical Experience

In this section I will draw on an argument from personal experience, by contrasting two clinical contexts in which I have worked with people who meet the criteria for personality disorders. I appreciate that this is an unusual approach to a philosophical argument, but I suggest that some degree of personal reflection – something that aims toward an amateur anthropology – may be able to reveal informative things about the nature of personality disorders.

In the early stages of my career, during my graduate studies and my post-doctoral clinical fellowship, I worked in psychodynamically oriented psychotherapeutic settings that were informed by a detailed relational psychodynamic theory of personality disorder. In these settings it was taken for granted that personality or character were important elements of mental health and our ability to engage with therapy. Supervisions and clinical group discussions included substantial attention to interpersonal themes: transference, countertransference, and the emotional experiences elicited by clinical encounters. The effect of all this was a clinical psychotherapeutic style that involved interventions targeted at mitigating the interpersonal difficulties that can arise in the context of highly emotionally charged discussions. I could see for myself that "putting a foot wrong" in a discussion with someone diagnosed with a personality disorder could lead to emotional flare up and interpersonal conflict. I could also see that anticipating such ruptures – and being able to address them directly in discussion – could significantly mitigate their frequency and intensity.

The upshot of this clinical experience for me was a fuller understanding of the ways in which the symptoms of personality disorder can be substantially mitigated/ameliorated by the work of the clinician. Although I hope I didn't harbor illusions about the possibilities afforded by competent milieu treatment, I did gain an appreciation of the power of interpersonal intervention to avert some of the more deleterious interpersonal consequences of emotional sensitivity coupled with a highly demonstrative interpersonal style. One of the results of this aspect of my training was an essay (Green, 2018) in which I tried to reformulate the interpersonal phenomenon of splitting in relational terms. Splitting is a psychological tendency to view the world as populated by individuals who are either good or bad (as opposed to understanding people's moral nuances). In treatment settings it can be associated with differential behaviors toward different staff members and contribute to a complex interpersonal phenomenon in which entire staff teams "split" (i.e., disagree about the treatment of patients). I tried to show that such interpersonal splitting must be consequent not only on the psychology of the individual with the disorder, but also on relational phenomena outside of their influence. This essay was thus an ameliorative intervention in the debate about personality disorder.

Since qualifying, I have worked clinically in acute healthcare settings, where therapeutically addressing the symptoms/interpersonal phenomena of personality disorder is not considered a central task. The service I work in does not exist to specifically treat personality disorders, and none of my colleagues considers themselves to have specialist competency in this area. Our main task in this department is to undertake neuropsychological assessment, and my role specifically is an inpatient role, which means that I work with people who are admitted to a general hospital after suffering acute injuries. These patients often require inpatient rehabilitation, and a significant part of the role is to ensure they receive appropriate referrals.

Some percentage of our caseload is made up of people who, in addition to their other symptoms, likely met criteria for personality disorders prior to their admission. Such patients can be referred for assessment and support from our liaison psychiatry team and receive subsequent admission to a psychiatric hospital if necessary. However, during the time that I see them they are in an acute general hospital ward and subject to the exigencies and emotional demands of an often stressful setting. People's characters are tested under these circumstances. As has been observed by generations of clinicians now, the interpersonal consequences of this state of affairs are often very striking. Patients with highly reactive and sensitive emotional reactions are liable to get involved in fraught exchanges with staff, to develop a pattern of liking and being liked by some staff and disliking/being disliked by other staff (splitting phenomena), and to become emotionally volatile. The result of all this is that our service receives significantly more calls for input in relation to these patients, often for assistance with capacity assessments related to impulsive decisions to self-discharge, to help with calming volatile situations, or to help "manage behavior." This state of affairs will be unsurprising to readers – have I not simply redescribed the familiar emotional and interpersonal phenomena that are constitutive of personality disorders?

The thing I want to draw attention to in all this is my experience of the difference between the two clinical contexts. In the first clinical context, where personality disorder was taken seriously as a phenomenon arising between patient and clinician in transference–countertransference patterns, it was possible to so substantially ameliorate the symptoms of personality disorder through adjustments to my own relational style that I began to wonder whether this was a category that even picked out anything meaningful. Are there really personality disorders, or are there only incompetent clinicians? I felt as if the clinician might – with enough training and supervision – become able to work with individuals with any degree of severity of personality disorder. If this was true, then it started to seem inappropriate to attribute the problems to the patient. It's not that people have personality disorders, it's that clinicians are not sufficiently able to empathize with everyone and become prone to being too emotionally reactive or defensive. The problem – I felt – did not reside in the people with the diagnosis, it was in the milieu which could not adequately recognize and accommodate their emotional needs. I now recognize this as an omnipotent fantasy, fostered by the experience of acquiring a particular set of skills.

The shift to working in a different setting was a dramatic change in perspective. Once my clinical task changed, it no longer seemed reasonable to me to expect of myself that I take on such extensive responsibility for the emotional tenor of a clinical encounter. Furthermore, working in a setting with a high turnover of patients (most of whom were diagnosable with no concomitant psychiatric disorder other than the effects of their brain injury), I acquired more experience of the way in which most people are trying to manage social and clinical situations in a way that avoids conflict, and which does not involve focus on the minutiae of social interaction. One effect of this was to think about the phenomenon of personality disorders differently. My model for what a personality disorder is changed. I became quicker to "spot" the dynamics that constitute this cluster of disorders, and more inclined to see them as something that some people simply have and other people simply do not. That is to say, I swung back toward a conventional/orthodox perspective of personality disorders as something that some people simply have and others don't.

The purpose of this autobiographical foray is to highlight something that most clinicians probably know but tend not to acknowledge. Different clinical settings have not only different clinical aims, but also create fundamentally different epistemic contexts. When it is your priority to detect and treat problems of sort *A*, and not problems of sort *B*, you necessarily become less proficient at detecting and formulating problems of form *B*. In the case of most physical medical illnesses, this is a primarily technical matter of detection. A stroke doctor specializes in the clinical semiology of stroke and is less well able to diagnose and manage kidney disorders. The structure of most medical specialties is such that this problem can be addressed by simply referring patients to the appropriate specialist. They can advise concrete measures (particular medications or laboratory investigations) that can be delegated to a medically competent managing team. There can be little doubt, though, that the total staff of a stroke ward will be less competent than a nephrology ward at detecting the subtle signs of deterioration in kidney function. The ward staff do not have the relevant training and experience.

This problem is of a different order of magnitude when the medical diagnosis in question is not closely tied to dysregulated biological functions but inheres in the interpersonal patterns and defensive styles of persons. Not only can personality disorders be (in some sense) poorly managed, they can be exacerbated and (a bolder suggestion I feel tempted toward) *even more fully brought into being* by the wrong sort of context.

13.3 The Dual-Aspect Approach to Personality Disorder

I have now, I hope, set the scene for the more substantive theoretical claim I want to make in this chapter. I will propose that these contextual differences in my experience of personality disorder, and the lively countervailing RA literature, are suggestive of something significant about the nature of personality disorders and indeed of personality itself.

Although psychological research on personality has been extremely successful on its own terms, producing an extensive (and highly replicable) body of literature, there is surprisingly little extant conceptual work on what a personality actually is. Contemporary personality research tends to take as its starting point the notions of traits. Traits are thought to be stable dispositions to act in a particular way and trait theorists have come to dominate personality research, and a specific model (the Big Five model) has been the most influential.

Clinical work on personality disorders focuses less on traits (although there are exceptions) and instead construes personality as being a matter of a characteristic pattern or style (e.g., Shapiro, 1965). Psychodynamic approaches to personality disorder posit a characteristic pattern of defenses, whereas cognitive behavioral therapies place more emphasis on schemas and coping strategies (e.g., Young et al., 2003).

The trait model and the clinical paradigms are primarily related to pragmatic programs of knowledge generation. It is possible (for research purposes) to define personality types by reference to a preponderance of traits, and personality disorders (for clinical purposes) by reference to a characteristic (putatively pathological) style. A trait description of a paranoid individual might invoke their having a high degree of trait neuroticism and low degrees of trait openness to experience and agreeableness. A formulation based on defensive styles would describe the same person in terms of (among other things) a tendency toward the frequent use of projection (attributing one's own negative emotions to others), a proneness to excessive hostility and rigidity. However, a comprehensive and satisfactory definition of what a personality is – and how we should think about the ontology of the emergent collection of phenomena that gets called "personality" – has not been widely agreed.

There have been some attempts by clinicians and personality researchers to rectify this. Michael Stone (1993) attempts a definition of personality by reference to the metaphor of a protective outer belt. Personality is, in this conception, the pattern of behaviors that we have developed to help us interact successfully with other people while keeping safe an inner feeling of integrity. For example, a cheerful, jocular veneer is an effective way to manage awkward interactions with unfamiliar people. What these various conceptions have usually under-emphasized is the extent to which there is a relational/interpersonal component involved in the creation of our personality.

When we talk about personality we are talking about something that arises out of (at least) two distinctive sorts of process. One important aspect of personality is the biology and psychology of the individual who "has" it. We can frame this in terms of existing views about the interaction between brain and character. I have a particular array of physiological "settings" that are the direct result of the calibration of my biology. I am to some degree novelty-seeking, cautious, conflict-averse, sensitive to noise, and so on, simply because my genetic makeup and particular ontogenetic history has produced a specific physiology. I express those features of my physiology in a repertoire of behaviors that I have acquired from my personal social history, embedded within a broader culture. The resulting combination is a more or less socially intelligible phenotype that gets called my "personality."

Critically, the expression of this complex phenotype is mediated directly by context. The array of physiological sensitivities that predispose me to conflict aversion feed into a pattern of behavior that is amenable and cooperative (high in "agreeableness" in trait language) when in the right context. When placed under particular conditions of duress (negotiating in a work context) the resultant personality style may become a problematic degree of pliability, even adding up to a reluctance that becomes traits of "dependent personality disorder."

The same combination of physiological and cultural contributors, I suggest, also operates in personality disorder. We must resist here the tempting pull towards a strong cultural determinism. The cluster of ameliorative approaches to personality disorder would appear to suggest that "there are no mad people, only mad societies!" (the familiar refrain of the psychiatric liberator). We need a model of personality disorder that does justice to both the reality of personality disorders (some people are simply suffering from interpersonal difficulties more often than others) and the fact that they are substantially constituted by how other people respond to them.

The resolution I suggest here is a concept of personality disorders, and in fact of personality wholesale, that explicitly avows the basically dual aspect of their nature. Personalities are the sort of things that are significantly determined by the biological, psychological, and historical facts about the people who have them. These facts do not evaporate and cannot be wished away. At the same time, personalities (and personality disorders) are the names we give to the way that people manifest these tendencies in the context of their interpersonal relationships. Personality is inherently relational; it not only responds to social context but is constituted by it. Personality (and personality disorder) exists at the point where the individual and the social meet.

This characterization points us toward a fundamentally dual reality at the core of personality disorders that has yet to be fully formulated. Personalities belong to people, who will still have tendencies and predispositions, even in the absence of a social context. This is a stubborn fact about humans as creatures with a nervous system and a history. These tendencies and predispositions don't entirely go away, even with the mitigation of a forgiving social context. Nonetheless, the milieu in which a person finds themselves has a significant effect on the expression of their personality. Indeed, this is part of the difficulty with personality disorders: if their manifestation were more predictable, they wouldn't be so difficult to address.

A good example of a partially ameliorative approach, which nonetheless takes account of the reality of personality disorder, is embodied in the work of Potter (2009). Her critical analysis of the construct of borderline personality disorder leads her to advocate for the cultivation – in clinicians – of particular virtues when working with patients who carry this diagnosis. These virtues allow for the creation of a relational context that is better able to provide patients with what they need, both in the clinical sense (what will be helpful for them in terms of their disorder) and in the moral sense (what they are entitled to expect interpersonally). Potter's analysis does not rely on the sort of polemical rejection or deconstruction of the notion of a disorder that sometimes accompanies sympathetic scholarly treatment of this group of patients. Nonetheless, she clearly views it as morally incumbent on clinicians to optimize the relational context for treatment of a personality disorder that is often characterized as especially "difficult" or conflictual. Taken further, Potter's approach potentially offers some of the resources required by a model of personality disorder that integrates the individual and the social.

13.4 Conclusion

I have proposed that we can discern two approaches to thinking about personality disorder. One places more emphasis on disorders that occur in people, the other on the society that produces (and labels) these disorders. There is sufficient divergence between these perspectives (in terms of political aims, clinical assumptions and broader philosophical commitments) that they can become split off from each other, and even openly antagonistic. The field of personality disorder, and of personality more generally, has struggled to provide a concise conceptual formulation that can account for the individual and social variables that constitute personality. The result is a failure to integrate two apparently contrasting views. I have tried to offer a brief sketch of such a formulation here.

References

Fricker, M. (2007). *Epistemic injustice: Power and the ethics of knowing*. Oxford University Press.

Green, H. (2018). Team splitting and the 'borderline personality': A relational reframe. *Psychoanalytic Psychotherapy*, *32*(3), 249–266.

Hacking, I. (1999). *The social construction of what?* Harvard University Press.

Herman, J. L. (1992). Complex PTSD: A syndrome in survivors of prolonged and repeated trauma. *Journal of Traumatic Stress*, *5*(3), 377–391.

Herman, J. L. (2015). *Trauma and recovery: The aftermath of violence – From domestic abuse to political terror*. Hachette UK.

Kernberg, O. F. (1984). *Severe personality disorders: Psychotherapeutic strategies*. Yale University Press.

Kernberg, O. F. (1992). *Aggression in personality disorders and perversions*. Yale University Press.

Linehan, M. M. (1993). *Cognitive-behavioral treatment of borderline personality disorder*. Guilford Publications.

Potter, N. N. (2009). *Mapping the edges and the in-between: A critical analysis of borderline personality disorder*. Oxford University Press.

Shapiro, D. (1965). *Neurotic styles*. Basic Books.

Stone, M. H. (1993). *Abnormalities of personality: Within and beyond the realm of treatment*. W.W. Norton & Co.

Young, J. E., Klosko, J. S., & Weishaar, M. E. (2003). *Schema therapy*. Guilford.

14 Network Architectures of Personality and Its Pathology

Annemarie C. J. Köhne and Adela-Maria Isvoranu

14.1 Introduction

The stance we take on the ontological status of mental disorders is at the heart of most controversy within the field of clinical psychology and psychiatry: What are mental disorders exactly? And, as a consequence, what is comorbidity, and how does it arise? Because the way we understand mental disorders determines our outlook on both research and treatment (e.g., if we hypothesize that major depression is a brain disorder, research would dedicate itself to finding the responsible brain anomaly, while treatment would focus on eradicating that anomaly), it is of the utmost importance that our ontological hypotheses are roughly correct. The ontological issue plays a vital role in debates around the comorbidity of mental disorders and personality disorders as well. These debates often revolve around the question whether this type of comorbidity is a socially constructed artifact of the *Diagnostic and statistical manual* (DSM) or a real existent phenomenon. The way we understand the comorbidity of mental disorders and personality disorders determines our treatment of patients, which makes a reflection of our conceptualization of this type of comorbidity highly relevant.

The DSM holds a categorical frame of thought and implies that DSM classifications like "major depressive disorder" and "borderline personality disorder" are naturally occurring, real existent and separable mental disorders that behave as discrete categories (see Figure 14.1). Critiques on the categorical nature of the DSM model are explicated in many works and can briefly be summarized as critiques on its non-empirical basis, reification effects, limited reliability, limited validity, and diagnostic instability (e.g., Hyman, 2010; Kapur et al., 2012; Kessler et al., 2005; Kotov et al., 2017; Krueger et al., 2014; Olbert et al., 2014; Skodol, 2012; Widiger & Shea, 1991).

An opposing view on the comorbidity of mental disorders and personality disorders is represented by dimensional trait models. A dimensional frame of thought implies that disorders should not be treated as categories that are qualitatively distinct from each other and from normalcy (e.g., the categories of depression and borderline personality disorder). Instead of categories, the

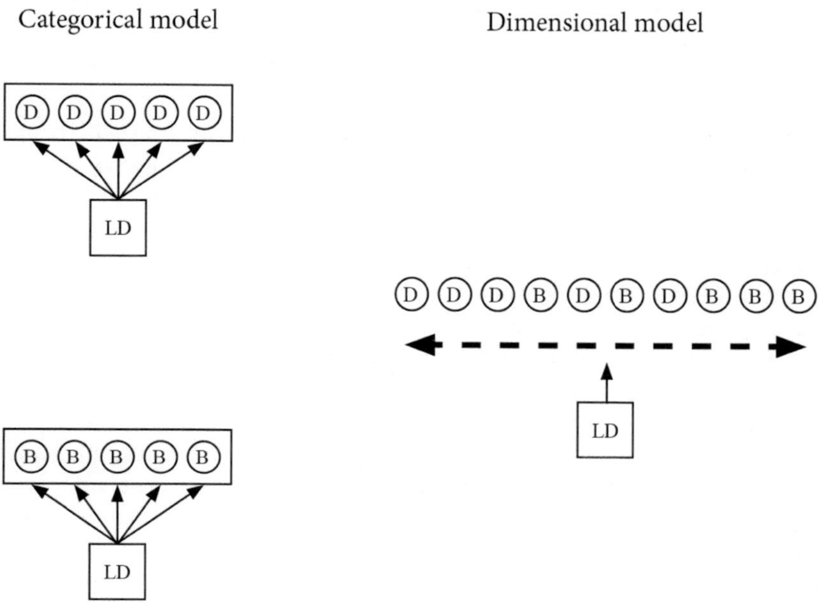

Figure 14.1 A visualization of the categorical model and the dimensional model in their understanding of mental disorder. In the categorical model the two disorders are thought to be distinct and qualitatively different. In the dimensional model the two disorders are composites of related symptom components/traits and belong to the subfactor Distress that belongs to the spectrum of Internalizing psychopathology. Both models assume a common cause/hidden factor/latent disorder (D, depression symptoms; B, borderline personality disorder symptoms; LD, latent disorder).

identifying features of all disorders are seen as existing and developing on continuous dimensions. For example, a depression symptom such as dysphoria and a borderline personality symptom such as affective instability are both located on the continuous dimension of distress. Some dimensional thinkers even argue that a differentiation of personality disorders from mental disorders is illusory (e.g., Widiger & Shea, 1991). The Hierarchical Taxonomy of Psychopathology (HiTOP) consortium understands symptoms to be "relatively transient forms of psychopathology, and maladaptive personality traits [to] form a more stable core of the clinical picture" (Kotov et al., 2017, p. 458). The consortium has built an alternative taxonomy that consists of hierarchically organized state–trait dimensions that move from the narrowest level of "symptoms" up to the broadest level of "super spectra" (very broad dimensions of multiple spectra; Kotov et al., 2017). The HiTOP consortium seeks to model the quantitative structure of psychopathology using factor analysis and does not make a firm distinction between personality pathology and all other psychopathology. The consortium aims to describe psychiatric phenomena dimensionally.

To sum up the above, within a dimensional frame of thought the underlying idea is that psychopathology develops on a continuum with normality and mental disorders are composites of related symptom components and traits. Within a categorical frame of thought disorder categories are traditionally seen as qualitatively distinct from normality and mental disorders and personality disorders are different kinds of disorders and are thought to be clearly separable from each other. Although these two conceptualizations of psychopathology differ with respect to the assumed "nature" of disorder, they have one thing in common: both adopt a latent disorder model (see e.g., American Psychiatric Association (APA), 2013, p. 20; Krueger, 1999). That is, they assume an underlying or hidden cause (e.g., "major depression") to act as the common cause of its observable symptoms (e.g., depressed mood, insomnia, and fatigue). Symptoms and or syndromes that occur at the same time are understood to co-occur because of this underlying disease entity often called "substrate" or "marker" and so on. Basically, three latent variable perspectives purport to explain the comorbidity between mental disorders and personality disorders: (a) personality disorders precede mental disorders (e.g., "the vulnerability hypothesis"; "the pathoplasticity hypothesis"), (b) mental state disorder precede personality disorders (e.g., "the scar hypothesis"; "the complication hypothesis"), or (c) mental disorders and personality disorders share common etiological grounds (e.g., Clark et al., 1994; De Bolle et al., 2012; Eurelings-Bontekoe et al., 2009; Klein et al., 2011). Although these three types of theoretical models differ with respect to their idea of causal direction, they all imply a latent variable perspective in which it is assumed that either personality disorders or mental disorders are latent variables that have certain causal relations (models (a) and (b)); or that, as in model (c), the etiology is in fact a common cause that leads to the symptomatology of both personality and mental disorders.

However, an enormous corpus of research into markers, brain regions, genes, and developmental precursors fails to prove the existence of an underlying disease entity (Borsboom, 2017; Borsboom et al., 2019; Kendler, 2012; McNally et al., 2015; Zachar & Kendler, 2007). As Adam (2013) puts it: "the genetic, metabolic and cellular signatures of almost all mental syndromes remain largely a mystery." In addition, biological and cognitive alterations associated with mental disorder are widely prevalent within the general population (Kendler, 2015; Brainstorm Consortium et al., 2018). People can have these neurobiological alterations without having a mental disorder, which means that these alterations are unlikely to determine what we regard as mental disorder (e.g., Ralston & Meynen, 2011; Zachar, 2000). The above raises the question whether there are other theoretical and methodological approaches to understanding the relationship between mental disorders and personality disorders.

In light of this, the current chapter will (i) challenge the current frame of thought and introduce an alternative frame of thought in understanding mental disorders, (ii) outline the network perspective on the comorbidity of personality pathology and mental disorders, (iii) provide an empirical illustration of a comorbidity network of symptoms of depression and borderline personality disorder, and lastly (iv) argue that embracing novel research perspectives may be beneficial and aid progress in the field of mental health, while also providing some recommendation for further research. The structure of this chapter will follow these aims.

14.2 Ontology: From Essentialism to Relationalism

The latent disorder frame of thought can be seen as an essentialist approach to psychopathology. In this context, essentialism broadly and basically refers to understanding or explaining mental disorder in terms of an underlying essence. A group of symptoms are thought to belong together and to co-occur because of this assumed underlying essence. And this essentialist frame of thinking becomes self-feeding and circular when the group of symptoms becomes an identifier of the assumed underlying disorder essence.

Because the latent disorder frame is embedded both in the categorical and dimensional models, both models employ essentialism. Yet, with this frame of thought, the possibility that symptoms may be constitutive of mental disorder is completely left out (e.g., McNally et al., 2015). Thus, we miss out on the possibility that symptoms of mental disorders and personality disorders could cause each other instead of that they reflect or indicate an underlying cause. The point here is not to explicate an anti-realist stance with regards to latent variables, but to explicate an anti-essentialist stance in understanding and explaining mental disorder. An anti-essentialist stance objects the view that clusters of symptoms reflect and should be explained by an underlying disorder essence. If our ontological understanding of psychopathology is essentialist and thereby not only reductionist but also narrowing our view, we may be working with a scientific frame of thought that will stagnate progress. We will thus have to search for fundamental innovation if we wish our field to move forward.

In this chapter, we wish to explicate an alternative ontological stance: relationalism. This idea basically refers to understanding and viewing things in their relational nature. Relationalism refers to an interpretation of reality in which particulars are only thought to exist and have meaning in their relationality. In this case: no symptom or feature of disorder is an island to itself; they are embedded in larger networks. It objects to explaining and understanding things in isolation but means to view things in their ontological interconnectedness. One translation of relationalism would entail to view the existence of a symptom or syndrome by its relation to other symptoms or syndromes. Instead of conceptualizing and studying particular symptoms and/or syndromes as isolated diseases that reflect underlying disease causes, relationalism entails that we understand psychiatric symptoms and/or syndromes as existing and functioning in relationship to each other. Within a relationalist ontology, mental state and personality traits become ontologically related systems (see also Köhne, 2020). With this approach, complex network models are invited into the picture.

14.3 Methodology: The Network Framework

Network theory harmonizes with a relationalist ontology and is accompanied by quickly developing psychometric models (Borsboom, 2017; Cramer et al., 2010, 2012). The first and central principle of the network theory is that mental disorders are complex systems: "[They] are multifactorial in constitution, aetiology, and causal background" (Borsboom, 2017, p. 7). The network theory holds that the relation between symptoms and diagnosis is mereological: symptoms are the particulars that are the diagnosis instead of that symptoms reflect an underlying disorder (Borsboom & Cramer, 2013). In analogy: jackals, coyotes, dogs, foxes, and wolves are not caused by the canine family, they are the parts that constitute it. Within the network approach, disorders are conceptualized as clusters of directly related symptoms (see Figure 14.2). Viewing and understanding comorbidity from a network perspective means that comorbidity arises from direct relations between symptoms of multiple disorders (Cramer et al., 2010). From the network perspective, the co-occurrence of two disorders is conceptualized as a symptom-to-symptom association between two disorders. For example, symptoms of major depression and generalized anxiety disorder may hang together in the following way: sleeping problems ➔ fatigue and agitation ➔ loss of interest in activities and people (Cramer et al., 2010). Here we see that in network theory, clusters of symptoms and/or syndromes do not derive from a latent cause, but are the product of forces, interactions, and flows in a network.

In response to the network theory, statistical tools – now known as the field of network psychometrics (Isvoranu et al., 2022) – have been developed, which allow investigating these particular associations between symptoms (Epskamp & Fried, 2018). Psychometric networks are constructed using nodes and edges. Nodes represent entities such as people, cities, theoretical constructs, or, in this

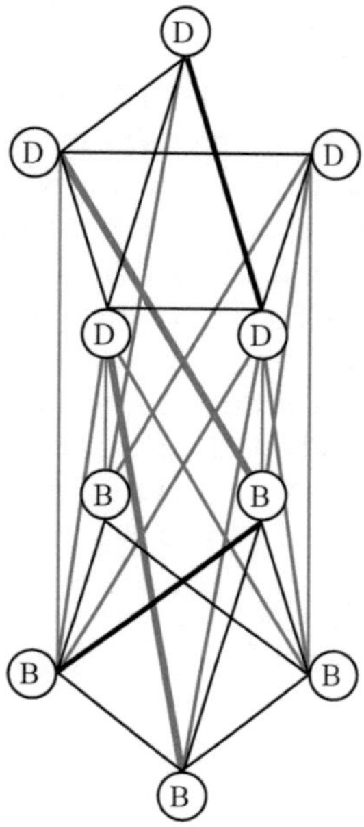

Figure 14.2 A visualization of the network model in which mental disorders are conceptualized as clusters of directly related symptoms (D, depression; B borderline personality disorder).

case, symptoms. Edges represent some sort of connection or relation between a pair of nodes like friendship, interaction, distance, or in this case, a statistical association. The activation of one node can transmit to other nodes, which in effect can alter the homeostasis of a network. A symptom like sleeping problems may activate other nodes like feeling tired, worry, or difficulty concentrating. In this way, symptoms may reinforce each other through feedback loops, leading to a prolonged state of symptom activation that we phenomenologically recognize as a mental disorder (Borsboom, 2017).

In the last decade, numerous studies investigated the network structures of a wide variety of mental disorders (Robinaugh et al., 2020), highlighting numerous associations between symptoms. Studies into the network architectures of personality have grown prominent as well (Cramer et al., 2012; Richetin et al., 2017). However, the investigation of joint network structures of mental disorders and personality disorders is not yet common. In this chapter we illustrate the network perspective on the comorbidity of mental disorders and personality disorders, with an example of a network structure on the symptom components of borderline personality disorders (BPD) that are related to symptoms of major depression disorder (MDD), in a clinical sample of patients suffering from co- and multimorbidity.

We focus on these two mental disorders (MDD and BPD) because they are well described, extensively studied, belong to the most prevalent of personality disorders and mental disorders, are known for their high disease burden, and are accompanied by high rates of mortality by suicide (e.g., Grant et al., 2008; Kessler & Bromet, 2013). Depression is projected to become the second cause of disability worldwide by the World Health Organization (e.g., Kessler & Bromet, 2013) and is characterized by loss of interest in activities and the presence of a sad, empty, or irritable mood, accompanied by somatic and cognitive changes that significantly affect the individual's capacity to function (APA, 2013). Lifetime prevalence of MDD in adults varies between 16 percent and to 25 percent (e.g., Patten, 2009). It is a highly recurrent mental disorder in which comorbidity with other mental disorders and substance use disorders is the norm rather than the exception. The disease burden of MDD is very high and from an economic and societal perspective, depression is perhaps one of the costliest mental disorders as well.

The disease burden of people with BPD is considerably high as well; it is associated with severe functional impairment and substantial treatment utilization (e.g., Grant et al., 2008). Borderline personality disorder is characterized by a pervasive, persistent, and pathological pattern of difficulties in the field of emotion regulation, impulse control and instability in relationships and self-image (APA, 2013; Skodol et al., 2002). In the United States the lifetime prevalence of BPD is about 6 percent (Grant et al., 2008). Of the people diagnosed with BPD, about 85 percent meet criteria for one or more mental disorders (trauma, addiction, and mood disorders are common) and about 74 percent also meet the criteria of another personality disorder (Coid, 2003; Grant et al., 2008; Lenzenweger et al., 2007; Zanarini et al., 1998). The rates of any 12-month mood disorder or MDD among respondents with lifetime BPD are about 51 percent and 31 percent, respectively, and the prevalence of BPD among respondents with mood disorders or MDD are about 29 percent and 19 percent, respectively (Grant et al., 2008).

14.4 An Empirical Illustration of a Comorbidity Network of Symptoms of MDD and BPD

This section will focus on an empirical illustration of a comorbidity network of symptoms of MDD and BPD, previously published online (Köhne & Isvoranu, 2021). We refer the reader to the published journal article for an extensive description of the technical methodological details, as this section will mainly focus on the results and their interpretation in light of network architectures of personality and its pathology.

To illustrate a comorbidity network of symptoms of MDD and BPD, data from 376 patients (67 percent male and 33 percent female) from the Dutch Healthcare institution *GGZ Momentum* who all had been hospitalized for 9 weeks of clinical treatment (123 women, 253 men, M age = 34.27, range: 18–72, SD = 9.90) were analyzed. The primary DSM classification for admission was an addiction of some sort and all patients suffered from co- and multi-morbidity. During the hospitalization of 9 weeks, patients were asked to complete a diagnostic screening assessment after 6 weeks of substance abstinence. This was done to facilitate and objectify descriptive diagnostics. The participants were assessed using four screening instruments; the Symptom Checklist (SCL-90; Derogatis & Unger, 2010), the Beck Depression Inventory – Second Edition (BDI-II; Beck et al., 1996), the Utrecht Coping List (UCL; Schreurs et al., 1993), and the Dutch questionnaire version of the Structured Clinical Interview for DSM-IV Axis II Personality Disorders (SCID-II; Weertman et al., 2003). For the current illustration, only data from the BDI-II and SCID-II measures were used. The SCID-II measures all DSM-IV criteria of all personality disorders and is composed of 119 items, of which 15 assess the nine BPD criteria (e.g., fear of abandonment, identity diffusion). Some of the nine criteria of BPD were measured by more than one SCID-II item. The BPD criterion "identity diffusion" is measured by four SCID-II items, the criterion "anger" by three SCID-II items, and the BPD criterion "self-harm/suicidality" is measured by two SCID-II items. All other BPD criteria are measured by only one item. We scored the BPD criterion positive if one or more of the corresponding items were scored positive. The BDI-II is one of the most widely used and empirically validated questionnaires for screening depression. The BDI-II is a self-report questionnaire measuring the symptoms (e.g., sadness, low energy) and severity (range: mild, moderate, severe) of depression with 21 items. Participants choose the statement that has been most representative of them in the past 7 days. Each item was rated on a 4-point Likert scale ranging from 0 to 3. To acquire higher statistical power to render the network analysis, this illustration only used the BDI-II items that matched best with the DSM criteria of MDD, resulting in a choice of 10 items. Thus, this analysis focused on core symptoms of depression and borderline personality disorder.

We constructed a network where each of the items is represented as a node and an edge between two nodes (i.e., items) denotes the partial correlation between them after controlling for all other items in the network. The nodes in the network model represent the symptom criteria of MDD and BPD and the edges represent the relationships between the symptom criteria (weighted and undirected associations). This comorbidity network structure of BPD and MDD was derived using the "graphical least absolute shrinkage and selection operator" (glasso) method that estimates a penalized maximum likelihood solution based on the extended Bayesian information criterion (EBIC; Chen & Chen, 2008). In this way, we were able to estimate a parsimonious ("sparse") network that accounts for most variance with the fewest number of edges. We used the EBICglasso regularization method, as implemented in the R software package *bootnet* version 1.4. (Epskamp, Borsboom, & Fried, 2018) and visualized the network structure using the R software package *qgraph* version 1.6.5. (Epskamp et al., 2012). The EBICglasso network estimation requires a tuning parameter, which was set to a default value of 0.5. Positive (negative) associations between symptom criteria (nodes) were represented as full (dotted) edges. The thickness of the edges represents the strength of the association. The thicker the edges between the nodes, the higher the partial correlation.

Figure 14.3 illustrates the network of relationships between the BPD symptoms and the MDD symptoms. An examination of the comorbidity network shows direct associations between the symptoms of MDD and BPD and shows that almost all connections are positive. The strongest positive link of this comorbidity network is the one between MDD sadness (BDI 1) and BPD emptiness (SBPD. C7). One could argue that sadness and emptiness measure a similar construct as patients that report severe depressive symptomatology may also report feelings of emptiness (Sharma & Copeland, 1989). If we, on the other hand, consider sadness and emptiness to represent dissimilar constructs, we may be able to formulate some other hypotheses. Previous studies show the BPD criterion of emptiness to be a robust predictor of depression (e.g. see Klonsky, 2008) and other studies reasoned that emptiness is a distinct characteristic in BPD patients with MDD (e.g. Silk, 2010).

If we form a hypothesis on this particular link with the empirically derived network model in mind, we may suppose that overwhelming feelings of sadness may (unconsciously) lead people to shut out their emotions, which leads to feelings of emptiness. This emptiness may sadden patients as they are devoid of emotions and purpose, which in effect nullifies the emptiness. This hypothesis is derived from and in line with the Schematherapy model to treat long-lasting symptoms of depression or anxiety and/or personality disorders: the "detached protector mode" trying to cope with the "vulnerable child mode" (Young et al., 2006). This hypothesis implies that the problem that manifests itself in this link is a troubled emotion regulation (overwhelm <-> detachment). In future research, it may be interesting to study whether therapies that address emotion regulation may not only help overcome BPD symptoms, but also have an indirect positive effect on symptoms of depression if this kind of comorbidity is present. Indeed, emotion regulation is found to be a transdiagnostic factor (e.g., see van Heycop ten Dam et al., 2014; Sloan et al., 2017). This may indicate a need to develop more integrated and unified treatments that target emotion regulation for individuals who present with depression and BPD.

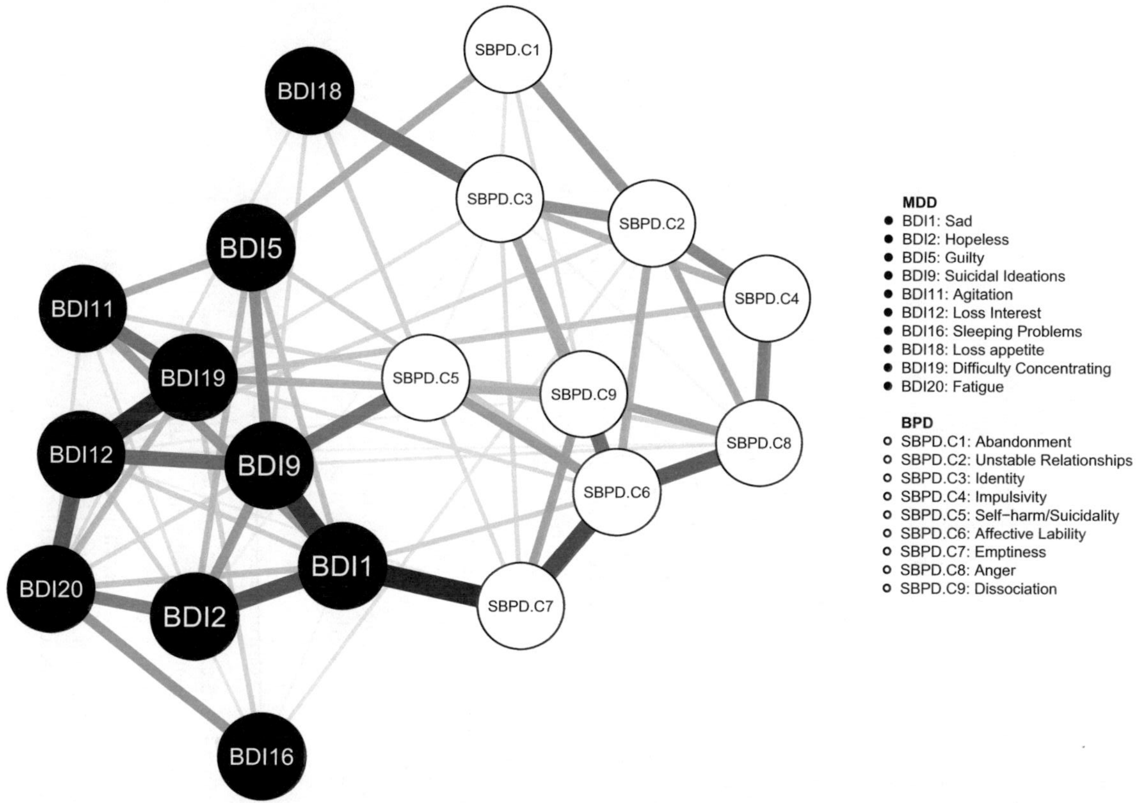

Figure 14.3 Network of the BPD and MDD symptoms. Symptom groups are differentiated by color. Each edge within the network corresponds to a regularized partial correlation between two individual symptoms, after controlling for all other symptoms in the network. The thickness of an edge represents the absolute magnitude of the correlation (thicker edges represent stronger links), whereas the color of the edge indicates the size of the correlation (full lines for positive links and dotted lines for negative links).

If we try to translate these outcomes to an individual patient, more depth into the clinical implications of this contribution may become apparent. For example, Emma experiences instability in her emotions and becomes very angry from time to time. Because of this, she experiences difficulties in relationships and as a result she often feels unconnected and empty. This makes her sad and she often experiences hopelessness. Emma feels guilty and ashamed of herself and hides these feelings to everyone in her surroundings which in effect augments her feelings of unconnectedness, emptiness, and depression. Contrary to common sense, it is innovative to understand these different symptoms as locally dependent. For in the common cause model, symptoms are thought to be locally independent when conditioned on the latent variable; in other words, they hang together and co-occur only because they are caused by the latent variable. However, if the symptoms of these two disorders are meaningfully connected, it may be relevant to identify and target the important links therapeutically. Whether this will lead to more effective treatment options for this type of comorbid psychopathology remains an interesting empirical question for future research.

Aligned with this frame of thought, theoretical models on the comorbidity of personality disorders and mental disorders may have to make room for an alternative understanding of how psychological disorders and the comorbidity between them arises. The comorbidity of personality disorders and mental disorders may arise from direct relations between symptoms of the two psychological disorders. We may not need latent variables or diseases to explain this type of comorbidity. Rather than MDD being secondary to BPD or the other way round (models (a) and (b)), the two disorders can be coupled together (in contrast to the view in the categorical model) and can be seen as maintaining each other with feedback loops instead of being explained by a common cause (model (c); in contrast to the view in the categorical model and dimensional model). Complexity-based approaches, explicated through an illustration of a network model, but not necessarily limited to the framework of network psychometrics, could pave a new road to follow in our attempt to understand the onset of mental disorders and their comorbidity.

14.5 Toward a Relationalist Perspective

This chapter aims to explicate an alternative ontological stance with regards to understanding mental disorder in general and the comorbidity of mental disorders and personality disorders specifically. We specifically argue for a relationalist ontology in which particulars are only thought to exist and have meaning in their relationality. This approach rejects the essentialist notion that is embedded in the categorical and dimensional model. Symptoms and/or syndromes are not to be viewed as separate particulars that derive from a latent cause, but particulars/entities which exist and function in relationship to each other. Within this relationalist frame of thought, mental states and personality traits are understood as ontologically related systems, rather than independent distinct mental disorders. This ontological conceptualization of mental disorder and personality disorder was illustrated by the construction of a network architecture of BPD and MDD. In sum, the analyses show associations within and between the symptom clusters of MDD and BPD. If we take the links in the network to be "substantive," it suggests a radical shift of our current dominant latent disorder conceptualization (a conceptualization heavily reliant on the DSM, especially in clinical care) of the comorbidity between mental disorders and personality disorders.

The example shows relationships between symptoms and relationships between syndromes (decompartmentalization of syndromes). This suggests leaving the idea that mental state disorders and personality disorders are clearly separable diseases (as they are represented in the categorical model) that are caused by underlying causes (as is the understanding in both the categorical and dimensional model). The psychiatric discourse is dominated by the latent disorder frame of thought, yet the links that we found between the symptoms and syndromes challenge this fundamental assumption: not only in terms of understanding the "cause and origin" of mental disorder ("non-essentialist"), but also in terms of understanding its "working mechanism" ("inner logic"). Again, this does not necessarily imply an anti-realist stance with regards to latent variables: some symptoms may be best explained by a latent factor, yet other symptoms may be best explained by forces and flows within the network.

However, our comorbidity network of cross-sectional data is still a "relatively static" representation of psychopathology. If we take the next step and consider mental well-being and the mind to be like a complex adaptive system, we have to take into account that symptoms may evolve and change over time and that equilibria are rare and temperate. In addition, we may have to move beyond the realm of symptoms and consider other aspects that play a role in symptom development and progression (e.g., risk factors). When it comes to treatment, it may therefore be more effective to focus on adapting to and dealing with changes within the mental system than to focus on the dissolution of particular symptoms.

The current illustration aimed to produce a relatively non-essentialist and bottom-up conception of psychopathology. Nonetheless, by using DSM symptom components within the analyses, we stick to a somewhat reductionist and essentialist frame of thought. Although the current example explicitly refrained from the reification of DSM syndromes and refrained from essentialist explanations, due to conventional measures it was restricted to using DSM symptom components in the analysis. Thereby the implicit assumption is that mental disorders can be ontologically described in terms of DSM symptoms. To be truly non-reductionist at heart means to transcend a mere (DSM) symptom-based account of mental disorders when building these kinds of comorbidity networks in future research.

This issue is more relevant than it may seem at first sight. Our current phenotypes are fuzzy and based on a single aspect (symptoms) of a human being that suffers from mental disorder. We seem to (implicitly) hold the idea that patients with similar symptomatic phenotypes form a homogeneous group. In analogy, this would mean to treat and feed a group of flowers on the basis of the color of their petals. As we realize we do not have clear phenotypes, nor can we equate these fuzzy phenotypes to genotypes, our field is currently faced with an enormous challenge. Patients may present with some of the same symptoms but may differ in terms of their neurobiological, psycho-experiential, and sociocultural factors (e.g., Jentsch et al., 2015). Thus, in a broader perspective, we are ready for new ontological descriptors and new building blocks in understanding psychopathology. This contribution did, however, intend to make a step toward a more representative frame of reference: from a conception of isolation toward a conception of complex integration of the DSM constructs of personality disorder and mental disorder. To fully grasp the mechanism of a patient's mental disorder, we may need building blocks other than symptom components. If we stick to the basic idea of a multifactorial constitution, it means we have to take into account the interacting layers of the neurobiological, psycho-experiential, and sociocultural when understanding the causes and mechanisms of mental disorder.

14.6 Conclusion

This contribution emphasizes the importance of embracing novel theoretical and methodological frameworks in the field of comorbidity research and brings an exemplification of this in the form of a network analysis of the links between symptoms of MDD and BPD. If the symptoms of mental disorders and personality disorders are indeed meaningfully connected, it may be relevant to identify and target the most important links therapeutically by which we may prevent this type of comorbidity in which one disorder activates the next disorder. For the field to progress, we argue that embracing a thinking frame that more adequately and accurately approximates the complexity of the human mind is imperative. It is thus important to look for new building blocks and ways to meaningfully integrate the interacting layers of the neurobiological, psycho-experiential, and sociocultural when understanding the causes and mechanisms of mental disorder.

References

Adam, D. (2013). On the spectrum: Research suggests that mental illnesses lie along a spectrum – but the field's latest diagnostic manual still splits them apart. *Nature, 496* (7446), 416–418.

American Psychiatric Association. (2013). *Diagnostic and statistical manual of mental disorders* (5th ed.).American Psychiatric Association.

Beck, A., Steer, R., & Brown, G. (1996). Beck Depression Inventory-II. San Antonio, 12–15. https://doi.org/10.1037/t00742-000.

Borsboom, D. (2017). A network theory of mental disorders. *World Psychiatry, 16*(1), 5–13. https://doi.org/10.1002/wps.20375.

Borsboom, D., & Cramer, A. O. J. (2013). Network analysis: An integrative approach to the structure of psychopathology. *Annual Review of Clinical Psychology, 9*(1), 91–121. https://doi.org/10.1146/annurev-clinpsy-050212-185608.

Borsboom, D., Cramer, A. O. J., & Kalis, A. (2019). Brain disorders? Not really: Why network structures block reductionism in psychopathology research. *Behavioral and Brain Sciences, 42*(e2), 1–63. https://doi.org/10.1017/S0140525X17002266.

Brainstorm Consortium, Anttila, V., Bulik-Sullivan, B., Finucane, H. K., Walters, R. K., Bras, J., . . . Murray, R. (2018). Analysis of shared heritability in common disorders of the brain. *Science*, 360(6395).

Chen, J., & Chen, Z. (2008). Extended Bayesian information criteria for model selection with large model spaces. *Biometrika, 95*(3), 759–771. https://doi.org/10.1093/biomet/asn034.

Clark, L.A., Watson, D., & Mineka, S. (1994). Temperament, personality, and the mood and anxiety disorders. *Journal of Abnormal Psychology, 103*, 103–116.

Coid, J. (2003). Epidemiology, public health and the problem of personality disorder. *British Journal of Psychiatry, 182*(44), 3–10.

Cramer, A. O. J., Van der Sluis, S., Noordhof, A., Wichers, M., Geschwind, N., Aggen, S. H., . . . Borsboom, D. (2012). Dimensions of normal personality as networks in search of equilibrium: You can' t like parties if you don' t like people. *European Journal of Personality, 26*, 414–431. https://doi.org/10.1002/per.1866.

Cramer, A. O. J., Waldorp, L. J., Van Der Maas, H. L. J., & Borsboom, D. (2010). Comorbidity: A network perspective. *Behavioral and Brain Sciences, 33*(2–3), 137–150. https://doi.org/10.1017/S0140525X09991567.

De Bolle, M., Beyers, W., De Clercq, B., & De Fruyt, F. (2012). General personality and psychopathology in referred and nonreferred children and adolescents: An investigation of continuity, pathoplasty, and complication models. *Journal of Abnormal Psychology, 121*(4), 958–970. https://doi.org/10.1037/a0027742.

Derogatis, L., & Unger, R. (2010). Symptom Checklist-90-Revised. In I. B. Weiner & W. E. Craighead (eds.), *Corsini Encyclopedia of Psychology* (pp. 18–19). Wiley.

Epskamp, S., Borsboom, D., & Fried, E. I. (2018). Estimating psychological networks and their accuracy: A tutorial paper. *Behavior Research Methods, 50*(1), 195–212. https://doi.org/10.3758/s13428-017-0862-1.

Epskamp, S., Cramer, A. O. J., Waldorp, L. J., Schmittmann, V. D., & Borsboom, D. (2012). qgraph: Network visualizations of relationships in psychometric data. *Journal of Statistical Software, 48*(4), 1–18. https://doi.org/10.18637/jss.v048.i04.

Epskamp, S., & Fried, E. I. (2018). Supplemental material for a tutorial on regularized partial correlation networks. *Psychological Methods*, *23*(4), 617–634. https://doi.org/10.1037/met0000167.supp.

Eurelings-Bontekoe, E., Snellen, W., & Verheul, R. (2009). *Handboek persoonlijkheidspathologie* (2nd ed.). Bohn Stafleu van Loghum.

Grant, B. F., Chou, P. S., Goldstein, R. B., Boji Huang, M. P. H., Stinson, F. S., Saha, T. D., . . . Ruan, W. J. (2008). Prevalence, correlates, disability, and comorbidity of DSM-IV borderline personality disorder: Results from the Wave 2 National Epidemiologic Survey on Alcohol and Related Conditions. *Journal of Clinical Psychiatry*, *70*(4), 383–385.

Van Heycop ten Dam, B., Hulsbergen, M., & Bohlmeier, E. (2014). *Transdiagnostische factoren. Theorie & praktijk*. Boom.

Hyman, S. E. (2010). The diagnosis of mental disorders: the problem of reification. *Annual Review of Clinical Psychology*, *6*, 155–179. https://doi.org/10.1146/annurev.clinpsy.3.022806.091532.

Isvoranu, A. M., Epskamp, S., Waldorp, L. J., & Borsboom, D. (eds.). (2022). *Network psychometrics with R: A guide for behavioral and social scientists*. Routledge, Taylor & Francis Group.

Jentsch, M. C., Van Buel, E. M., Bosker, F. J., Gladkevich, A. V., Klein, H. C., Oude Voshaar, R. C., . . . Schoevers, R. A. (2015). Biomarker approaches in major depressive disorder evaluated in the context of current hypotheses. *Biomarkers in Medicine*, *9*(3), 277–297. https://doi.org/10.2217/bmm.14.114.

Kapur, S., Phillips, A. G. & Insel, T. R. (2012). Why has it taken so long for biological psychiatry to develop clinical tests and what to do about it? *Molecular Psychiatry*, *17* (12), 1174–1179. https://doi.org/10.1038/mp.2012.105.

Kendler, K. (2015). A joint history of the nature of genetic variation and the nature of schizophrenia. *Molecular Psychiatry*, *20*(1), 77–83. https://doi.org/10.1038/mp.2014.94.

Kendler, K. S. (2012). The dappled nature of causes of psychiatric illness: Replacing the organic–functional/hardware–software dichotomy with empirically based pluralism. *Molecular Psychiatry*, *17*, 377–388. https://doi.org/10.1038/mp.2011.182.

Kessler, R. C., & Bromet, E. J. (2013). The epidemiology of depression across cultures. *Annual Review of Public Health*, *34*, 119–138. https://doi.org/10.1146/annurev-publhealth-031912-114409.

Kessler, R., Chiu, W., Demler, O., & Walters, E. (2005). Prevalence, severity, and comorbidity of twelve-month DSM-IV disorders in the National Comorbidity Survey Replication (NCSR). *Archives of General Psychiatry*, *62*(6), 617–627. https://doi.org/10.1001/archpsyc.62.6.617.

Klein, D. N., Kotov, R., & Bufferd, S. J. (2011). Personality and depression: Explanatory models and review of the evidence. *Annual Review of Clinical Psychology*, *7*(1), 269–295. https://doi.org/10.1146/annurev-clinpsy-032210-104540.

Klonsky, E. D. (2008). What is emptiness? Clarifying the 7th criterion for borderline personality disorder. *Journal of Personality Disorders*, *22*(4), 418–426. https://doi.org/10.1521/pedi.2008.22.4.418. PMID: 18684053.

Köhne, A. C. J. (2020). The Relationalist Turn in understanding mental disorders: From essentialism to understanding dynamic and complex relations. *Philosophy, Psychiatry and Psychology*, *27*(2), 119–140.

Köhne, A. C. J., & Isvoranu, A. M. (2021). A network perspective on the comorbidity of personality pathology and depression: A symptom-level approach. *Frontiers*, *12*, 1–9.

Kotov, R., Krueger, R. F., Watson, D., Achenbach, T. M., Althoff, R. R., Bagby, R. M., . . . Zimmerman, M. (2017). The Hierarchical Taxonomy of Psychopathology (HiTOP): A dimensional alternative to traditional nosologies. *Journal of Abnormal Psychology*, *126*(4), 454–477. https://doi.org/10.1037/abn0000258.

Krueger, R. (1999). The structure of common mental disorders. *Archives of General Psychiatry*, *56*, 921–926. https://doi.org/10.1001/archpsyc.56.10.921.

Krueger, R. F., Hopwood, C. J., Wright, A. G. C., & Markon, K. E. (2014). DSM-5 and the path toward empirically based and clinically useful conceptualization of personality and psychopathology. *Personality and Psychopathology*, *21*(3), 245–261. https://doi.org/10.1111/cpsp.12073.

Lenzenweger, M. F., Lane, M. C., Loranger, A. W., & Kessler, R. C. (2007). DSM-IV personality disorders in the National Comorbidity Survey Replication. *Biological Psychiatry*, *62*(6), 553–564. https://doi.org/10.1016/j.biopsych.2006.09.019.

McNally, R. J., Robinaugh, D. J., Wu, G. W. Y., Wang, L., Deserno, M. K., & Borsboom, D. (2015). Mental disorders as causal systems: A network approach to posttraumatic stress disorder. *Clinical Psychological Science*, *3*(6), 836–849.

Olbert, C. M., Gala, G. J., & Tupler, L. A. (2014). Quantifying heterogeneity attributable to polythetic diagnostic criteria: Theoretical framework and empirical application. *Journal of Abnormal Psychology*, *123*(2), 452–462. https://doi.org/10.1037/a0036068.

Patten, S. B. (2009). Accumulation of major depressive episodes over time in a prospective study indicates that retrospectively assessed lifetime prevalence estimates are too low. *BMC Psychiatry*, *9*, 2–5. https://doi.org/10.1186/1471-244X-9-19.

Ralston, A., & Meynen, G. (2011). Zeven visies op een psychiatrische stoornis. *Tijdschrift Voor Psychiatrie*, *53*(12), 895–902.

Richetin, J., Preti, E., Costantini, G., & De Panfilis, C. (2017). The central role of identity in Borderline Personality Disorder: Evidence from network analysis. *PLoS One*, *12*(10), e0186695. https://doi.org/10.1371/journal.pone.0186695.

Robinaugh, D. J., Hoekstra, R. H., Toner, E. R., & Borsboom, D. (2020). The network approach to psychopathology: A review of the literature 2008–2018 and an agenda for future research. *Psychological Medicine*, *50*(3), 353–366.

Schreurs, P. J. G., van de Willige, G., Brosschot, J. F., Tellegen, B., & Graus, G. M. H. (1993). *Utrechtse Coping Lijst*. Pearson.

Sharma, V. K., & Copeland, J. R. M. (1989). Presentation and assessment of depression in old age. In K. Ghose (ed.), *Antidepressants for elderly people*. Springer.

Silk, K. R. (2010). The quality of depression in borderline personality disorder and the diagnostic process. *Journal of Personality Disorders*, *24*(1), 25–37. https://doi.org/10.1521/pedi.2010.24.1.25.

Skodol, A. E. (2012). Personality disorders in DSM-5. *Annual Review of Clinical Psychology*, *8*(1), 317–344. https://doi.org/10.1146/annurev-clinpsy-032511-143131.

Skodol, A. E., Gunderson, J. G., Pfohl, B., Widiger, T. A., Livesley, W. J., & Siever, L. J. (2002). The borderline diagnosis I: Psychopathology, comorbidity, and personality structure. *Biological Psychiatry*, *51*, 936–950.

Sloan, E., Hall, K., Moulding, R., Bryce, S., Mildred, H., & Staiger, P.K. (2017). Emotion regulation as a transdiagnostic treatment construct across anxiety, depression, substance, eating and borderline personality disorders: A systematic review. *Clinical Psychology Review*, *57*, 114–163. https://doi.org/10.1016/j.cpr.2017.09.002.

Weertman, A., Arntz, A., Dreessen, L., van Velzen, C., & Vertommen, S. (2003). Short-interval test–retest interrater reliability of the Dutch version of the Structured Clinical Interview for DSM-IV personality disorders (SCID-II). *Journal of Personality Disorders*, *17*(6), 562–567. https://doi.org/10.1521/pedi.17.6.562.25359.

Widiger, T. A., & Shea, T. (1991). Differentiation of Axis I and Axis II disorders. *Journal of Abnormal Psychology*, *100*(3), 339–406.

Young, J. E., Klosko, J. S., & Weishaar, M. E. (2006). *Schema therapy: A practitioner's guide*. The Guilford Press.

Zachar, P. (2002). The practical kinds model as a pragmatist theory of classification. *Philosophy, Psychiatry, & Psychology*, *9*(3), 219–227.

Zachar, P., & Kendler, K. S. (2007). Psychiatric disorders: A conceptual taxonomy. *American Journal of Psychiatry*, *164*(4), 557–565. https://doi.org/10.1176/appi.ajp.164.4.557.

Zanarini, M. C., Frankenburg, F. R., Dubo, E. D., Sickel, A. E., Trikha, A., Levin, A., & Reynolds, V. (1998). Axis I comorbidity of borderline personality disorder. *American Journal of Psychiatry*, *155*(12), 1733–1739. https://doi.org/10.1176/ajp.155.12.1733.

15 From Paul Tillich's *The Courage to Be* to Radical Acceptance and Radical Openness

Or Spiritually Based Dialectical Approaches to Neurotic Character

Konrad Banicki

Among the accusations most frequently directed at biomedical approaches in psychiatry is that of reductionism. The latter can be understood either methodologically or ontologically. Or, as is often the case, these two aspects can be somehow conflated. A set of useful tools to address the very idea of reduction was originally provided by logical positivism including a crucial distinction between reduction of terms and reduction of laws, as well as relatively strict and empirically meaningful accounts of both of them (e.g., Hempel, 1966). What makes these instruments especially valuable is that they seem to be relatively unbiased and allow the possibility of both successful and unsuccessful reductive attempts. In fact, they provide specific criteria intended to help one decide how scientifically fruitful a particular reductive model is. What seems to be lacking in these positivist and post-positivist approaches, however, are conceptual vehicles that would allow criticism of more existential or ontological character. The criticism, in other words, that would go essentially beyond comprehensive assessment of, say, descriptive, explanatory, and predictive power.

An example of an approach that can serve as a useful corrective to strictly empirically oriented positivist frameworks is a model provided by the Austrian psychiatrist, Viktor Emil Frankl (1969) under the label of *dimensional anthropology and ontology*. Frankl's framework, inspired by the contributions of Nicolai Hartmann and Max Scheler, is founded on the idea of *ontological difference* between body, mind, and spirit and the notion of *anthropological unity* of a human creature. It is precisely in order to do justice to both of these fundamental assumptions that Frankl employs the image of geometrical figures located in three-dimensional space as an analogy allowing a coexistence of qualitative differences and the unity of structure. Such a conceptual framework is an elegant way of addressing isomorphism or, as one of the "laws" of dimensional ontology has it, the fact that different phenomena when "projected out of their own dimension into one dimension lower than their own" (Frankl,

1969, p. 22) – that is, when reduced to a lower dimension – might lose their qualitative specificity and become indistinguishable. Just like a cylinder, a cone, and a ball of the same radius when projected onto a two-dimensional surface become identical as three disks, phenomena as fundamentally different as, say, psychotic episode, religious or mystical epiphany, and psychedelic experience may become indistinguishable when projected into lower dimensions of the biomedical, or even biopsychosocial, model (cf. Fulford & Jackson, 1997).

To do justice to all ontological features characteristic of human existence, a conceptual space of sufficient number of dimensions is needed. Arguably, an interesting example of such a space has been provided by the scholar immersed in the very same cultural milieu from which Frankl's model arises, Paul Tillich (1962). The multidimensional framework of dialectical ontology provided by this existential philosopher and Lutheran theologian will be briefly discussed that not only is capacious enough to contain the matters of body, mind, and spirit, but also, and crucially in the present context, provides a conceptual apparatus directly applicable to the domain of personality disorders. This includes both the ontologically thick account of being and non-being and the Neo-Freudian notion of anxious/neurotic character rooted in it. The latter, which is of significance, is not only impressively consistent and insightful, but also supplemented with a comprehensive account of existential courage required to live meaningfully (cf. Linehan, 2021) despite all those terrifying and painful aspects of reality one can justifiably be afraid of or avoid. It is nothing less than such a dialectical account of being and non-being, of anxiety and neurotic character, and of the courage needed to live "in-spite-of" that will be subsequently referred to more recent psychological frameworks developed to address personality-related psychopathology.

More specifically, it is Marsha Linehan's (1993) dialectical behavior therapy (DBT) and Thomas R. Lynch's (2018a, 2018b; cf. Lynch et al., 2015) radically open dialectical behavior therapy (RO-DBT) that will be explored. Such an exploration will first be made in the context of their explicitly dialectical character and the way in which the latter is an attempt to address the very same kind of dynamic Tillich wanted to make sense of. Then, in turn, the notions of radical acceptance (Linehan) and radical openness (Lynch) will be brought to the fore together with their spiritual background of Zen Buddhism and contemplative Christianity in the former case and Malâmati Sufism in the latter. Finally, some concluding remarks will be made to emphasize how a strikingly parallel ontological and existential structure appears to be employed by approaches as different as Lutheran theology of Tillich and essentially secular psychotherapeutic models of Linehan and Lynch and how non-trivial differences between DBT's radical acceptance and RO-DBT's radical openness adequately reflect the existential and clinical specificity of Cluster B (Linehan) and Cluster A and Cluster C (Lynch) personality disorders.

15.1 Avoiding Non-Being by Avoiding Being: Paul Tillich on Neurotic Anxiety

The ontological model developed by the author of *The courage to be* can be most easily introduced in terms of its fundamental and irreducible dialectics between being and non-being. It is, especially, the importance of the latter that should not be overlooked. In particular, not only are philosophical views that aspire to the complete removal of non-being from philosophical discourse (with Parmenides being the most striking example) found totally insufficient by Tillich, he is also not content with the kind of a reductive and derivative account allowed by those who acknowledge non-being only in a form of the negative judgment. What matters to him are not negative judgments per se, but rather what the fact of such judgments being so deeply entrenched in our language tells us about the deepest ontological structure of reality. What is revealed is that "non-being is ontologically as basic as being" (Tillich, 1962, p. 41). In other words, just like two primitive notions in an axiomatic system, both being and non-being require an independent status and none of them can be explained away in terms of the other.

Such a fundamentally philosophical assumption might seem to be very distant from clinical theory and practice, but, as a matter of fact, it has both a straightforward psychological meaning and direct psychological consequences. Just like non-being is fundamental and irremovable from any valid ontological account, its psychological correlates of anxiety, fear, despair, and courage will also need to remain at the very center of any existentially meaningful psychological framework. Or, to make this point a bit more specific, anxiety, fear, and despair are not just pathological and, thus, ontologically accidental phenomena to be eradicated with a sufficient amount of therapy employed. Rather, according to Tillich at least, it is the very nature of being human that makes them unavoidable dimensions of our experience.

What is remarkable about Tillich is not only that he was acquainted with Neo-Freudian authors such as Karen Horney and Erich Fromm, but also that he seems to be familiar with a kind of dimensional thinking so characteristic of our contemporary conceptualization of personality pathology. And even if, strictly speaking, he did not think that the ideas of "neurotic elements in everybody" (Tillich, 1962, p. 72) and of the difference between mental health and psychopathology being only quantitative are ontologically sufficient, he did provide an account in which anxiety of both existential and neurotic kind have the same ontological root and, thus, belong to the very same substantially human dynamic.

Anxiety is defined by Tillich (1962, p. 44) as "the existential awareness of non-being . . . [of] finitude, experienced as one's own finitude." The non-being at place can express itself in three ways depending on the endangered aspect of being (ontic, spiritual, or moral) and, what is more, can have either a relative or an absolute form. Respectively, it can strike one ontologically as *fate* and *death*, spiritually as *emptiness* and *meaninglessness*, and morally as *guilt* and *condemnation*. All these phenomena are related to anxiety as far as they are of global and existential nature: as far as they are rooted in non-being as such. When they become more concrete, mostly by acquiring a specific object, they become *fears*. "The sting of fear is anxiety, and anxiety strives toward fear," as Tillich (1962, p. 46) has it.

Specific fear, in opposition to existential anxiety per se, "can be faced . . . One can act upon it and in acting upon it participate in it – even if in the form of struggle" (Tillich, 1962, pp. 44–45). That "participation, struggle and love" (Tillich, 1962, p. 45) with respect to fear are possible is most generally reflected in the phenomenon of *courage* as ontological, spiritual, and moral self-affirmation "'in-spite-of', that is in spite of that which tends to prevent the self from affirming itself" (Tillich, 1962, p. 41).

It is nothing else than such an "in-spite-of" dialectics of being and non-being that provides a conceptual background against which a crucial difference between "the normal self-affirmation of the average personality" (Tillich, 1962, p. 73) and pathological or neurotic self-affirmation can be introduced. Both, interestingly, are only fragmentary and relative. Both "the average personality" and a neurotic person avoid extreme situations and react with despair when facing them. The difference lies somewhere else. The healthy self-affirmation, even if fragmentary, is relatively extensive and diversified. The individual's energy, in other words, is invested at many places and in many meaningful projects. As such, it is much more flexible, resilient, and, in fact, adjusted to the complex and multidimensional reality.

The neurotic self-affirmation, on the other hand, is substantially limited and, in consequence, distorted and fragile. It still counts as a genuine affirmation, but one "on a limited scale" characteristic of self-confinement and of "*avoiding non-being by avoiding being*" (Tillich, 1962, p. 71). The lack of extensiveness and flexibility proper to "the normal self-affirmation" is compensated by intensiveness and rigidity of local involvements, the features most easily recognizable in cases of obsessive-compulsivity. The intensity, fixation, and locality of the self-affirmation in question are reflected in its unrealistic character, in "a distorted relation to reality as a whole" (Tillich, 1962, pp. 71–72). The neurotic "castle . . . and the imaginary world behind it" (Tillich, 1962, p. 73), in other words, are the price to be paid for the surrendering of the project of more thorough self-affirmation. And even if the reward of relative security and comfort is gained, it "is comparable to the security of a prison" (Tillich, 1962, p. 79).

The surrendering in question as well as the distorted relation to reality it entails can be revealingly conceived of in terms of what Linehan (1993) will later call a "dialectical failure" (see below). The neurotic person does not succeed at existentially implementing a dialectical "in-spite-of" dynamic or, more specifically, "does not succeed in taking his anxiety courageously upon himself" (Tillich, 1962, p. 71). It is nothing else than such an ontologically fundamental failure that Tillich (1962, p. 73) refers to when he says that "neurotic is sick and needs healing."

Having made this point it might be helpful to emphasize that the domain he refers to as "sick" and as in need of healing is not, strictly speaking, that of the DSM's Axis I anxiety disorders, of, say, general anxiety disorder or social anxiety. To use a more psychoanalytic parlance, it is not just so-called symptom neurosis in which he is ultimately interested. Rather, what he is after is the phenomenon Wilhelm Reich (1933/1972) once called character neurosis (*Charakterneurose*). The latter term was introduced to address those cases in which the conceptual framework specific to discrete and egodystonic (i.e., seen as problematic by the very person affected) symptom neuroses turned out to be insufficient, calling for a much more comprehensive account required to understand egosyntonic (i.e., recognized as an obvious or natural way of being/reacting) symptoms typical of "a character permeated by neurotic pattern" (McWilliams, 2011, p. 63). As made clear by McWilliams (2011, p. 63), the age-old distinction "lives on in the DSM" with analysts' symptom neuroses usually classified as "disorders" and neurotic characters more typically being called "personality disorders." It is nothing less than the domain of the latter that Paul Tillich explores in existentially rich terms of the experiential world of an anxiety-ridden "castle" or "prison" (cf. Reich's character armor, *Charakterpanzer*).

15.2 Interrelatedness, Opposition, and Change: The Dialectical "Dance of the World"

Among the ways in which the age-long insights concerning personality psychopathology made by Tillich might be reformulated and revitalized is the reference to contemporary dialectical approaches of Marsha Linehan and Thomas R. Lynch. The dialectical behavior therapy (DBT) of the former and the radically open dialectical behavior therapy (RO-DBT) of the latter, respectively, would substitute the Neo-Freudian background against which this German author originally worked and, by the same token, make his philosophical and existential contributions refurbished in the context of more up-to-date clinical knowledge.

A bridge that makes such a reference possible and conceptually coherent is dialectics, which not only describes the relationship between being and non-being and can be employed to explain the nature of neurotic character in Tillich, but also is brought to the fore by DBT and RO-DBT. These approaches are explicitly "dialectical" both in the ways they address the pathodynamics of the conditions they are designed to treat and in terms of particular remedies they recommend. Only dialectical solutions, in short, can be relied on to successfully address problems of a fundamentally dialectical nature.

Linehan's DBT, for the time being at least, seems to be a relatively broad-spectrum approach and has been applied to clinical phenomena as diverse as, say, substance abuse, eating disorders, and post-traumatic stress disorder (PTSD). Initially, however, it was developed to address suicidal and parasuicidal behaviors commonly connected with the diagnosis of borderline personality disorder. Linehan (1993, p. 35) quite explicitly suggests that "borderline behaviors can be viewed as results of dialectical failures." What she gestures toward, more specifically, are phenomena typically labeled as splitting by psychoanalytically oriented clinicians or as dichotomous thinking by those of more cognitive leaning. Irrespective of whether these are intra- or interpersonally reflected (usually, they will be visible on both levels), it is a strictly dialectical remedy that is required: "The resolution of conflict requires first the recognition of the polarities and then the ability to rise above them ... seeing the apparently paradoxical reality of both and neither" (Linehan, 1993, pp. 35–36). What is meant here by "the polarities" are intentional phenomena of both cognitive and affective nature: "positions, wishes ... and so on always going through a very characteristic process of a frequent vacillation "between rigidly held yet contradictory points of view."

As for Linehan, interestingly, it seems that she had worked dialectically before even coming across the very notion in question. It took "a Marxist philosopher at the university" as well as his wife to make her realize that her treatment "is dialectical." And the creator of the DBT frankly admits that it was "like an epiphany, like learning what intuitively ... [she] already knew to be true" (Linehan, 2021, pp. 226–227).

When discussing the notion of *dialectics* explicitly, Linehan makes quite a lot of references mentioning, not surprisingly, such figures as Socrates and Plato. At the same time, it seems that it is mostly Zen Buddhism (Linehan herself is a Zen master) and more recent post-Hegelian authors dealing with developmental psychology (Basseches, 1984) and evolutionary biology (Levins & Lewontin, 1985) that inform her notion of the dialectical. Dialectics as understood by Linehan is, importantly, something more than a set of particular therapeutic techniques, as a superficial reading of more pragmatically oriented manuals (e.g., Linehan, 2014; McKay et al., 2019) could make one think. Also, it is not only a logical and conceptual framework or "a coherent system of exploring and understanding our world" (Robins et al., 2004, p. 32). Rather, it is nothing less than "a view of the fundamental nature of reality" (Heard & Linehan, 1994, p. 60), adhering to which is expected to substantially change "one's experience of the world and activities therein" (Robins et al., p. 32). It is exactly because of such a deeply ontological character that the dialectical perspective of Linehan is directly comparable with that of Tillich.

The dialectical philosophy at hand can be accounted for in terms of "three primary characteristics" (Heard & Linehan, 1994; cf. Fruzzetti, 2022; Robins et al., 2004) of interrelatedness or unity, opposition or heterogeneity, and continuous change. (1) The feature of *interrelatedness*, to begin with, "emphasizes relationships, the complexity of causal connections, and the whole as opposed to the parts" (Heard & Linehan, 1994, p. 60). As such it goes substantially beyond the classical behaviorist stance of exploring the environment in search of controlling stimuli and contingencies of reinforcement. Rather, with its explicit claim that parts and wholes are not just broadly interrelated, "not a mere collision of objects with fixed properties and immutable boundaries," what this perspective posits is that differing parts do not hold any independent significance (or essence) and, thus, need to be "defined in relation to one another" (Robins et al., 2004, p. 33). When one adds that also the whole cannot be reduced to the mere sum of its elements, it is a position very close to the spirit of classical German Gestalt psychology, systemic thinking (Von Bertalanffy, 2010) and, obviously, many Eastern proposals such as that of Zen Buddhism that is yielded.[1]

(2) *Opposition*, in turn, is understood in terms of a metaphysical thesis that reality "is not static but is comprised of opposing forces in tension" (Heard & Linehan, 1994, p. 61). What is meant here, importantly, is not "some dynamic balance," homeostasis, or an easy equilibrium. "The white yin and black yang of eastern philosophies," as Robins and colleagues have it (2004, p. 24), "do not combine to form a tepid, gray mush, but rather continue to oppose one another, surging here and receding there as they respond to both internal and external forces." It is this very feature of reality that, on the psychological level, is experienced as conflict and ambivalence and that, in therapeutic process, expresses itself in the form of "the central opposition . . . between change and acceptance" (Heard & Linehan, 1994, p. 62).[2]

[1] Among the references made by Linehan, that need to be admitted, one can find neither such authors as Köhler, Koffka, or Lewin, nor von Bertalanffy. What she mentions, instead, is Fritz Pearl's Gestalt therapy.

[2] In her work with highly disturbed suicidal patients Linehan became painfully aware that not only traditional behavioral emphasis on changing the patient's behavior but also the focus on acceptance might prove highly inadequate when applied in isolation. The former, to begin with, can turn out to be received as simply invalidating and, even more so, as invalidating not only a particular thought, emotion, or behavior, but also as invalidating the person as such. The

(3) The characteristics of *change*, finally, concern universal impermanence constituting not only "the very essence of experience," but also "a fundamental aspect of reality" (Heard & Linehan, 1994, p. 64). It is "the complex interplay of opposing forces" or the dialectical "dance of the world" (Robins et al., 2004, p. 34), in other words, which governs not only ontologically superficial levels of direct experience, but also the very nature of things. The vacillation between contradictory subjective perspectives, so characteristic of the individuals Linehan works with, in consequence turns out to be an expression, even if a very extreme one, of the forces built into in the very matrix of things. And even if Linehan, just like Hegel or Zen Buddhism, does not provide a systematic or definitive list of the "opposing forces" at play, one may hypothesize that a significant part of what has in mind concerns the oppositions such as those of life and death, self-identity and unity with others, isolation/alienation and relatedness. In other words, the very same polarities her patients tend to struggle with so painfully (cf. Linehan, 1993, pp. 35–36).

The recognition of such a radically dynamic reality, interestingly, is very directly reflected in the way in which successful therapy is to be conducted. Reflected not only in the therapeutic frame, which is much more flexible in DBT than any traditionally psychoanalytic approach would allow, but also in particular techniques such as those pertaining to skills training (see Linehan, 2014; McKay et al., 2019) directed at either changing reality (change-related skills: emotion regulation and interpersonal regulation) or at learning to cope with it changing in directions we are not at all happy about (acceptance-related skills: mindfulness and distress tolerance).[3]

15.3 Radical Acceptance, or "Giving up Tantrums"

According to Tillich's account, as one might remember, non-being intrinsically and unavoidably present at the very core of reality endangered one's ontic, spiritual, and moral self-affirmation as reflected, respectively, in the terrifying experiences of fate and death, emptiness and meaninglessness, and guilt and condemnation. And it was nothing else than "participation, struggle and love"

humanistic unconditional acceptance, in turn, may suggest the disregard for the patient's problems and, respectively, might seem "to discount the desperation" of the person concerned. It can, in consequence, "paradoxically . . . also invalidate" (Heard & Linehan, 1994, p. 64).

[3] The "three primary characteristics" of Linehan's dialectics can be interestingly compared with the three Buddhist marks of existence involving: impermanence (*anicca*), suffering (*dukkha*), and the non-self doctrine (*anattā*). The first is obviously directly included in her account, whereas the third, even if not explicitly referred to, would belong to the variety of phenomena summarized under the general heading of interrelatedness. Suffering, finally, seems to be the very *raison d'etre* of her project at large (cf. her own personal "vow to God that I would get myself out of hell and that, once I did, I would go back into hell and get others out," Linehan, 2021, p. 29 as well as Mahayana Buddhism's ideal of *bodhisattva* as one devoted to ending the suffering of all sentient beings).

(Tillich, 1962, p. 45) as courageous ways of facing them that allowed the one and only self-affirmation available to the human being: self-affirmation "in-spite-of."

Interestingly, this very same general structure can be found in Linehan and Lynch. The dialectical reality of interrelatedness, opposition, and change, to begin with, constitutes a significant challenge to us as certified not only by the Buddhist First Noble Truth: life is suffering (*dukkha*, see footnote 3), but also by the experience of conflict and ambivalence omnipresent in therapeutic offices and outside of them. For Tillich it was courage that allowed one to seek self-affirmation "in-spite-of" all those forces that endangered it. What would be its counterpart in DBT and RO-DBT? A short answer to this question is not difficult and sounds, respectively: radical acceptance and radical openness. To make it meaningful, however, a longer story needs to be told.

Linehan's notion of radical acceptance, importantly, was not the very first version of her answer to the question: How to face the constantly changing and ontologically unstable reality of all too human suffering? Rather, it was the concept of *willingness* that she took from Gerald May (1982), the psychiatrist and theologian as well as the brother of the existential psychologist Rollo May.[4] Willingness is obviously a phenomenon of psychological and existential character. At the same time, it is hard to omit its deeply and fundamentally ontological nature: "Willingness is about opening yourself to what is. It is about becoming one with the universe, participating in it, doing what is needed in the moment" (Linehan, 2021, p. 201). Willingness is all about allowing "the world to be what it is" and, in a truly Tillichian in-spite-of spirit, to agree to participate in it "no matter what it is" (Linehan, 2021, p. 253). It is nothing less than such an indiscriminative "what is" to which one is to react with a unifying act of "becoming one," with "doing what is needed in the moment" and with letting go of at least some of the struggles: "It is doing the dishes when needed, helping someone up who has fallen, letting go of battles you will never win and even some you could win" (Linehan, 2021, p. 201). Such an act, importantly, with all its existential seriousness and depth, has some quite simple and very down-to-earth consequences: it is, at the end of the day, about "giving up tantrums" (Linehan, 2021, p. 202).

It was May's concept of willingness that turned Linehan in the direction that eventually yielded the notion of *radical acceptance* so crucial to the final form DBT took. Radical acceptance is acceptance, and it is radical, and it is such

[4] The mixture of Zen-related inspirations and those belonging to Christian contemplative traditions is as characteristic of Linehan as it was of her teachers and spiritual directors: Willigis Jäger and Patrick Hawk who, apart from being Zen masters, were also a Benedictine monk and a Catholic priest, respectively. It was the latter who made Linehan a Zen master herself (Linehan, 2021).

a twofold structure that might help to elaborate its meaning. Mere or non-radical acceptance, to begin with, is somehow local and in a sense confined, both in terms of the depth and exhaustiveness of the act of acceptance (of the *way* of accepting) and in terms of this acceptance's object (of *what* is accepted). It might, for instance, consist of the cognitive or intellectual (but not emotional) acknowledgment of some facts and of letting go of one's behavioral efforts to change a selected aspect of reality. Contrary to a relatively common misconception, such acceptance does not amount to liking or being happy about the facts in question, to positive evaluation of them as something good or welcome. When one realizes that the reality at hand may include such external circumstances like that of having been fired or subjective phenomena of the kind characteristic of emotional anguish (Fruzzetti, 2022), it would not only be absurd, but often, simply speaking, inhuman to expect anything like that. Rather, acceptance is all about acknowledging, listening to, and doing justice to what there is to acknowledge, listen to, and do justice. It is to emphasize this character of the act in question that some prefer to talk about "radical acknowledgment" (Linehan, 2021, p. 250), "radical truth" (Linehan, 1993, p. 517), or accepting things "descriptively" (Fruzzetti, 2022, p. 568).

To acquire its whole existential meaning as "radical," the kind of acceptance summarized above needs to embody the completeness of the commitment made and the fullness of its scope. In short, not only does it need to be made "from deep within," but also needs to be "*complete*" (Linehan, 1993, p. 148). The quality of being made "from deep within" can be easily rephrased in anthropological terms as being made "all the way, with your mind, your heart, and your body" (Linehan, 2021, p. 250; cf. the multidimensional model of Frankl referred to at the beginning of the chapter). Or, in formally negative terms, as being made "without distortion, without adding judgment of good and bad." Without, as the analysts would have it, "defense" (Linehan, 1993, p. 517). The exhaustiveness of the commitment's scope, in turn, can be understood as non-discriminativeness of the act. The acceptance sought for, in particular, "does not choose what to accept and what not to accept." Only when made in such a total way can it be deemed "radical" and placed on a par with May's willingness and Tillich's courage to be.

Acceptance as meant by Linehan, interestingly, is not recommended *instead of* change. Rather, as already mentioned, both factors remain in a strictly dialectical relationship. In other words, it is not only the case that acceptance understood as providing a firm footing on reality is required for change and constitutes the first step toward it. Also, the very act of accepting what there is to be acknowledged might, at least sometimes, amount to a non-trivial existential and experiential shift. Just like in Zen or mindfulness practice, where even if there is no explicit intention to change anything, the very commitment to "simply observe how feelings, thoughts, and overt behavior, both pleasant and aversive, naturally come and go" (Heard & Linehan, 1994, p. 65) can, when implemented with serious commitment, naturally lead to the substantial rearrangement of the way one experiences the world.

15.4 From Radical Acceptance to Radical Openness

The above account of dialectics and radical acceptance has been based on the writings of Linehan and, respectively, one should give it some consideration before automatically applying it to Thomas R. Lynch's (2018a, 2018b) RO-DBT. And it is especially so if one recalls that the philosophico-spiritual underpinning of Linehan is Zen Buddhism and Christianity, whereas for Lynch it is Malâmati Sufism (see Seale, 1968; Toussulis, 2010) that has provided a framework of that kind. And, even if both Zen and Christianity (or, at least, those aspects of Christianity Linehan is interested in) and Malâmati Sufism can be accurately described as contemplative or mystical in spirit, it would be not only too hasty, but simply false to reduce them to the same thing.

Even the very source of the term "Malâmati" should already alert one of potential and non-trivial differences at place. The term in question is rooted in the Arabic "malāmah" or "blame" and, indeed, the Malâmatis (those involved in the movement) have always emphasized the importance of criticism or blame (hence, the "Malāmatīya" or the "way of blame"). And it was nothing else that their own carnal self (Ar. *nafs*) that was a default object of such a critical stance: "The self was their great enemy . . . a cunning creature, forever setting traps, [and] seeking to snare them." The one, in consequence, that "had to be subdued, humiliated and punished at all costs" (Seale, 1968, p. 12). The language employed by Lynch (2018a, p. 187) is considerably weaker. What he refers "malāmah" to is the "practice of sustained self-observation and healthy self-criticism in order to understand one's true motivations." But even after such a non-negligible adaptation is made the whole formula is clearly normative and can be understood as including judgment and, as a result, dualism. When read along such lines it would certainly occupy a very different conceptual space than that of non-dualism proper to Zen Buddhism and some branches of contemplative Christianity. It is exactly because of this discrepancy that the potential differences between DBT and RO-DBT need to be carefully scrutinized.

As for dialectics, the issue at hand turns out to be relatively straightforward, both as far as the general concept is understood and in the way it is applied to comprehend and alleviate the conditions treated by DBT and RO-DBT. The "three primary characteristics" of Linehan, to begin with, seem to be directly reflected in Lynch's (2018a, pp. 297–298) "five key concepts or assumptions." This should not come as a surprise, because Lynch, just like Linehan, develops his account on the basis of a broadly Hegelian approach. His *Assumption 1* that everything "is transient and finite" explicitly acknowledges the very same reality Linehan explored under the heading of change, and it is nothing less than the latter that is then further specified in terms of the inevitability of "crises and turning points" (*Assumption 3*) and the "continual and transactional" nature of the processes in question (*Assumption 5*). *Assumption 2*, in turn, is Linehan's principle of opposition rephrased as a thesis that all important things in life are "composed of contradictions" or "opposing forces." *Assumption 4*, finally, introduced as a tenet that the "world is holistic, and everything is connected and in relationship" is a reflection of DBT's interrelatedness.

Also, the very general structure of the dialectical failure and the dialectical remedy seems to be replicated by Lynch. His approach is mostly addressed to people struggling with overcontrol understood in terms of inhibition and delay of gratification. As highly socially valued and, indeed, highly functional these two might be, when employed in a too extreme and too rigid way they seriously detriment one's self-affirmation and especially so in regard to interpersonal and social functioning. Even if overcontrol, as Lynch (2018a, p. 8) has it, "works well for sitting quietly in a monastery or building a rocket ... it creates problems when it comes to social connectedness." Once again, just as the deficits at place can be understood in terms of falling short of the full acknowledgment of the dialectical reality of truly human life, also the antidote offered is strictly dialectical in nature. A *thesis* that "inhibition is useful," so characteristic of many of those treated by Lynch (2018a, p. 297), is not, in consequence, just to be substituted by an *antithesis* that "disinhibition is useful," but transgressed and solved on the level of "a *synthesis* ... which ideally results in higher-order functioning, not simply in a compromise."

Linehan's dialectics and Lynch's dialectics, as shown above, seem to share not only their most fundamental assumptions, but also the general dialectical-remedy-to-dialectical-problem applicatory structure. Some closer attention, however, needs to be paid to RO-DBT's concept of radical openness and the way in which it relates to that of radical acceptance. *Radical openness* as a "core philosophical principle and core skill" (Lynch, 2018a, p. 177) pertaining to RO-DBT is defined in terms of "the confluence of three core capabilities" (Lynch, 2018a, p. 186) including receptivity, flexibility, and intimacy/connectedness. (1) *Receptivity*, to begin with, consists of one's openness to new experience and, especially, to that characteristic of disconfirming feedback. As such, it is connected with an ability and readiness to adapt to that kind of experience and, thus, constitutes a condition of possibility of learning. (2) *Flexibility*, in turn, refers to the capacity of maintaining self-control without simultaneously decreasing one's ability of reaction and adaptation to the changing environment. (3) *Intimacy* and *connectedness*, finally, are specified in terms of maintaining close connection with "at least one other person." The examples of these capabilities provided by Lynch (2018a, pp. 186–187) illustrate very vividly how truly dialectical they are. One is recommended, for instance, to "strive for perfection" unless it is "counterproductive or damaging a relationship," to "be rule-governed . . . except when breaking the rules is needed," or "to be polite and cooperative . . . yet be bad-tempered if the situation calls for it."[5]

The common dialectical core of RO-DBT and DBT, however, should not make one neglect the difference of emphasis between Lynch's radical openness and Linehan's radical acceptance. The difference, importantly, the former (Lynch, 2018a, p. 190) is ready to explicitly acknowledge. Radical acceptance of Linehan is rooted in a Zen-flavored attempt to see reality as it is or "without illusion." And it is exactly in the context of such an attempt that letting go of the fight with reality or "giving up tantrums" take place. The starting point of RO-DBT as inspired by Malâmati Sufism is considerably different and it is, using a philosophical parlance, more epistemological. What Lynch (2018a, p. 190) invites us to challenge, more specifically, is nothing less than "our *perceptions of* reality" and what he advances is, actually, a thesis that "we are unable to see things as they are but instead see things as we are" (Lynch, 2018a, p. 190). It is exactly in reference to such a general skeptical viewpoint, specified later in psychological terms of cognitive biases negatively influencing our ability to open and learn, that RO-DBT encourages "the cultivation of self-enquiry and healthy self-doubt" (Lynch, 2018a, p. 190). Indeed, it is in a genuine spirit of the Malâmatis that the very first non-graphic handout of the RO-DBT skills training manual (Lynch, 2018b, p. 62) invokes such normatively and, actually, theologically laden notions as "humility," "fallibility," and "responsibility." What one is constantly reminded of is "that the *truth hurts*" and that it is "more than mindful awareness" (Lynch, 2018a, p. 187) that is needed.

15.5 Courage to Be, Radical Acceptance, and Radical Openness: Toward a Conclusion

The analyses conducted above can be summarized and concluded in two ways. A conceptual and philosophical structure, to begin with, might be identified providing a kind of a common denominator connecting Tillich's model on the one side and Linehan's and Lynch's approaches on the other. The core of such a structure is metaphysical or ontological in character and is constituted by a dialectical framework proper to Tillich's account of being and non-being and, for DBT and RO-DBT, by a broadly Hegelian elaboration of the notion of dialectics. It is such a core that is, subsequently, applied to address all the "why"

[5] A very similar and truly dialectical or, if one prefers, phronetic (Gr. *phronesis*, practical wisdom) recommendation has been made once by the German chess master, Siegbert Tarrasch: "Always put the Rook behind the Pawn . . .. Except when it is incorrect to do so" (as quoted in Soltis, 1997, p. 129).

questions related to suffering of not only those who struggle with mental health issues but of all human creatures as such. Even if, as seems to be the case of Tillich (see above), these accounts are not technically speaking dimensional, they certainly operate within a conceptual and existential framework in which any kind of human suffering, whether conceived of in terms of a formal nosological diagnosis or devoid of any such reference, has ultimately the very same ontological root of the dialectical nature of reality and human being as such.

Importantly, the answers to the "why" questions provided by Tillich, Linehan, and Lynch are not of an explanatory kind proper to causal scientific hypotheses. What they seek to provide, in other words, is not Dilthey's *Erklären* (explanation). Rather, what they make possible to construe are meaningful and meaning-given structures characteristic of this philosopher's *Verstehen* (understanding): sense-making worldviews we all so deeply need. Of the same meaning-related, rather than cause-related, order are ultimate "recipes" devised by all these accounts: courage, radical acceptance, and radical openness. It may merit a mention that all three of them, irrespective of the non-trivial differences at place, maintain the "in-spite-of" structure Paul Tillich so neatly captured. It is always only via facing and challenging, rather than via avoidance and withdrawal, that any meaningfully human self-affirmation might be sought for.

The second important point to make concerns the sources and meaning of the difference between radical acceptance and radical openness or, to formulate it in somewhat broader terms, of the difference between DBT and RO-DBT. It might be tempting to not only describe but also to explain the latter in terms of Linehan being inspired by Zen Buddhism and some currents of contemplative Christianity and Lynch being rooted in Malâmati Sufism. But even if, as shown above, such an interpretive framework can yield some valuable results, if implemented as the main or even exclusive heuristic tool it would be not only too far-reaching (both DBT and RO-DBT are, after all, applied and clinical endeavors, rather than those belonging to contemplative spirituality) but also simply unnecessary.

It is because a relatively straightforward step of devoting some attention to the respective projects' target groups might reveal the reasons for which it is radical acceptance that is exactly "what is needed" for DBT and radical openness what is required by RO-DBT. *Both* DBT and RO-DBT are mainly addressed to people diagnosed with personality disorders or, to use a somewhat anachronistic parlance of Tillich and Reich, to those of neurotic character. And it is exactly for this reason that radical acceptance and radical openness emphasizing the dangers of getting stuck with inflexibility and dualistic thinking are so well suited for both of these projects. At the same time, however, within the broad and very heterogeneous category of personality disorders these are relatively distant, if not simply opposing, subclasses of Cluster B on the one hand and Clusters A and C on the other that are Linehan's and Lynch's respective areas of interest. DBT is directed at individuals struggling with emotional dysregulation (or *undercontrol*) and quite literally seeking the way "out of hell" (Linehan, 2021, p. 328). It is in the context of such an intolerable anguish that the priority given to emotion regulation and acceptance skills such as mindfulness or distress tolerance is often simply a life-saving necessity. RO-DBT, on the other hand, is addressed to those who can be characterized in terms of *overcontrol* and a kind of anxiety-driven experiential, cognitive, and interpersonal avoidance and rigidity. Rather than hell, as it seems, it would be an area of safety guaranteed by Tillich's (1962, p. 79) "prison." For this group including avoidant, paranoid, schizoid, and, first of all, obsessive-compulsive personality disorders it is exactly an invitation to radically open and actively seek "those areas of our lives that we want to avoid or may find uncomfortable," to attend to "the very place we don't want to go" (Lynch, 2018a, p. 187) that might sound like a good recommendation. "When hungry, eat; when tired, sleep" (quoted in Watts, 1989, p. 99), as a famous Zen saying has it.

Acknowledgments: I am deeply grateful to Ela, Lena, and Bartek for all their patience, support, and inspiration.

References

Basseches, M. (1984). *Dialectical thinking*. Ablex.

Frankl, V. E. (1969). *The will to meaning: Foundations and applications of logotherapy*. World Publishing.

Fruzzetti, A. E. (2022). Dialectical thinking. *Cognitive and Behavioral Practice*, *29*(3), 567–570.

Fulford, K. W. M., & Jackson, M. (1997). Spiritual experience and psychopathology. *Philosophy, Psychiatry, & Psychology*, *4*(1), 41–65.

Heard, H. L., & Linehan, M. M. (1994). Dialectical behavior therapy: An integrative approach to the treatment of borderline personality disorder. *Journal of Psychotherapy Integration*, *4*(1), 55–82.

Hempel, C. G. (1966). *Philosophy of natural science*. Prentice-Hall.

Levins, R., & Lewontin, R. (1985). *The dialectical biologist*. Harvard University Press.

Linehan, M. M. (1993). *Cognitive behavioral treatment of borderline personality disorder*. Guilford Press.

Linehan, M. (2014). *DBT skills training manual*. Guilford Publications.

Linehan, M. M. (2021). *Building a life worth living: A memoir*. Random House Trade Paperbacks.

Lynch, T. R. (2018a). *Radically open dialectical behavior therapy: Theory and practice for treating disorders of overcontrol*. New Harbinger Publications.

Lynch, T. R. (2018b). *The skills training manual for radically open dialectical behavior therapy: A clinician's guide for treating disorders of overcontrol*. New Harbinger Publications.

Lynch, T. R., Hempel, R. J., & Dunkley, C. (2015). Radically open-dialectical behavior therapy for disorders of over-control: Signaling matters. *American Journal of Psychotherapy, 69*(2), 141–162.

May, G. G. (1982). *Will and spirit: A contemplative psychology.* HarperCollins Publishers.

McKay, M., Wood, J. C., & Brantley, J. (2019). *The dialectical behavior therapy skills workbook: Practical DBT exercises for learning mindfulness, interpersonal effectiveness, emotion regulation, and distress tolerance.* New Harbinger Publications.

McWilliams, N. (2011). *Psychoanalytic diagnosis: Understanding personality structure in the clinical process.* Guilford Press.

Reich, W. (1933/1972). *Character analysis.* Farrar, Straus & Giroux.

Robins, C. J., Schmidt, H. III, & Linehan, M. M. (2004). Dialectical behavior therapy: Synthesizing radical acceptance with skillful means. In S. C. Hayes, V. M. Follette, & M. M. Linehan (eds.), *Mindfulness and acceptance: Expanding the cognitive-behavioral tradition* (pp. 30–44). The Guilford Press.

Seale, M. S. (1968). The ethics of Malāmatīya Sufism and the Sermon on the Mount. *The Muslim World, 58*(1), 12–23.

Soltis, A. (1997). *Grandmaster secrets endings. Everything you need to know about the endgame.* Thinkers' Press.

Tillich, P. (1962/1952). *The courage to be.* Collins.

Toussulis, Y. (2010). *Sufism and the way of blame: Hidden sources of a sacred psychology.* Quest Books.

Von Bertalanffy, L. (2010). General systems theory. In D. Hammond (ed.), *The science of synthesis: Exploring the social implications of general systems theory* (pp. 103–142). The University Press of Colorado.

Watts, A. (1989). *The way of Zen.* Vintage Books.

16 Personality "Disorder" and the Incapacity to Self-Regulate

Answering Practical and Metaphysical Questions

Garson Leder and Tadeusz Zawidzki

16.1 Introduction

There is an unresolved debate about whether the ways of being currently identified by the DSM-5-TR Cluster B personality disorders (i.e., narcissistic, antisocial, borderline, and histrionic) should be considered genuine mental disorders or normal (if often serious) problems of living.[1] This issue is a microcosm of a larger debate about whether psychiatry is overextending itself and overmedicalizing many of life's hardships. Our goal in this chapter is to show that the resolution of the first debate can inform the second, larger, question. To this end, we will examine Louis Charland's influential arguments (2004, 2006, 2010) that the Cluster B personality disorders are "really moral, and not medical, conditions" (2004). Charland offers two arguments in support of this conclusion. The first, the Argument from Identification, argues (roughly) that we cannot identify Cluster B "disorders" without explicit reliance upon moral terms; thus these disorders are not genuine medical conditions. The second, the Argument from Treatment, posits (again, roughly) that we cannot treat these "disorders" without something like a "moral conversion"; thus these disorders are not genuine medical conditions (2004). In this chapter we show that while both of Charland's arguments are flawed (and, thus, do not directly support this conclusion), Charland's Argument from Treatment is on to *something*. Namely, Charland is right in arguing that a focus on how and why mental health treatments achieve their effects should inform our views about what ways of being should properly be considered "mental disorder," he is just mistaken about what mental healing consists of.

In this chapter, we argue that skilled metacognitive self-regulation is a necessary component to mental healing. We offer two lines of argument for this claim: (1) the practice of psychotherapy necessarily involves enabling such

[1] For example, see: Kendell (2002), Charland (2004, 2006, 2010), Pickard (2009), Zachar and Potter (2010), Reimer (2013), and Banicki (2018).

metacognitive, self-regulatory skills; (2) such skills are necessary for reasons responsiveness – a plausible necessary condition on mental health. Expanding on the latter line of argument, we argue that a Davidsonian approach to reasons responsiveness is best suited for the purpose of characterizing mental health and distinguishing medical from moral conditions. Our focus on the role played by skilled self-regulation in healing partially vindicates Charland's argument. The Cluster B personality disorders are not *necessarily* "moral conditions," although some instantiations will be. We also show that the current definitions of personality disorders (in both the DSM-5 and ICD-11) are both overly *inclusive* and overly *exclusive*, allowing moral judgments to drive diagnosis. Finally, we conclude by showing that this focus on the role of skilled action in psychological healing can help distinguish between mental disorders and normal problems of living, full stop.

16.2 Personality Disorders

The DSM-5 definition of personality disorder is as follows (with the ICD-11 offering a similar definition):

> A personality disorder is an enduring pattern of inner experience and behavior that deviates markedly from the expectations of the individual's culture, is pervasive and inflexible, has an onset in adolescence or early adulthood, is stable over time, and leads to distress or impairment . . . Only when personality traits are inflexible and maladaptive and cause significant functional impairment or subjective distress do they constitute personality disorders. (APA, 2013)

Note that this definition is not meant to supersede either of the DSM's or ICD's definitions of mental disorder. Both the DSM and ICD adopt definitions of disorder that require "dysfunction" in the "psychological, biological, or developmental processes that underlie mental and behavioural functioning" (WHO, 2021). So, according to both manuals, behavior that deviates from expected norms would not count as a mental disorder unless it also resulted from a "dysfunction." This "dysfunction" requirement is supposed to help differentiate normal (although possibly serious) problems of living from mental disorders. Problematically, neither manual offers a definition of "dysfunction," and this term is used ambiguously in both texts.

This term is sometimes used in reference to dysfunctions within the person (e.g., dysfunctions of "processes that underlie mental and behavioral functioning"), and sometimes in reference to impairments in persons' interactions with the world (e.g., social or occupational dysfunctions). This latter usage of "dysfunction" is operational in both the DSM-5's and ICD-11's requirements that personality disorders cause either "clinically significant distress or impairment in social, occupational, or other important areas of functioning" (APA,

2013).[2] Personality disorders, then, according to the dominant diagnostic manuals in the Americas, Europe, and much of the rest of the world, require not only pervasive and stable patterns of norm-transgressing experience and behavior that cause subjective distress or functional impairment, but this experience and behavior must also be the result of a "dysfunction."[3]

Also note that the issues addressed in this chapter are largely orthogonal to the question of whether personality disorders are best conceptualized as dimensional rather than categorical diagnostic entities. The DSM-5 has retained the categorical conception of personality disorders from its previous iterations (while also suggesting a dimensional alternative in an "emerging measures and models" section), whereas the ICD-11 has adopted a dimensional construction of personality disorders (and, thus, does not contain the specific diagnostic labels used in the DSM). However, all the ways of being identified by the Cluster B disorders are also reconstructable under these dimensional models. The focus here, then, is whether these ways of being (whether identified categorically or dimensionally) are best conceptualized as mental disorders or normal problems of living.

Finally, note that this chapter is focused on a subset of personality disorders that fall under the DSM-5 label of "Cluster B" personality disorders. The DSM-5 divides personality disorders into three clusters: Cluster A (paranoid, schizoid, and schizotypal), Cluster B (antisocial, borderline, histrionic, and narcissistic), and Cluster C (avoidant, dependent, and obsessive-compulsive). These clusters are often referred to, respectively, as the "mad," "bad," and "sad" clusters. Although insensitive, these labels do point toward an important point. Many of the "symptoms" listed for the Cluster B personality disorders (e.g., "deceitfulness," "reckless disregard for the safety of self or others," "inappropriate sexually seductive or provocative behavior," "interpersonally exploitative," and "arrogant") do consist in behavior commonly considered to be *bad* (or otherwise somehow morally problematic). The question, then, is what differentiates normal "bad" behavior from pathologically "bad" behavior?

[2] The ICD-11 wording differs slightly. It reads: "The disturbance is associated with substantial distress or significant impairment in personal, family, social, educational, occupational or other important areas of functioning" (WHO, 2021).

[3] Note that while both the DSM-5's and ICD-11's general definitions of "mental disorder" do not make distress or functional impairment a *necessary* condition for disorder (they use "usually associated with" as a modifier), both documents' specific definitions of "personality disorder" do. There is one exception: the ICD-11 proposes that the diagnosis of "*Mild* Personality Disorder" *may* (rather than necessarily must) be associated with distress or functional impairment "that is either limited to circumscribed areas (e.g., romantic relationships; employment) or present in more areas but of milder severity" (WHO, 2021). Note also that the DSM-5's alternative model for personality disorders uses slightly different wording than the main text. Specifically, it replaces "impairment" with "disability" and "functioning" with "pursuits." We do not take these rewordings to reflect a substantive change in meaning.

16.3 Medical or Moral?

This chapter will attempt to answer this question by first examining Louis Charland's influential claim that the ways of being currently identified by the Cluster B personality disorders are wrongly identified as mental disorders.[4] In a series of papers (2004, 2006, 2010), Charland argues that Cluster B personality disorders "are not genuine medical kinds; they are really moral kinds" (2004). Charland, here, is not claiming that these ways of being are not (often serious) problems; they are just not medical problems.

According to Charland, what sets the Cluster B's apart from genuine medical disorders is that their identification and treatment both logically necessitate moral judgments. To see the motivation for Charland's argument, consider, for example, the DSM-5 diagnostic criteria for Narcissistic Personality Disorder (NPD):

Diagnostic criteria: A pervasive pattern of grandiosity (in fantasy or behavior), need for admiration, and lack of empathy, beginning by early adulthood and present in a variety of contexts, as indicated by five (or more) of the following:

1. Has a grandiose sense of self-importance (e.g., exaggerates achievements and talents, expects to be recognized as superior without commensurate achievements).
2. Is preoccupied with fantasies of unlimited success, power, brilliance, beauty, or ideal love.
3. Believes that he or she is "special" and unique and can only be understood by, or should associate with, other special or high-status people (or institutions).
4. Requires excessive admiration.
5. Has a sense of entitlement (i.e., unreasonable expectations of especially favorable treatment or automatic compliance with his or her expectations).
6. Is interpersonally exploitative (i.e., takes advantage of others to achieve his or her own ends).
7. Lacks empathy: is unwilling to recognize or identify with the feelings and needs of others.
8. Is often envious of others or believes that others are envious of him or her.
9. Shows arrogant, haughty behaviors or attitudes.

Differential diagnosis (reads in part): Many highly successful individuals display personality traits that might be considered narcissistic. Only when these traits are inflexible, maladaptive, and persisting and cause significant functional impairment or subjective distress do they constitute narcissistic personality disorder.

[4] Charland's arguments were made in reference to DSM-IV, but apply equally to the DSM-5 (and the dimensional reconstructions of the Cluster B's in the ICD-11).

In addition to "lack of empathy," we also find wording such as "grandiose sense of self-importance," "requires excessive admiration," "envious," "arrogant," and "haughty" (APA, 2013). Charland is certainly right that this language *is* often used to reflect morally disvalued behavior. It is difficult, then, to see how the identification or treatment of this condition can be made without necessary reference to ways of being that are commonly considered moral shortcomings. Charland extends this line of reasoning to all of the Cluster B's. For example, Charland (2006) argues:

> consider very briefly the nature of the individual Cluster B disorders. Antisocial personality disorder is said to involve a "pervasive pattern of disregard for and violation of the rights of others" (APA, 1994, p. 649), and narcissistic personality disorder is said to involve a "lack of empathy" (p. 661). The moral nature of histrionic personality is more implied than explicit but is clear nonetheless; here the "excessive attention seeking" and "inappropriate sexually seductive and provocative behavior" is flatly inconsistent with a pattern of empathy and regard for others (APA, 1994, p. 657–658). Finally, the "inappropriate, intense anger" and "instability in interpersonal relationships" cited in the diagnostic criteria for borderline personality disorder again imply clear moral deficits in empathy and regard for others . . . There is therefore no escaping the conclusion that, either by explicit mention or by implication, persons diagnosed with Cluster B personality disorders exhibit morally objectionable and reprehensible behavior toward others. That moral aspect of their condition is logically inseparable from their having the condition. Without it, the diagnosis cannot be applied. (p. 122)

Before addressing the plausibility of Charland's arguments in support of the purported ineluctable moral nature of the Cluster B's, we should first note its scope. This is not a broad antipsychiatry argument; Charland is not arguing that mental disorders are not "real" or that there is no substantive difference between genuine and spurious applications of the term "mental disorder" (Charland, 2010). Charland, for example, accepts that the other personality disorder diagnoses may represent genuine "medical" kinds (2004, 2006). Charland is also not merely making the claim that the Cluster B's are *value-laden*. Rather, Charland's argument is that the values in play in the Cluster B's are primarily *moral* values. Charland's point, here, is that the *moral* aspect of the Cluster B's are *necessarily* connected to both treatment and identification, whereas *moral* evaluations are only sometimes associated in other conditions (even if they may be otherwise value-laden). In contrast, the other clusters of personality disorders are supposed to be "morally neutral" (2004). This necessary "moral nature" of the Cluster B's is what is supposed to set them apart from genuine "clinical" disorders.

The question, then, is whether this hypothesized necessary moral nature of the Cluster entails that they should not be considered genuine mental disorders. Charland offers two arguments in support of this claim: the Argument from Identification, and the Argument from Treatment. We will address both in order.

16.4 The Argument from Identification

Charland's Argument from Identification can be formulated as such:

(1) In order to identify the putative disordered ways of being identified by the Cluster B's, we necessarily have to focus on "morally reprehensible behavior" (2006).

(2) Therefore, the Cluster B's are moral, rather than medical, kinds.

This is the weaker of Charland's two arguments. The biggest problem here is that it is unclear why the patterns of behavior and inner experience that Charland identifies as "morally reprehensible" should not be symptoms of a disorder. If being morally reprehensible was all there is to the identification of a disorder, then Charland would clearly be right. But that's not necessarily all there is to it. The DSM-5 definition of "mental disorder" is explicit that: "Socially deviant behavior (e.g., political, religious, or sexual) and conflicts that are primarily between the individual and society are not mental disorders unless the deviance or conflict results from a dysfunction in the individual" (APA, 2013). Charland provides no argument for why morally reprehensible behavior that is the result of a dysfunction (or some other cause) should *not* be identifying criteria for genuine medical disorder (Reimer, 2013). And there is good reason to think that there are at least some instances where this type of behavior should be considered disordered. Consider, for example, morally problematic behavior that results, in part, from a brain tumor, a brain injury, delirium, or florid psychosis. Although there may be some debate about moral responsibility in these cases, there is little doubt that these conditions may reflect genuine medical disorders (assuming, as Charland does, that medical kinds exist).

Note that we are not arguing that the Cluster B's *are* the result of a "dysfunction" (this is an open empirical question), nor are we arguing that the DSM-5 definition of mental disorder is correct (we don't think it is). The point here is that Charland does not provide an argument for why the *cause* of morally problematic behavior is not relevant to its status as a medical kind. This is especially problematic given that Charland is explicitly critiquing the conception of personality disorders proposed in the DSM, which posits that the cause *is* relevant in these cases. The Argument from Identification, then, is (at least) undermotivated. We will return to this point in the next section.

16.5 The Argument from Treatment

Charland's Argument from Treatment can be formulated as such:

(1) It is impossible to imagine a successful treatment for the Cluster B disorders that does not involve a moral conversion or change.

(2) Therefore, the Cluster B's are moral, rather than medical, kinds.

This is the stronger of Charland's two arguments and is worth considering in detail. According to Charland:

> The central issue is whether there exists a *moral willingness* to change together with a sustained readiness to make the *moral effort* to make and sustain that change. Thus it is impossible to imagine a successful "treatment" or "cure" for those conditions that does not involve some sort of conversion or change in *moral character*. On this basis, it can be argued that these are fundamentally moral conditions and, consequently, that their treatment requires a sort of *moral treatment* . . . A full cure requires moral willingness, moral change, and moral effort. (2004)

> Successful treatment in this case is tantamount to a moral conversion . . . . What emerges from these considerations is that, unless the moral problems and behaviors associated with the Cluster B disorders can be overcome or eliminated, successful treatment and cure is impossible . . . . What this philosophical analysis shows is that the Cluster B personality disorders are fundamentally moral conditions. (2006)

Charland's method here is "to work back from the possibility of treatment to the nature of the kinds that are allegedly treated" (2004). According to Charland, a focus on the potential treatments for the Cluster B's leads us to the conclusion that whatever relevant change is effected by successful treatment will be *moral* change. If treatment is effective, according to this argument, it is effective only insofar as it makes one a morally "better" person; thus, the conditions are hypothesized to be primarily moral in nature, not medical.

Although we think that Charland's method of argumentation is promising, there are serious problems. Notably, the argument does not work as a logical necessity claim. Premise 1 is false. If we take "successful treatment" or "cure" to mean a person no longer meets the diagnostic criteria for a disorder (and this does appear to be Charland's view), then it is logically possible that a person could be successfully treated while the "symptoms" of the Cluster B's remain *exactly the same* and all that changes is whether they cause distress or functional impairments. Recall that the DSM-5 definition of personality disorders is explicit in requiring that the enduring patterns of behavior and inner experience that mark the specific personality disorders are only *disordered* when they cause "clinically significant distress or impairment in social, occupational, or other important areas of functioning" (APA, 2013). This distress-or-impairment requirement is, for example, part of what is supposed to differentiate between "many highly successful individuals [who] display personality traits that might be considered narcissistic" with individuals properly diagnosable with NPD. Thus, at least as a matter of logical necessity, a person diagnosed with NPD (and the other Cluster B's) could be successfully treated by merely altering their circumstances (e.g., so they become more "successful" or less distressed). No moral conversion or change is necessary here.

Charland's Argument from Treatment, then, does not support his conclusion about the moral nature of the Cluster B personality disorders. However, it is instructive to examine what goes wrong with this argument. It is possible that Charland disagrees with the DSM's (and ICD's) "distress" or "functional impairment" criteria. This *does* appear to be Charland's view (at least in relation to Cluster B's). Charland's (implicit) argument seems to be something like this: Of course, treating others in morally reprehensible ways may alienate individuals from society and this may be distressing, but being distressed that others don't like your behavior does not make that behavior a disorder (unless it becomes something like a mood disorder). Charland's argument does become more plausible if we drop the distress or impairment requirement. Indeed, as we will argue later, it is a serious problem for these diagnostic manuals that a "successful" sociopath may be considered "disordered" for something as arbitrary as being "caught" committing some wrongdoing (and thus suffering the functional impairment, and corresponding distress, of being imprisoned or otherwise sanctioned).

However, even if we drop the distress and functional impairment clauses, we will still run into the same problem encountered by the Argument from Identification. Namely, Charland provides no argument for why it should necessarily be the case that "morally reprehensible behavior" that is the result of some dysfunction (or other cause) should not be considered a medical problem. As noted earlier, there are at least some instances (e.g., antisocial behavior precipitated by delirium) where we have strong reason to believe immoral behavior should be considered reflective of a medical problem. Successful treatment, in cases such as these, will likely involve moral change, but such treatments (e.g., correcting metabolic disturbances in the case of some instances of delirium) require nothing like moral conversion or moral effort. Causes do seem to matter here.

What else might have gone wrong with Charland's argument? It is possible that Charland is assuming that "successful" treatment or "cure" requires no longer experiencing *any* of the core phenomena categorized as "symptoms" of a disorder (in addition to dismissing the dysfunction and distress requirements). If so, then Charland's argument again becomes more plausible. For example, the core feature of DSM-5 criteria for antisocial personality disorder (APD) is described as "a pervasive pattern of disregard for and violation of the rights of others," whereas the essential feature of NPD is "a pervasive pattern of grandiosity, need for admiration, and lack of empathy" (APA, 2013). If successful treatment entailed that individuals no longer had these enduring patterns of behavior and inner experience, then successful treatment may plausibly be described as entailing moral conversion. For example, successful treatment of APD would require a person no longer disregarding and violating the rights of others; this certainly appears to be a *morally* changed person.

But this conception of "successful" treatment is far too demanding. Such a view of healing would end up wrongly pathologizing a wide range of normal human differences. The core phenomena or symptoms of mental disorders are not uncommon in the general population (Leder & Zawidzki, 2023). For example, prolonged depressed mood can be both a symptom of a disorder or a normal response to life-stressors, whereas auditory hallucinations may be both symptomatic of a disorder or benign (Horwitz & Wakefield, 2007; Baumeister et al., 2017). The presence or absence of any particular "symptom" (or group of symptoms) does not, by itself, explain why certain states are disordered and others not. Regarding Cluster B's such as NPD and APD, sometimes people are just jerks, and we should not pathologize this. And to return to the "mad," "bad," "sad," language: sometimes individuals just consistently act badly. This is not necessarily pathological.

16.6 The Revised Argument from Treatment

Charland's Argument from Treatment is underdeveloped, but it does point toward a way to resolve the question of the metaphysical status of personality disorders. Namely, a focus on how and why people mentally heal can help us better understand what the problem is that is being healed. Charland was just mistaken about what successful treatment consists of. We argue that mental healing necessarily involves (re)gaining the skill of metacognitive self-regulation, and that a focus on this skill can resolve the debate over the metaphysical status of the personality disorders. In this section, we offer a revised argument from treatment:

The Revised Argument from Treatment:

(1) Successful treatment necessarily involves patients (re)gaining the ability to metacognitively self-regulate.
(2) Thus, ways of being will be mental disorders only if they involve inabilities to metacognitively self-regulate.
(3) Some ways of being that fall under the umbrella of Cluster B personality disorders will involve inabilities to metacognitively self-regulate.
(4) Some ways of being that fall under the umbrella of Cluster B personality disorders will not involve inabilities to metacognitively self-regulate.
(5) Therefore, although some ways of being that fall under the umbrella of Cluster B disorders may be disordered, others will not.

Successful treatment for mental disorders necessarily involves either gaining or regaining skill at metacognitive self-regulation. This idea has been around (in one form or another) since at least the 1980s (although, usually only implicitly). An early articulation of this idea is Marvin Goldfried's (1980) claim that therapy just is a "vehicle for training clients in coping skills." Goldfried's conception of "coping skills" is admittedly vague and is defined as "any class of cognitive or overt behavior patterns that would deal effectively with problematic situations" (1980, p. 110). Goldfried's point seems to be that therapy is not just about symptom elimination or reduction; the symptoms matter, but so does what an individual is able to do in response to these symptoms. We usually cannot eliminate all life-stressors and we cannot completely control the content of our own minds. But, Goldfried notes, we can develop coping skills to help us manage these problems of living.

We believe that Goldfried's view about "coping" can best be understood, in part, as a claim about self-regulation. Self-regulation, here, is defined as the process of altering or controlling how one responds to stimuli in order to align with one's goals or standards (Baumeister et al., 1994; Fujita, 2011). The focus is on the ability to regulate (to one's own standards) how one *responds* to exogenously and endogenously generated stimuli, not necessarily whether one is able to completely eliminate the generation of such stimuli. In the context of mental healing, all successful treatments involve patients either gaining or regaining this ability to self-regulate or "cope" (DeYoung & Krueger, 2018; Leder, 2019; Zawidzki, 2019; Leder & Zawidzki, 2023). No plausible conception of healing requires the complete elimination of symptoms associated with a disorder. And, if one can be healthy (or at least not disordered) while experiencing ways of being that may also be symptoms of a disorder, then healing must involve the ability to "cope" with them in some way.

16.7 Skilled Metacognitive Self-Regulation and Reasons-Responsiveness

One can reasonably wonder why acquiring or restoring skilled metacognitive self-regulation plays such an important role in mental healing. As we have argued, it is an important component of all successful psychotherapies; however, this does not necessarily show that it is necessary or sufficient for mental health. Perhaps learning how to cope with symptoms is merely a temporary "crutch," enabling functionality in the absence of a cure. This characterization of the skills learned in psychotherapy is natural from a functionalist perspective: skilled metacognitive self-regulation may permit social functionality, while leaving the underlying biological dysfunction untreated. But only once the biological dysfunction is successfully treated is mental health restored.

Our perspective is part of a broader, contemporary response to the inadequacies of theories that view mental disorders as biological dysfunctions (Dembić, 2023; Leder & Zawidzki, 2023). According to this broader alternative, mental disorders involve inabilities to respond to one's available reasons. As Dembić puts it, "[w]hen we ascribe a mental disorder to an individual, we basically ascribe to them that they 'cannot' (in the relevant sense) respond adequately to some of their available reasons. There are reasons for (or against) attitudes such as beliefs and emotions; as well as reasons for (or against) actions" (2023, p. 12). This perspective is motivated by the well-known inadequacies of views according to which mental disorders are biological dysfunctions: the latter seem neither necessary nor sufficient for the former (e.g., Lilienfeld & Marino, 1995; Garson, 2022). For example, there are good reasons to think that the symptoms of major depressive disorder and generalized anxiety disorder are biologically functional, that is, normal responses for which relevant neural mechanisms were selected in evolution. On the other hand, many behaviors that may be considered biologically dysfunctional, for instance homosexuality, asexuality, a love of unnecessarily risky behaviors like extreme sports, are not symptomatic of mental disorders. Our point here is not to endorse any particular theory of normal function; rather, the point is that a focus on skilled metacognitive self-regulation and reasons-responsiveness obviates the need to address these (potentially unanswerable) questions. The inability to respond adequately to one's available reasons is a promising alternative characterization of mental disorder: intuitively, in all cases of mental disorder, the person has good reasons for a certain course of behavior, or pattern of cognition and conation, reasons that they themselves should (ideally) recognize, upon which they are unable to act. The anxious or depressed patient should recognize the reasons why their anxiety or depression are inappropriate, yet they are unable to act on them. The deluded patient should recognize that there is no evidence for their delusions yet is unable to act on this evidence. The addicted person should recognize their reasons to stop or minimize their addictive behavior yet is unable to act on these reasons. It is reasonable to suppose that such inabilities can be characterized as breakdowns in metacognitive, self-regulatory skill: those suffering from mental disorders cannot skillfully regulate their own cognitive, conative, and behavioral reactions in ways that respect the available reasons they recognize.

The plausibility of this perspective depends on what, precisely, is meant by "reasons-responsiveness," and one's "available reasons." There are stronger and weaker possible interpretations. According to the stronger interpretation endorsed by Dembić, call it "thick reasons-responsiveness," one's available reasons are:

> The practical normative reasons rational creatures have for . . . [their actions], that is, . . . the facts (or true propositions) that count in favour of some action φ of ours to be good or worthwhile of pursuit. We can deliberate on the pro tanto reasons we have for or against some action φ, weigh these reasons against one another, and settle the question on whether we have, all things considered, sufficient (or decisive) reason to φ. Attitudes such as beliefs or emotions are rationally evaluable (1) with respect to whether they "fit together", that is, whether they are consistent or coherent with one another and (2) with respect to the situations we are in, that is, with respect to the facts (or true propositions)

that count in favour of the belief being true or the emotion being objectively adequate. (Dembić 2023, p. 17)

On Dembić's view, such reasons are "available" to a subject if they know them (Dembić, 2023, p. 18). But this understanding of reasons-responsiveness is inadequate for understanding mental health, as it overpathologizes difference. It is plausible that being *unable* to respond appropriately to *true* propositions (relevant to one's actions and cognitive and conative attitudes) is fully compatible with mental health. Consider "terror management theory" (Becker, 1973), according to which mental health *requires ignoring* unpleasant truths that one knows, for example about mortality, the risk of disease and suffering, and so on. Or, supposing science is roughly right about the nature of the world, consider all the true propositions known yet ignored in favor of false, supernatural propositions, in the regulation of behavior and psychological attitudes, by countless human beings who appear mentally healthy. Such examples can be multiplied indefinitely. The point is that there is no necessary connection between mental health and the ability to respond adequately only to *true* propositions relevant to regulating one's behavior and psychological attitudes; often responding adequately to *false* propositions, that is, comforting myths, while actively ignoring or compartmentalizing distressing true propositions seems more compatible with mental health.[5] The problem with thick reasons-responsiveness is that it risks conflating mental health with ideal practical rationality, where this involves believing only action-relevant *truths* and desiring only justifiable goals.

What is needed is a weaker understanding of the ability to respond to one's available reasons – a "thin reasons-responsiveness." Fortunately, there is a well-known alternative to Dembić's characterization, according to which reasons-responsiveness does *not* require being able to respond to *true* propositions that count in favor of available actions, that is, ideal practical rationality: Davidson's (2001) idea that to act for a reason is to have one's behavior caused by a belief and "pro-attitude" pair.

[5] A way out for Dembić: "Only if the individual is harmed, their condition is 'clinically relevant', that is, worthy of psychiatric or psychotherapeutic concern. Only then are they in the clinically relevant sense 'unable' to respond adequately to some of their available reasons" (2023, p. 13). However, harm is a slippery notion. On some views, just living one's life so beholden to illusions is inherently harmful. And if such illusions function to maintain people in poverty, as Marxists maintain, there are many practical harms in addition. Finally, as we pointed out above, regarding harmful social consequences of personality disorders, making harm a necessary condition on mental illness seems to imply that one can succumb to or be cured of a mental illness simply in virtue of changes in surrounding social attitudes that render one's dispositions more or less harmful, with no relevant change in one's internal constitution. For instance, a person unable to respond adequately to anything but false, supernatural beliefs would not be harmed in a religious society but would suddenly be subject to harm if that society had a successful Marxist revolution.

According to Davidson, behavior constitutes action, that is, is reasons-responsive, just in case it is caused by a belief/pro-attitude pair, where "pro-attitudes" include desires, goals, preferences, intentions, and any other states that favor some counterfactual state of the world. Thus, for example, reaching for an apple constitutes a reasons-responsive action if it is appropriately caused by a belief that the apple is within reach and a desire to retrieve the apple, for example in order to eat it. This is an extremely weak version of reasons-responsiveness, as it makes no assumption about the status of the reasons causally implicated in action. Beliefs causing actions need not be true, and pro-attitudes causing actions need not be justified in terms of survival, reproduction, or any practically rational ideal. As Davidson puts it:

> Whenever someone does something for a reason, therefore, he can be characterized as (a) having some sort of pro attitude toward actions of a certain kind, and (b) believing (or knowing, perceiving, noticing, remembering) that his action is of that kind. Under (a) are to be included desires, wantings, urges, promptings, and a great variety of moral views, aesthetic principles, economic prejudices, social conventions, and public and private goals and values in so far as these can be interpreted as attitudes of an agent directed toward actions of a certain kind ... Giving the reason why an agent did something is often a matter of naming the pro attitude (a) or the related belief (b) or both" (2001, pp. 3–4)

Thus, for example, a medieval ascetic's decision to starve herself because it is an appropriate expression of her devotion to God (Davis & Nguyen, 2014) counts as reasons-responsive, on Davidson's view: it is the product of (probably false) beliefs about the nature of God, and highly contestable private goals and values, but this is enough, on Davidson's view, to render it reasons-responsive. Similarly, the distress-free narcissist's decision to exploit even his closest family members counts as reasons-responsive, as it is the product of (similarly questionable) beliefs and desires. It follows that, if we use Davidsonian weak reasons-responsiveness to distinguish mental health from disorder, such behaviors do *not* count as symptoms of mental disorder: whether or not the relevant beliefs and pro-attitudes are legitimate or justifiable, their playing appropriate causal roles in the generation of behavior is sufficient to make the behavior reasons-responsive. It seems, therefore, that distinguishing mental health from disorder in terms of Davidsonian weak reasons-responsiveness avoids the overpathologization problems that plague biological dysfunction views, and strong reasons-responsiveness views (that appear to conflate mental health with ideal practical rationality).

There is a risk, however, that the appeal to Davidsonian weak reasons-responsiveness throws the baby out with the bathwater. For, one might wonder, is it not too cheap? Is it not possible to interpret almost any behavior, including symptoms of paradigmatic mental disorders, as reasons-responsive in the Davidsonian sense? Patients with generalized anxiety disorder, or major depressive disorder, feel and behave the way they do for reasons. The reasons may not be justified (indeed, patients themselves typically see them as unjustified); however, the whole attraction of Davidsonian weak reasons-responsiveness as an alternative to Dembić's strong reasons-responsiveness is that it allows that behavior can count as reasons-responsive (and hence, not disordered) even if it is appropriately caused by unjustified reasons. Davidson has addressed essentially this question in the context of explaining how his theory of reasons-responsive action can account for *akratic* behavior (Davidson, 2001, pp. 21–42). In explaining how "weakness of the will" is possible, Davidson endeavors to show that behavior can be subjectively irrational, yet still intentional, that is, done for *a* reason. Since Socrates, this possibility has seemed paradoxical, as it is hard to see how someone might act against their avowed better judgment intentionally. Davidson's discussion inaugurates a voluminous contemporary discussion of this problem, the gist of which is the following: human agents often have multiple, conflicting reasons for acting, and sometimes, in the competition to control behavior, the reasons they explicitly endorse lose out to conflicting reasons. These are *akratic* actions: intentional because caused by reasons; however, subjectively irrational because at odds with explicitly endorsed reasons.

The Davidsonian approach to *akrasia* is relevant to distinguishing mental health from disorder, as Heather and Segal have recognized in discussions of addiction (2013, 2015). The reason is that it makes room for behavior that, although intentional because done for a reason, is subjectively irrational, because it goes against the explicitly avowed beliefs and desires of the agent. As Davidson puts it:

> Why would anyone ever perform an action when he thought that, everything considered, another action would be better? If this is a request for a psychological explanation, then the answers will no doubt refer to the interesting phenomena familiar from most discussions of incontinence: self-deception, overpowering desires, lack of imagination, and the rest. But if the question is read, what is the agent's reason for doing A when he believes it would be better, all things considered, to do another thing, then the answer must be: for this, the agent has no reason. We perceive a creature as rational in so far as we are able to view his movements as part of a rational pattern comprising also thoughts, desires, emotions, and volitions. (In this we are much aided by the actions we conceive to be utterances). Through faulty inference, incomplete evidence, lack of diligence, or flagging sympathy, we often enough fail to detect a pattern that is there. But in the case of incontinence, the attempt to read reason into behaviour is necessarily subject to a degree of frustration … What is special in incontinence is that the actor cannot understand himself: he recognizes, in his own intentional behaviour, something essentially absurd. (2001, p. 42)

This is precisely the kind of reasons-responsiveness that is appropriate to distinguishing between mental health and disorder in terms of skilled, metacognitive self-regulation.[6]

What matters is not whether an individual meets some ideal of practical rationality or whether they are functioning properly relative to biological imperatives like survival and reproduction, but rather whether their behavior is rationally interpretable *by their own lights*. On the Davidsonian view, the *akratic* fails to be reasons-responsive in an important sense, even though the relevant behavior is caused by reasons (and hence intentional), because the relevant behavior is not caused by their explicitly avowed reasons, and this renders their overall pattern of behavior uninterpretable. In terms of skilled, metacognitive self-regulation, the *akratic* is incapable of regulating their own mental states and behavior such that their avowed reasons are in control. The same can be said for victims of paradigmatic mental disorders: chronically anxious or depressed or obsessive patients should view these patterns of belief, affect, and behavior as irrational by their own lights. The problem is that they are *incapable* of the kind of skilled metacognitive self-regulation required to control them.

Thus, an appropriately modified Davidsonian conception of weak reasons-responsiveness is well suited to distinguishing mental health from disorder, while, at the same time, making clear why skilled metacognitive self-regulation is constitutively linked to mental health. The key to mental health, on this view, is that an agent's behavior is rationally interpretable *by their own lights*, that is, controlled by their avowed best judgments regarding the reasons for which they should act. This avoids the overpathologization of biological dysfunction views, as well as strong reasons-responsiveness views which appear to conflate mental health with ideal practical rationality. What matters is what individuals themselves take to be legitimate reasons for acting, not objectively legitimate reasons for acting. The Davidsonian perspective also explains why behavior that might be biologically adaptive, for example, on some theories, depressed or anxious behavior, might nonetheless be disordered: afflicted individuals cannot make sense of it in terms of their own best judgments about the reasons for which they ought to act. Finally, it is clear that in this view, the relevant failures in mental disorder involve a lack or breakdown in skilled metacognitive self-regulation: patients are unable to

[6] As Alfred Mele argues in a particularly thoughtful and systematic development of the Davidsonian paradigm: "[s]elf-control . . . involves both motivation to act as one judges best and, typically, a collection of *skills* and powers of resistance . . . this motivation and exercises of these *skills* and powers may influence one's motivational condition at the time of action and, therefore, one's intentional behavior. Through an exercise of self-control . . . an agent may intervene in his own motivational processes, generating a motivational balance favorable to continent action" (1987, p. 108, emphasis added).

skillfully regulate their own cognition, conation, and behavior to respect their own explicitly endorsable reasons or goals.

16.8 Medical or Moral, Redux

So, are Cluster B personality disorders genuine mental disorders? It depends. A focus on the metacognitive skill of self-regulation shows that the Cluster B's, as currently formulated in the DSM, are both overly inclusive *and* overly exclusive. Regarding the over-inclusivity, the ways of being diagnosable as Cluster B's can involve no inability to skillfully self-regulate but may still be considered "disordered" because of the "functional impairment" clause. For example, a contented and successful sociopath may be diagnosable with APD just because they got caught performing an antisocial act and thus add a functional impairment to the presence of their antisocial personality traits matching the essential features of APD. Similarly, a contented and successful narcissist may be diagnosable with NPD just because the world changed and they got "canceled" (leading to functional impairment).[7] In both cases, the functional impairment clause makes it the case that whether an individual's enduring pattern of behavior and inner experience is properly judged to be pathological will depend (in large part) on the reactions of *others*; this is absurd. Charland is right that this functional impairment clause does smuggle in moral values (if this was his view). Cases like these would reflect the wrongful pathologization of normal differences (if there were no failure of skilled self-regulation).

However, all the Cluster B's can also capture genuine inabilities to self-regulate (and, thus, capture genuine disorders). For example, individuals meeting the diagnostic criteria for NPD may genuinely be unable to regulate their responses to others not admiring them sufficiently, individuals meeting the criteria for APD may be unable to regulate how they respond to their impulsivity, individuals meeting the criteria for BPD may be unable to regulate their responses to chronic feelings of emptiness, and individuals meeting the diagnostic criteria of HPD (histrionic personality disorder) may be unable to regulate their responses to their discomfort in not being the center of attention. The diagnostic criteria for all the Cluster B's, although sometimes capturing normal human difference, often will also capture individuals who are unable to skillfully regulate their responses to endogenously and exogenously created stimuli.

The Cluster B's, as currently formulated in the DSM, are also overly exclusive. Specifically, the "dysfunction" requirement is unnecessary. Recall that both the DSM-5 and ICD-11 require a psychological, biological, or developmental "dysfunction" for a way of being to be identified as disordered. So, the

[7] Note that this point is specific to the current DSM-5 and ICD-11 diagnostic criteria with the noted exception of the diagnosis of "Mild Personality Disorder" in the ICD-11 (see footnote 3).

debate about the pathological status of the Cluster B's comes down, in large part, to whether they are the result of a "dysfunction." This is wrongheaded. As noted earlier, we agree that the cause of the behaviors and mental events associated with the symptoms of these disorders does matter in adjudicating their status as medical or moral kinds. However, as argued above, function and dysfunction are the wrong place to focus. The pathological status of the Cluster B's is best assessed by a person's ability to skillfully self-regulate.

To conclude: Charland's analytic method (i.e., working back from the possibility of treatment to the nature of the kinds being treated) was on the right track. Charland was just mistakenly focused on the role played in treatment by the alteration of mental content (i.e., "moral conversion"). The presence or absence of any particular mental content does not explain why certain states are disordered and others not. People can, and do, differ greatly in the content of their mental states. This variation only reflects a disorder when people are no longer able to regulate their responses to these mental states (Leder & Zawidzki, 2023). So, what does successful therapy do? It enables folks to "skillfully cope" or skillfully self-regulate. If there is no inability to skillfully cope/skillfully self-regulate, then there should be no disorder. Sometimes this inability applies to folks who fall under the current DSM-5 diagnostic criteria, sometimes it does not. So, what does a focus on "the possibility of treatment" show us about the "nature of the kinds that are allegedly treated"? The boundary between disordered and non-disordered mental states is drawn by what individuals are able to do, not just what they do.

References

American Psychiatric Association. (1994). *Diagnostic and statistical manual of mental disorders* (4th ed.). American Psychiatric Association.

American Psychiatric Association. (2013). *Diagnostic and statistical manual of mental disorders* (5th ed.). American Psychiatric Association.

Banicki, K. (2018). Personality disorders and thick concepts. *Philosophy, Psychiatry, & Psychology*, 25(3), 209–221.

Baumeister, D., Sedgwick, O., Howes, O., & Peters, E. (2017). Auditory verbal hallucinations and continuum models of psychosis: A systematic review of the healthy voice-hearer literature. *Clinical Psychology Review*, 51, 125–141.

Baumeister, R. F., Heatherton, T., & Tice, M. (1994). *Losing control*. Academic Press.

Becker, E. (1973). *The denial of death*. The Free Press.

Charland, L. C. (2004). Character: Moral treatment and the personality disorders. In J. Radden (ed.), *The philosophy of psychiatry* (pp. 64–77). Oxford University Press.

Charland, L. C. (2006). Moral nature of the DSM-IV Cluster B personality disorders. *Journal of Personality Disorders*, *20*(2), 116–125.

Charland, L. C. (2010). Medical or moral kinds?: Moving beyond a false dichotomy. *Philosophy, Psychiatry, & Psychology*, *17*(2), 119–125.

Davidson, D. (2001). *Essays on actions and events: Philosophical essays volume 1*. Clarendon Press.

Davis, A. A., & Nguyen, M. (2014). A case study of anorexia nervosa driven by religious sacrifice. *Case Reports in Psychiatry*, 2014, 512764. http://dx.doi.org/10.1155/2014/512764

Dembić, S. (2023). Mental disorder: An ability-based view. *Philosophy and the Mind Sciences*, *4*, 2. https://doi.org/10.33735/phimisci.2023.9630

DeYoung, C. G., & Krueger, R. F. (2018). A cybernetic theory of psychopathology. *Psychological Inquiry*, 29(3), 117–138.

Fujita, K. (2011). On conceptualizing self-control as more than the effortful inhibition of impulses. *Personality and Social Psychology Review*, 15(4), 352–366.

Garson, J. (2022). *Madness: A philosophical exploration*. Oxford University Press.

Goldfried, M. R. (1980). Psychotherapy as coping skills training. In M. J. Mahoney (ed.), *Psychotherapy process: Current issues and future directions* (pp. 89–119). Springer US.

Heather, N., & Segal, G. (2013). Understanding addiction: Donald Davidson and the problem of akrasia. *Addiction Research & Theory*, *21*(6), 445–452.

Heather, N., & Segal, G. (2015). Is addiction a myth? Donald Davidson's solution to the problem of akrasia says not. *International Journal of Alcohol and Drug Research*, *4* (1), 77–83.

Horwitz, A. V., & Wakefield, J. C. (2007). *The loss of sadness: How psychiatry transformed normal sorrow into depressive disorder*. Oxford University Press.

Kendell, R. E. (2002). The distinction between personality disorder and mental illness. *The British Journal of Psychiatry*, 180(2), 110–115.

Leder, G. (2019). What does it mean to have a meaning problem? Meaning, skill, and the mechanisms of change in psychotherapy. *Philosophy, Psychiatry, & Psychology*, *26* (3), E35.

Leder, G., & Zawidzki, T. (2023). The skill of mental health. *Philosophy and the Mind Sciences*, *4*, 3. https://doi.org/10.33735/phimisci.2023.9684

Lilienfeld, S. O., & Marino, L. (1995). Mental disorder as a Roschian concept: A critique of Wakefield's "harmful dysfunction" analysis. *Journal of Abnormal Psychology*, *104*, 411–420.

Mele, A. R. (1987). *Irrationality: An essay on akrasia, self-deception, and self-control*. Oxford University Press.

Pickard, H. (2009). Mental illness is indeed a myth. In L. Bortolotti & M. Broome (eds.), *Psychiatry as cognitive neuroscience: Philosophical perspectives*, pp. 83–101. Oxford University Press.

Reimer, M. (2013). Moral disorder In the DSM-IV?: The Cluster B personality disorders. *Philosophy, Psychiatry, & Psychology*, *20*(3), 203–215.

World Health Organization (2021). International statistical classification of diseases and related health problems (11th ed.). https://icd.who.int/

Zachar, P., & Potter, N. N. (2010). Personality disorders: Moral or medical kinds – or both? *Philosophy, Psychiatry, & Psychology*, 17(2), 101–117.

Zawidzki, T. (2019). Metacognitive skill and the therapeutic regulation of emotion. *Philosophical Topics*, *47*(2), 27–51.

Part IV

Exploring Negative Consequences of Diagnosing Personality Disorder

17 Aversive and Antagonistic Personality Disorder

A Post-Colonial Analysis

Grant Gillett and Armon J. Tamatea

> Just as a grizzly bear cannot be separated from its larger context – metaphorically it is 5% claws, teeth, fur, and bone and 95% forest, salmon rivers, ocean beach, and alpine meadow – so too, we are very much emergent properties comprising both biophysical and societal contexts. (Taylor et al., 2010, p. 81)

The complex phenomenon of criminality, violence, and antisocial behaviour is far too readily linked to individuals and to their biologically determined psychology. Such a link undoubtedly exists and affects criminal propensities, but it is overly simplified by being thought of in terms of the internal neuropsychological dispositions of the individual. That view is slowly being moderated and these reflections applaud and offer an Indigenous voice to politically informed research and enquiry into the development of human behaviour through infancy, upbringing, and early adult experience. That voice is required and timely in rethinking an overtly 'Western' formulation and individualistic view of this mental discontent (as suggested by the label 'personality disorder'). However, such a re-formulation does not negate the extensive empirical research now available on the underlying neural dimensions of personality function (Gillett & Glannon, 2023) but merely adds sophistication to that ongoing neuroscientifically informed work by acknowledging the top-down neurocognitive elements in personality development and behavioural integration.

These potentially more inclusive factors operate in the light of overarching variables operating in human ethology. The child's self-formation in a post-colonial setting is often a very different project for individuals from a marginalised group such as Indigenous people. In popular culture, *Boy*, a film directed by Māori filmmaker Taika Waititi, explores this cultural phenomenon: that potentially adverse developmental factors are often exaggerated by socioeconomic disadvantage, family instability, and financial hardship, all of which disrupt taking a well-functioning place in society. In that 'synthetic' and inclusive mode of doing neurophilosophical and neurocognitive research in the philosophy of psychiatry, we can consider the post-colonial situation of many of the young people who become involved in crime and social dysfunction and are over-represented in the relevant statistics.

The brain is an associative neural network that develops holistic patterns of sensorimotor and cognitive activity adapted to an ethological environment. For the human organism this site has a feature that is found in many species but exaggerated in our own to the point of making a qualitative difference between the human world and that of other creatures. That feature is the sociocultural character of the lived human world replete with its abstract constructions, such as various aspects of culture, human relations, ethics, and the law (which is itself based on a culture and its multiple situated histories). In many cases in which post-colonial thought needs to be considered, the relevant post-industrial socioculturally inflected thinking arises in a developed post-industrial culture such as that of Europe or the United Kingdom or other developed colonising powers.

In developed-world contexts, post-colonial analysis forms an oft-neglected strand of thinking and critique that concerns historical contacts between a colonising culture and an Indigenous or (prehistorically originating) culture in a given geographical area with a complex history (Burney, 2012). As a result of that history young people in such contexts are sometimes torn by conflicting ways of being. Just such forces are found with New Zealand Māori, Aboriginal and Torres Strait Islanders (Indigenous Australians), or First Nations people in North America. Two very different sets of rhythms of life intersect and sometimes mismatches or conflicts occur that result in psychosocial dysfunction and an 'othering' narrative. Young people from Indigenous groups lose their psychosocial roots and the loss is reflected in crime statistics (Anthony & Blagg, 2022). These authors remark that across identified settler colonies such as Australia, Aotearoa New Zealand, Canada, and the United States, the colonial drive to conquer land and remove Indigenous peoples has left deep scars on Indigenous communities and compromised bonds to kin, culture, and nationhood. The authors lament the breakdown in human psychology and relationships that this causes among Indigenous populations whose own values can be dramatically disrupted or marginalised. The 'lost' values could otherwise (albeit counterfactually) form a powerful antidote to the post-colonial effects, even in the unjust context of colonial history. The intersections between these factors with crime and youth unrest are complex and multifaceted, but should cause us to rethink an overly simplistic and biologically individualistic relationship between neuroscience and personality as it is theorised and researched to *cause* disorders that contribute to antisocial behaviour and violence.

17.1 Neurodynamics, Indigeneity, and Personality Formation

In all human societies, including those of the lands from which the colonisers came, the rhythms of life have incorporated reciprocity, the formation of group bonds, the binding together of families as the basis for society, and the roles of leadership incorporating protection of those who fall under the authority of the leader or chief, in the face of a sometimes 'cruel' nature (Sawyer, 1978). This basic human pattern built into our rhythms of life and society is recognisable even in the modern world and it is interesting to notice that it predates that world and the sociopolitical influences which have shaped scholarship within it. It is time to apply a post-colonial correction to that very contemporary strand of thinking in personality theory and psychology in general. In fact, individualistic and somewhat biologically reductive thought about neuroscientific tendencies that held sway in an earlier age should not be allowed to distort neuroscience and psychiatry after the ground-breaking work of thinkers such as John Hughlings-Jackson, Alexander Luria, and Walter Freeman.

Hughlings-Jackson combined extensive clinical experience with an approach to neuroscience deeply affected by Darwinian theories of adaptation and evolution in a holistic context (Gillett & Franz, 2016). The resultant form of dynamic neuroscience did not easily merge with thinking under a post-industrial (or quasi-mechanistic) model of neuroscience as Hughlings-Jackson kept his eye informed and directed by evolutionary thinking and offered an organic understanding of the brain and its realisation of the rhythms of life that was inclusive and subtly antireductive.

Vygotsky – and then Luria – added to this much earlier work bringing an orientation towards social function and the holism of psychology in the light of human language. They examined and considered psycholinguistics as an advanced adaptive feature of human neurocognition distinguishing the human species and articulating human intelligence in a distinctive way. They thereby added a sophisticated and structured form of socioculturally situated cognition and knowledge to human adaptation.

Walter Freeman added to neurobiology a dynamic orientation in neuroscience by experimenting on live intact animals using sophisticated neuroimaging. He adapted Aristotle's naturalistic theory as laid out by Aquinas (Freeman, 2008), which aimed to include language and sociopolitical function in the development of a distinctively human phenotype. Language, of course, must be regarded as a hybrid feature of a human being – both biological and sociopolitical. This was a distinctive (and partly epigenetic, in the broadest sense) function and not merely a somatic contribution to evolutionary fitness. Just as Freeman wished to retain a deeply Aristotelian orientation and avoid the philosophically problematic and unnecessary complexities of cognitive dualism, we can acknowledge the profound contribution of language and social factors in the human personality as being both inclusively and non-biologically 'epigenetic'.

Between them, these thinkers and contemporary neuroscientific and psychological literature, developing new experimental programmes aided by neuroimaging, have reformed our understanding of the relationship between neuroscience and psychology in its broadest scope. Northoff, Howhy, and others have also remodelled the relationship between neuroscience and the mind using such a combination of clinical neuroimaging and experimentation. Northoff focuses on the development of a coherent sense of personal being as an individual located in a certain time and spatiotemporal domain in whom is formed a sense of oneself as a coherent psychological individual (e.g., Hamilton & Northoff, 2021). He notes that this sensate being is severely disrupted in psychotic states where thought is subject to all kinds of disorders and affective anomalies. Through the work of neurodynamic thinkers and clinical scientists, we now possess the theoretical and scientific groundwork to apply contemporary findings to personality research (Hanegraaf et al., 2023). In their study, Hanegraaf and collaborators found 'a consilience between neurobiological and trait-based factors ... affecting social functioning'. This interesting result did not explicitly look at the sociopolitical and post-colonial inflections of social functioning, which is our concern, and it would be entirely consistent with that focus for more biological personality factors to interact significantly with post-colonial influences.

Personality development and maturation in the human neurocognitive/neuropsychological system must therefore be considered to be a holistic phenomenon incorporating the diverse factors noted by Hughlings-Jackson, Luria, and, in the 1970s, Neisser. Neisser (1976) critiqued trait-based personality and psychological factors by exploring the complexity and fluidity underlying many accounts of human cognition in the real world, and suitably updated psychological theory to include a nod to contemporary advances in cognitive neuroscience. We must now examine, with an eye to post-colonialism, the relation between familial and social disruption and wider factors in personality formation that will result in antisocial tendencies and a sense of marginalisation in many young people.

We acknowledge the intricate interplay between genetics and the widest possible range of epigenetic factors, including not only intracellular factors but also those that act on the organism as a whole. These factors influence the total context of biological function and the way it forms psychological characteristics. This does nothing to undermine the importance of biological traits associated with personality disorders but merely allows *complexity* to enter into psychological aetiology.

Complexity has long been suspected of being an important conceptual factor in properly assessing psychiatric research. In his extended review,

Butz (1997) acknowledges the effect on human psychology of a changing menu that has to be dealt with by multiple psychological and personal adjustments sometimes resulting in psychiatric disturbance. He notes that the complexity of the human associative system is in evidence here and that psychotherapists involved with those who are casualties of this complex change must take maximal account of the fluidity and multiple responsiveness of the human neurocognitive and neuropsychological system when we assess social adaptation. For instance, the so-called aversive-antagonistic 'dark core' of personality, which is variously factored into anything from 16 traits (Cattell, 1978) to five (Costa & McCrae, 1992), or even as few as three (Eysenck, 1967), is said to be an intrapersonal and possibly biological element in the constitution of an individual human subject predisposing that person to antisocial behaviour and criminality. This conceptualisation, one could argue, harks back to an earlier model of psychology as an internal set of characteristics of an individual that developed in the social context but was largely determined by neurobiological and humoral factors. The malleability of behaviour in the face of operant conditioning cast doubt on this early view and one of the authors of this work (G.G.) was involved in an experiment which inadvertently revealed that, even in rats, factors which could be described as personality were vulnerable to the contingencies to which the individual was exposed (Gillett & Webster, 1975). Despite that demonstration, the dominance of the functional model driving behaviourism caused the authors not to realise what had happened even when faced with ethological indicators of an alternative hypothesis with potentially broad social significance.

The rats had clearly developed phenomena that indicated psychological dysfunction such as aggression, loss of body condition, fear of the experimental setting, and hostility towards those conducting the experiment who were taking them to a 'learning' session. However, these did not fit with the paradigms being followed and so were not appreciated until years later when the full import of ethology and training in psychiatric medicine had enabled the experience to be reflected upon anew. In the light of that reflection it is interesting and instructive to read contemporary work on the adverse or 'dark' factors in personality and even more interesting to begin to discern the relationships between that work and post-colonial analyses of social behaviour (Hilbig et al., 2021).

Contemporary scholarship in developed societies indicates that the disruption of families and communities has a complex interaction with criminal behaviour and the psychological tendencies that predispose to it (Wong, 2011). That fact radically disrupts any tendency to link antisocial behaviour and its legal correlates or consequences merely (and simplistically) to intra-individual factors which orientation can ignore sociopolitical realities particularly in mixed-ethnicity and post-colonial contexts.

In fact, there is a confused literature – the interpretation of which tends to confine itself, by overuse of the biomedical model, and under-analyse socially deviant and destructive behaviour; that perspective does not help with understanding the problems faced by Indigenous communities. On the other side of the personality 'coin', factors to do with empathy and humility seem to form a corrective to the dark side of personality and its expression and clearly fit within social functioning both in their genesis and expression (Posick, 2013). The relevant study showed a complex overlap between sociopolitical phenomena such as victimisation and subsequent criminal offending. Following the Soviet tradition of Luria and Vygotski, it is not surprising to find that wider sociocultural factors to do with family, community, and empathy play an important role in the genesis of crime and an effective policing so that empathy, again, must be jointly analysed in terms of the psychological traits of the individual and a community context (or human ecology). This corrective contextualisation of personality theory in the light of contemporary neurophilosophy and philosophical psychology allows us to re-evaluate the rather harsh statistical evidence about criminality that can be so skewed by the biomedical model.

Northoff and his group (2013) have explored many aspects of neurodynamic function in relation to different areas of psychological adaptation. They note that the brain is a holistic associative system constantly reconfiguring itself and its dispositions in the light of situated ethological activity. This results in the formation of a conscious, psychologically complex 'self' who must be analysed in an inclusive and naturalistic manner that can be traced back to Aristotle (Gillett, 2018). Such a contemporary conceptualisation re-introduces the sociocultural and political context into the analysis and that relativises intra-individual factors to a partial role in antisocial behaviour and crime, although it does nothing radical to alter the contribution of neuropathology and neurohumoral effects on behavioural tendencies. These neurobiological and medically accessible factors coexist with the autopoietic self-formation of the individual under diverse contextual conditions.

17.2 Neurodynamics: Philosophical Psychology, Ethics, and Youth Crime

We have already noted the need to update our post-industrial and individualistic methods and concepts in neuropsychology so as to incorporate wider sociopolitical contexts, which have a profound effect on individual psychological function. Neurophilosophy has not been backward in this venture and the new holistic neurodynamics allows us to advance the analysis in the light of contemporary scientific evidence and philosophical analyses of psychological function (Gillett & Glannon, 2023).

During life, a human being develops, as we have outlined, culturally inflected rhythms of sensorimotor and cognitive interaction, each connected with their sociocultural and physical context. These rhythms form *hexes* or complex dispositions to respond within a given space of action and thought. The neurocognitive formation of the child is cumulative and progressive, so that there is progress towards mastery of an adult way of acting within a culture and society that results in the *sociocultural formation* of the child to the point where the attainment of adult masteries can be signalled in some culturally appropriate manner – such as a 21st birthday party, a vigil, or some other performance which can be followed by a coming-of-age ceremony, or a name change into an adult form (such as ‘Mr Jones’). All cultural settings have a means of marking such transitions. At the stage of life where childhood ends and adult rhythms are being formed, other things are happening to the embodied being; we often think of adolescent hormones, but there are many other changes in adolescents, for instance they are expected to begin to create relationships across the sexes rather than solely with the companions of their youth. The neurocognitive states that thereby develop under adolescent patterns of relationship are therefore quite different; the rough and tumble of youth have to become inflected by maturity and a growing sense of responsibility or answerability for one’s actions and decisions within/to families and wider contexts.

The philosophy of adolescence is complex because there we see factors that have operated on personality formation in childhood (which include neurobiological factors such as minimal brain damage and neurohumoral factors) further complexified and their expression by the many adjustments and changes that mark the transition to adulthood in any society. In particular, Indigenous societies reflect the respect and emulation of adult behaviour as being disrupted by post-colonial factors whereby the adults are rendered ineffective or marginalised and sometimes deeply dysfunctional in ways that affect their child-rearing practices and ethological competencies. The disruption of tribal and ancestral structures and community bonds (such as those that bind together families) is hugely confounding for adolescent identity development. Problems such as alcoholism, drug addiction, antisocial behaviour, or the formation of disruptive collectives such as gangs are common and offer some amelioration for the disordered ethological situation. Various of these results or sociopolitical elements are more ascendant in various post-colonial settings depending on multiple interacting factors.

In short, alienation and socialisation form a problematic intersection. We can express the philosophical problem here by means of a syllogism:

(1) Personality is considered to be an 'individual' psychological characteristic.
(2) Personality is a result of psychologically relevant factors and wider effects on human development.

Considering (3): Those psychological factors include sociopolitical ethology.
(4) Sociopolitical ethology acts on and not only within an individual.

Therefore (1) as stated, if taken to imply that personality is an 'intra-individually determined' characteristic, is false. We have developed the alternative idea that antisocial and personality disorder must be understood as a phenomenon (or complex mix of phenomena), analysed in biopsychosocial terms (Bolton & Gillett, 2019).

17.3 Identity Development: An Indigenous View

The imposition of a 'personality disorder' as part of a psychological diagnosis that carries with it a presumption of treatment and correction is an affront to Māori and other Indigenous notions of *identity*. Thus, there are critical tensions between Indigenous ways of being and becoming and the medical model that underlies psychiatry in most post-colonial psychiatric and medical science and particularly in its understanding of personality disorder.

Although a description of the Māori World is beyond the scope of this chapter – indeed, there is no single Māori reality (Durie, 1998) – it will be worth noting a couple of points to reflect the conceptual and social challenges of traversing between worldviews. For Marsden (1992), there are relational and transcendental dimensions to consider, but he warns that an abstract rational and empirical approach to understanding Māori culture is inadequate to grasp the 'concrete act of existing which is fragmentary, paradoxical and incomplete' (p. 136), adding that the integration of an individual as a full member of a community takes place over a long time – not through formal schooling, but via experience in the cultural milieu.

Furthermore, and in acknowledgement of the complexity involved in identity development, renowned Indigenous healer Wiremu NiaNia and colleagues (2017) offer three practical concepts to help non-Māori mental health practitioners to navigate an Indigenous world. (1) *Mauri* refers to a 'life force' (p. 3). This has a transcendent function and reflects one's connectedness to Te Kaihanga (the Creator); (2) *Tapu* reflects the sacredness of that relationship – which can signal whether the state of something is forbidden or sacred (e.g. person, place, object, or ritual); and (3) *Mana* refers to the spiritual authority, energy, or power embodied in a person or their whanau (family) by virtue of their relationship with Te Kaihanga and other significant relationships.

Māori, like other Indigenous groups, have been susceptible to socioeconomic disempowerment resulting from colonisation, economic dislocation, and the imposition of alien legal, educational, health, and religious systems (Lee, 1995). On an everyday level, many Māori are subject to multiple prejudices in relation to: (1) criminal histories and associations (e.g. gangs), (2) lower socioeconomic status and poverty, and (3) racism. Furthermore, Māori have traditionally been marginalised in national decision-making about issues of health and economic autonomy, usually as a result of low political influence or consideration (Cox, 1993). These social biases and structures have resulted in young Māori males being disproportionately represented in the youth and adult justice system in New Zealand. Commonly, young Māori who offend have (Department of Corrections, 2007):

- experienced neglect and abuse;
- been exposed to interpersonal violence;
- been exposed to and/or used alcohol, drugs and other substances;
- poor literacy/numeracy skills and limited/poor engagement with education;
- untreated mental health and/or behavioural difficulties; and/or,
- limited access to consistent and prosocial supports.

In addition to the risk factors above, a significant proportion of these youth have histories of early involvement with government agencies for care and protection due to personal safety from abuse and neglect, multiple placements during growth and development, and consequent complex disruptions of family connections.

Stereotypes about Māori are easily accessible – they inform and contribute to cultural distortions about what is considered to be essentially Māori and what is 'other'. Many young Māori draw narratives about who they are *as Māori* from racial stereotypes and in an absence of other information may perpetuate behaviours and practices which maintain the status quo. The opportunity to change is also fraught with difficulty – movement away from particular positions implies an acceptance or rejection of certain senses of Māori identity (Tamatea & Waipara-Panapa, 2022).

By way of example, in the early 2000s the second author (A.T.) had just entered the New Zealand correctional service as a practicum psychologist stationed at a medium-security facility for young people who had seriously offended. Most of these young boys were Māori or Polynesian by descent. Although the facility was then-state of the art with regard to security and well-being considerations in the design itself (i.e. no shared cells, private showers and toilets, large and deliberative spaces for work (horticulture), play (basketball), education (literacy and numeracy), and therapy (group-based and criminogenic in focus)), it was not uncommon for many of those young people to express a strong desire and aspiration to work their way to Paremoremo (Auckland) prison – the only maximum-security prison in New Zealand, and one with formidable formal and informal histories of violence. To do so traditionally required an act of serious violence, sexual violence, kidnapping, or serious assaults on custodial officers, among other things. The setting was widely known as dangerous and largely occupied by gang members. However, the appeal for many of the young prisoners was not only to attain reputation ('no one f*cks with you when they know you've been up there') but also proximity to criminalised whanau (family) members – usually fathers, uncles, and cousins – who were held therein.

These two sociopolitical phenomena combine in many alienated youth to blunt their empathy for other people affected by their crimes. If we accept that the ongoing self-remaking that is part of one's psychological life during youth requires a supportive affective and disposition-shaping environment then it follows that the worst place for these malleable young minds is a context in which resistance, opposition, and self-protection form part of a survival strategy. This is the brew that ferments a vintage of self-serving and wary individuals always looking for an 'edge' (multiple senses) within their dealings with others. That 'edge' can take many forms, but may often include being feared for who one is or a nested member of a prominent grouping.

17.4 Personality Disorders

The psychological dysfunctions called 'personality disorders' can be viewed as internal to the psychology of the individual all too easily seen as reflecting biological variations underlying social and psychological function, and thus as intrapersonal before being (causally) interpersonal in their characteristics. There are undoubtably biological and possibly genetic factors in the mix but there is a profound effect of relationships and sociocultural factors in the psychological functioning of the individual such that the individual's self-formation and cognitive/affective functions are often compromised. The 'internal' psychological disruptions that result then affect the well-being of the person who suffers from the anomalies comprising the 'personality disorders' and the lack of flexibility in integration of the internal rhythms of self-control and adaptation to the human milieu. Indigenous societies are often more settled in their ways of socialising and integrating their younger members through flexible village-based nurturing. A combination of cultural rituals, folkways, and opportunities for formative activity, with socially recognised markers guiding young people towards an adult role in society and well-recognised contexts of family formation and stable breeding partnerships, help form characteristic ways of being part of an Indigenous social context.

When those of an ethnic or cultural group are marginalised within their sociopolitical context as happens to many adolescents in Western urban contexts, such individuals struggle in terms of the accepted norms of post-industrial society and its sociopolitical arrangements. These often focus on instrumental and individual benefit for its members as economic individuals, so it is no wonder that alternative value systems gain social prominence among those individuals in that setting. This ethos marginalises more 'natural' and ethological human relationships and cultural groups that highly value them. Modern medical approaches to personality disorders have, far too often, adopted the medical model and its founding of psychiatric disorder on neurocognitive characteristics as revealed by post-Enlightenment neuroscience. This tradition conceals a complex relationship between neurodynamics, post-colonialism, identity formation, and crime. That complex relationship needs to be examined from a more inclusive and holistic Indigenous understanding in the post-colonial world we all inhabit.

A recent study by the Justice Department in New Zealand showed that Māori are more likely to be convicted of crime than Pakeha (NZ European), are more likely to be imprisoned for a similar crime, are more likely to reoffend after release from prison, and receive harsher sentences than Pakeha for a similar crime (McIntosh & Workman, 2017). The same is true for First Nations people in Canada (Department of Justice Canada, 2019) and Aboriginal people in Australia (Australian Bureau of Statistics, 2016). In every case we have a post-colonial setting and government institutions, even those committed to impartial justice, where there is clear evidence that the key markers of dysfunctional psychological life are disproportionately represented in the colonised population. It is much too easy for a relatively affluent and middle-class dominated society to associate this with internal psychological disruption and take the focus away from post-colonial injustices of diverse kinds. These show up in various ways, such as addiction, family disruption, antisocial behaviour, educational under-achievement, and violence of many kinds including self-harm and intrafamilial abuse.

17.5 Postcolonial Psychology and Its Discontents

Indigenous people in postcolonial settings find themselves labouring under a number of disruptions. Their life-world is changed from the one in which they have developed rhythms of life or folkways which were adaptive and fitting to the environment they inhabited before colonisation. In the environments created by the colonisers all the ills of urban life and a history of colonial disruptions of Indigenous communities are brought into the rhythms of life, its relationality, and social structures. Within this context their language and their 'ways of going on' – to use Wittgenstein's (1958) phrase – are both rendered dysfunctional for the purposes of everyday life.

Unfortunately, the result of Western individualist philosophy is to attribute dysfunction and crime to the internal constitution of the individual and neglect the sociopolitical factors to which worldwide research should alert us. This is particularly tragic for Indigenous children and youth who were raised with a distorted self-image in which the language is regarded as an anomaly and the ways of being in community are relegated to irrelevance. Thus, there is no support for becoming a person who can fruitfully, productively, and creatively live your heritage for an Indigenous person. The damage this does as we develop is incalculable and ramifies through every aspect of life. Where postcolonial inequities abound, there is no way to be a proud and self-valuing young Māori, First Nations person, Aboriginal Australian, or Inuit. That is one of the many losses that will distort your life.

We acknowledge, then, that the factors which contribute to aversive-antagonistic personality patterns cannot be considered in a superficial way as merely lifestyle choices, behavioural quirks, or cultural issues. Rather, they are manifestations of the complex interplay of historical, socioeconomic, and political circumstances that impact on health and justice outcomes as well as uneven access to appropriate and adequate services designed to medicalise problems that are largely social in nature. We would further argue that solutions to problems (medical or otherwise) are influenced – and limited – by how they are *conceptualised*. So, a quasi-medical formulation of aversive-antagonistic personality patterns such as psychopathic, antisocial, and borderline personality disorder indicates individual pathology where the person is the source of the problem (and blame), which in turn, implies a quasi-medical solution (e.g. prison-based offender rehabilitation programmes) complete with a pre-packaged language that speaks of 'treatment' and 'dosage'.

By contrast, the concerns of a post-colonial analysis involve decentring the orientations of the Coloniser (as reflected in mainstream health, justice, and social services), and reclaiming an epistemological space for Indigenous persons whose position has been marginalised and whose perspective has been ignored due to being represented as 'exotic' at best or 'unsophisticated' at worst. Whereas many critical and reflective analyses focus on literary texts (e.g. Said, 1978), it is argued that psychiatric practices are informed by diagnostic schemes that are themselves derived from specific research traditions (e.g. clinical trials, individual differences) that promote categorical and disaggregating approaches to personhood. This means notions of representation – how the person is framed in psychiatric/psychological discourse – are imposed with signifiers of psychopathology emanating from centralised bases of power (the mental health professions and institutions) to a passive periphery (service users, patients, clients). In jurisdictions where colonial baggage and 'difficult knowledge' (Pitt & Britzman, 2003, p. 755) is a salient feature of the personal and collective context, it is prudent to consider practices and texts with a post-colonial lens. Interrogating texts and practices by means of identifying the prominence of one group (e.g. colonizers) over the other (colonized), the reproduction – or criticism of – stereotypes, and highlighting *how* a group is oppressed individually or are oppressed collectively can be made visible.

In the context of personality disorders, antagonistic and aversive personality patterns are most frequently observed and acutely experienced in psychiatric and criminal justice contexts. In this sense, they reflect patterns of behaviour that negatively impact on the safety and well-being of others. Instead of starting from – and unquestioningly validating – the pathology, a post-colonial perspective takes relationality as a point of entry (Kirkness & Barnhardt, 2001; Wilson, 2008). For instance, the *law* and *culture* would be seen here as two significant forces that influence and shape the conduct and values of individuals, communities, and societies. According to Rosen (2006), these are a society's means of expressing a sense of order. The law provides a framework for maintaining order and stability in society by defining and regulating behaviour and setting consequences for violations, in order to deter wrongful conduct. By contrast, culture shapes human behaviour by providing a collective sense of meaning and purpose through shared traditions, beliefs, values and customs. However, conflicts between the law and a person's cultural heritage can raise issues that bear significant consequences in judicial settings, especially where Indigenous identity and cultural practices are concerned. In order to illustrate the importance of considering and unpacking layers of cultural information to facilitate clarity in 'a case', the following is an example that briefly describes where Indigenous and colonial realities collided in a judicial setting. It does not rest on a diagnosis of 'personality disorder' but raises cogent points inspiring reflection about 'world views' and medical diagnosis in psychological medicine.

On 12 October 2007, Janet Moses, aged 22 years, of Wainuiomata died consequent to attempts to lift a *makutu*.[1] The eight people accused of killing her were all *whānau*.[2] A media account reported that 'the whanau believed Ms Moses had been possessed by demons'. The family performed a mākutu-lifting on Ms Moses that involved 'forcing water into her mouth and eyes to flush out the demons and lift the makutu' (*New Zealand Herald*, 2009b).

Although this case presents an extreme example of Indigenous practices, the case of Janet Moses (*R v Rawiri*) raises important issues when considering behavioural and personality issues in a post-colonial context. First, a primary task is to *understand the context of the behaviour*. The judge commented on why a mākutu might be considered a contributing factor for Ms Moses' concerning behaviour that preceded these tragic events:

> Some Māori people, as indeed do many other people, believe in the existence of spirits, which can be good or evil. Makutu is a particularised form of such beliefs. It is the practice of deliberately imposing a curse on a person. As I understand the evidence at

[1] In this context: a curse, spiritual possession by malevolent forces.
[2] Family or blood relations.

trial, in very general terms it was a belief that existed more generally in Māori in centuries past, but has declining acceptance. However, there remain some or many Māori who still believe in its existence. The accused in this trial, and many of their wider whanau, fall within that group. They believe that at other times in their lives other family members have also been afflicted by a makutu. [15]

Paterson's (2011) study of Māori responses to mākutu in the nineteenth and early twentieth centuries described the Māori world as being comprised of many elements that would be deemed – and perhaps dismissed – as spiritual or supernatural nowadays. He comments that 'second sight, omens, tapu ... malignant spirits, demons, monsters, various other supernatural beings and makutu ... were accepted phenomena that impacted on the lived experience of individuals and communities' (p. 175). Furthermore, Paterson notes that this world was mediated by *tohunga* – a holder of specialist knowledge and skill in ritual, healing, or sorcery. The experience of mākutu, its effects, and remedial activity establishes a relevance in this context that may not otherwise be understood if this historical link was not appreciated.

A second task is to determine whether the defendants' behaviour was *consistent with cultural norms*:

The family, and these are of course generalisations, also have a firm belief in the healing and protective powers of water. Again this is a belief not unique to them or to Māori. Water is obviously symbolic in many rituals, such as baptism for example. Many members of the family follow a practice of doing their waters, which is an extended process of blessing themselves with water in a set order of movements. Some do it daily; others when thinking that they are going into situations that might be unsafe. [16]

The judge acknowledged that Māori have a close relationship with water in all its forms, spiritually and physically, and is a *taonga*[3] of huge significance to iwi (a confederation of tribes). The link of water to personal health and the health of the iwi is closely linked to the health of water bodies. As such, water is seen to have a vital role in health and healing practices.

A third task is to formulate the case and *make the situation intelligible* for a just decision to be determined and administered. A psychiatric assessment had emphasised Ms Moses' behaviour as being consistent with Western notions and diagnostic criteria for psychosis and paranoid delusions. Drawing this all together, the judge commented that:

... It is not to excuse but the events were in part the product of several features coming together in timing: the recent death of Mrs Rawiri, the theft of the lion[4], Janet's mental

[3] Treasured item, artefact.

[4] The makutu was reported to have begun after Ms Moses' sister allegedly stole a stone lion statue from outside a Greytown Hotel (*Sydney Morning Herald*, 2007). Further, after they brought the statue home, the family's children were observed to have taken ill and were unsettled. Following advice from a kaumatua (elder) in Porirua, the family drove to return the statue to the place it was

> ill-health and the way in which her utterances and actions were capable of reinforcing the family's view, together her own belief that she had been cursed, the confirmation by the tohunga of makutu being the cause, the confusion over his advice on the Tuesday night, his subsequent unavailability through hospitalisation, and Janet's deterioration after that time. [99]

In this instance, the defendants were sentenced to community-based sentences, supervision, and a range of special conditions, such as undertaking a Māori culture course, counselling, or psychiatric assessment as directed by the probation service.

In some cases, consideration of culture, as it applies to legal cases, calls for an examination of knowledge and practices about which there is restricted (or even marginal) 'knowledge' (e.g. mākutu). The subject matter drastically reduces the pool of experts who could likely assist with any enquiries. Psychiatrists and psychologists are not likely to have the cultural knowledge to deal effectively with such issues. However, in the wake of major health inquiries such as *He Ara Oranga* (Government Inquiry into Mental Health and Addiction, 2018) and *He Puapua* (Technical working group on a plan for the UN Declaration on the Rights of Indigenous Peoples, 2019), there is growing demand for mental health practitioners to recognise and attend to *cultural* issues. Although this is positive and has been a much-needed area of growth, what can also exist is a distortion in defining cultural knowledge – and imposing misunderstandings – by some practitioners that can be detrimental for clients. It is worth remembering that for now '*culture*' remains posited in mainstream psychology as '*other*'.

To endorse a 'dark core' of personality traits suggests an innate malevolence that is biologically determined. An Indigenous view in a post-colonial context recognises (1) connectedness between the individual, community, and the wider environment (think 'tangata whenua' – 'people of the land'); (2) the primacy of relatedness and the nature and quality of social environment as a resource – a process as well as a set of structures; and (3) the community as a unit of analysis. The individual is a product of complex social processes that shape behavioural expectations and interpersonal conduct as well as connection to the wider environment and a cosmology that explains origins and order. In this sense, personality is a matter of (4) fitness. That is, how well a person 'fits' into their environment, or how they modify the environment around them to suit their needs. Looked at in this way, a so-called dark core of personality – antagonistic, malevolent, or socially aversive behaviour (Moshagen et al., 2020) – can be seen as a set of strategies (extractive, combative, etc.) that serve the individual's needs, albeit in a manner that negatively impacts others in the community.

stolen from. However, disruptions to the trip home violated the instruction for the family to travel together. Ms Moses' behaviour deteriorated from this point (*New Zealand Herald*, 2009a).

17.6 Conclusion

The end of our psychosocial journey must be to return us to what Dylan calls 'The man who died a criminal's death'. Jurisprudence can live according to an eye for an eye and a tooth for a tooth (to use two old formulae) and emerge stained red. Alternatively it could aim to be restorative rather than Pharisaic. 'Restorative justice' aims to be just that: to heal and restore rather than condemn (Schmidt, 2001; Brookbanks, 2015). In the latter NZ Government outline, taking responsibility, apologising, putting things right as much as you can, and taking steps to try and prevent yourself reoffending are the main features of the programme.

Indigenous people in postcolonial settings find themselves labouring under a number of disruptions. Their life-world is changed from the one in which they have developed rhythms of life or folkways which were adaptive and fitting to the environment they inhabited before the colonisation. In the environments created by the colonisers all the ills of urban life and a history of colonial disruptions of Indigenous communities are brought into the rhythms of life, its relationality, and social structures. Within this context their language and their 'ways of going on' (to use Wittgenstein's phrase (1958), #183, 202–203) are both rendered dysfunctional for the purposes of everyday life.

An Indigenous life in a post-colonial setting grows 'uprooted' (albeit in situ) and therefore both undernourished and highly sensitive to adversities, of which there are many for any human being: childhood vulnerabilities and naivety must be overcome and grown out of, adolescent urges and sensitivities must be endured, a resilient adult self able to bear 'slings and arrows' must be forged, relationships have to take shape and endure for the sake of all affected by them, and mature reflection must grow and take its place in the collective that fosters being fully human. This task is both demanding and enduring and a lifelong project if one is to mature and play a part in the fulfilment of human potential in one's tribe (or to use a telling pun, 'pride'). We are an apex species that brings every adaptation its own mountain top but unfortunately for some of us that is threatened and has in some cases been excluded by an unheimlich sociopolitical context.

References

Anthony, T., & Blagg, H. (2020). Hyperincarceration and indigeneity. In E. Erez & P. Ibarra P (eds.), *Oxford encyclopedia of international criminology*. Oxford University Press.

Australian Bureau of Statistics. (2016). Summary of findings: Persons in corrective services. Retrieved from www.abs.gov.au/AUSSTATS/abs@.nsf/Lookup/4512.0Main+Features1December%20quarter%202016

Bolton, D., & Gillett, G. (2019). *The biopsychosocial model of health and disease: New philosophical and scientific developments*. Palgrave.

Brookbanks, W. (ed.). (2015). *Therapeutic jurisprudence: New Zealand perspectives*. Thomson Reuters.

Burney, S. (2012). Conceptual frameworks in Postcolonial Theory: Applications for educational critique. *Counterpoints*, *417*, 173–193.

Butz, M. (1997). *Chaos and complexity: Implications for psychological theory and practice*. CRC Press.

Cattell, R. B. (1978). *The use of factor analysis in behavioral and life sciences*. Plenum.

Costa, P. T., & McCrae, R. R. (1992). The five-factor model of personality and its relevance to personality disorders. *Journal of Personality Disorders*, *6*(4), 343–359.

Cox, L. (1993). *Kotahitanga: The search for Māori political unity*. Oxford University Press.

Department of Corrections. (2007). *Over-representation of Māori in the criminal justice system: An exploratory report*. Department of Corrections.

Department of Justice Canada. (2019, May). Indigenous overrepresentation in the criminal justice system. *JustFacts*. Retrieved from www.justice.gc.ca/eng/rp-pr/jr/jf-pf/2019/may01.html

Durie, M. (1998). *Whaiora: Māori health development*. Oxford University Press.

Eysenck, H. J. (1967). *The biological basis of personality*. Thomas.

Freeman, W. (2008). Non-linear brain dynamics and intention after Aquinas. *Mind and Matter*, 2008, *6*(2), 207–234.

Gillett, G. (2018). *From Aristotle to cognitive science*. Springer.

Gillett, G., & Franz, E. (2016). Evolutionary neurology, responsive equilibrium, and the moral brain. *Consciousness and Cognition*, *45*, 245–250.

Gillett, G., & Glannon, W. (2023). *The neurodynamic soul*. Palgrave MacMillan.

Gillett G. R., & Webster, D. M. (1975). Mediodorsal nucleus and behavior regulation in the rat. *Physiology & Behavior*, *14*, 883–885.

Government Inquiry into Mental Health and Addiction. (2018). *He ara oranga: Report of the government inquiry into mental health and addiction*. Crown.

Hamilton, A., & Northoff, G. (2021). Abnormal ERPs and brain dynamics mediate basic self disturbance in schizophrenia: A review of EEG and MEG studies. *Frontiers in Psychiatry*, *12*, 642469–642469.

Hanegraaf, L., Paton, B., Hohwy, J., & Verdejo-Garcia, A. (2023). Combining novel trait and neurocognitive frameworks to parse heterogeneity in borderline personality disorder. *Journal of Personality*, *91*(6), 1344–1363.

Hilbig, B. E., Thielmann, I., Klein, S. A., Moshagen, M., & Zettler, I. (2021). The dark core of personality and socially aversive psychopathology. *Journal of Personality*, *89* (2), 216–227.

Kirkness, V. J., & Barnhardt, R. (2001). First Nations and higher education: The four R's – Respect, relevance, reciprocity, responsibility. In R. Hayoe & J. Pan (eds.), *Knowledge across cultures: A contribution to dialogue among civilizations* (pp. 1–21). Comparative Education Research Centre, University of Hong Kong.

Lee, N. (1995). Culture conflict and crime in Alaskan native villages. *Journal of Criminal Justice*, *23*, 177–189.

Marsden, M. (1992). God, man and universe, a Māori view. In M. King (ed.), *Te Ao Hurihuri: Aspects of Māoritanga*. Reed.

McIntosh, T., & Workman, K. (2017). Māori and prison. In A. Deckert & R. Sarre (eds.), *The Palgrave handbook of Australian and New Zealand criminology, crime and justice* (pp. 727–735). Palgrave Macmillan.

Moshagen, M., Zettler, I., & Hilbig, B. E. (2020). Measuring the dark core of personality. *Psychological Assessment*, *32*(2), 182–196.
New Zealand Herald. (2009a, June 9). Woman slain in exorcism acted 'like a lion'. Retrieved from www.nzherald.co.nz/kahu/woman-slain-in-exorcism-acted-like-a-lion/67J6CBSL372HWODZCAWXV6NIIY/
New Zealand Herald. (2009b, June 13). Five guilty in exorcism case. Retrieved from www.nzherald.co.nz/nz/news/article.cfm?c_id=1&objectid=10578192
Neisser, U. (1976) *Cognition and reality*. Freeman.
NiaNia, W., Bush, A., & Epston, D. (2017). *Collaborative and Indigenous mental health therapy: Tātaihono – Stories of Māori healing and psychiatry*. Routledge.
Northoff, G. (2013). Brain and self: A neurophilosophical account. *Child & Adolescent Psychiatry and Mental Health*, *7*, 1–12.
Paterson, L. (2011). Government, church and Māori responses to Mākutu (sorcery) in New Zealand in the nineteenth and early twentieth centuries. *Cultural and Social History*, *8*, 175–194.
Pitt, A. J., & Britzman, D. P. (2003). Speculations on qualities of difficult knowledge in teaching and learning: An experiment in psychoanalytic research. *Qualitative Studies in Education*, *16*(6), 755–776.
Posick, C. (2013). The overlap between offending and victimisation among adolescents: Results from the second self-report delinquency study. *Journal of Contemporary Criminal Justice*, *29*(1), 106–124.
R v Rawiri [2009] CRI 2007–032–5294.
Rosen, L. (2006). *Law as culture: An introduction*. Princeton University Press.
Said, E. W. (1978). *Orientalism*. Pantheon Books.
Sawyer, P. H. (1978). *From Roman Britain to Norman England*. Methuen.
Schmidt, D. (2001). *Restorative justice in New Zealand: A model for US Criminal Justice*. Axford.
Sydney Morning Herald. (2007, November 13). Exorcism: 14-year-old nearly dies. Retrieved from www.smh.com.au/world/exorcism-14-year-old-nearly-dies-20071113-gdrl2i.html
Tamatea, A. J., & Waipara-Panapa, A. (2022). Māori, psychology, and the law: Challenges and opportunities for practitioners. In F. Seymour, S. Blackwell, & A. J. Tamatea (eds.), *Psychology and the law in Aotearoa New Zealand* (3rd ed., pp. 11–41). New Zealand Psychological Society.
Taylor, D. M., Segal, D., & Harper, N. J. (2010). The ecology of adventure therapy: An integral systems approach to therapeutic change. *Ecopsychology*, *2*(2), 77–83.
Technical working group on a plan for the UN Declaration on the Rights of Indigenous Peoples. (2019). *Report of the Working Group on a plan to realise the United Nations Declaration on the Rights of Indigenous Peoples: He Puapua*. Crown.
Wilson, S. (2008). *Research is ceremony: Indigenous research methods*. Fernwood.
Wittgenstein, L. (1958). *Philosophical investigations*. Blackwell.
Wong, S. K. (2011). Reciprocal effects of family disruption and crime: A panel study of Canadian municipalities. *Western Criminology Review*, *12*(1), 43–63.

18 Right to Be Angry

Affective Injustice and Borderline Personality Disorder

Astrid Fly Oredsson and Kasper Lippert-Rasmussen

18.1 Introduction

Borderline personality disorder (BPD) has a bad reputation, in healthcare and society at large. This is something persons diagnosed with BPD such as one of the authors of this chapter cannot help but be(come) acutely aware of. To navigate the healthcare system with a BPD diagnosis means having to navigate a sea of negative stereotypes. It means being alerted to the fact that many of the people you encounter moving through the healthcare system – nurses, doctors, social workers – think of you as "manipulative, demanding, attention-seeking, and violent," as another one of "the service users 'no one likes'" (Pickard, 2011, p. 210) or, more colloquially, a "pain in the ass" (anonymous psychiatrist as cited by Sulzer, 2015, p. 85).

In their review of research into clinicians' responses to the BPD diagnosis, Sansone and Sansone note that "with few exceptions, most researchers have found that the majority of participants in various studies harbor negative feelings about and attitudes toward patients with BPD" (2013, p. 42). This included viewing patients with the diagnosis as dangerous and unrelenting and feeling uncomfortable with and manipulated by them (Bodner et al., 2015; Brodsky, 2018; Lamont & Dickens, 2021; New & Triebwasser, 2018). Further, these attitudes were linked with defensiveness and anger as well as expressions of less helpfulness and empathy toward patients with a BPD diagnosis. This is put into sharp focus in interviews conducted by Sulzer (2015) where one healthcare provider jokes, "how do I treat Borderline Personality Disorder? I try to find another clinician [laughter]" (p. 86).

In this chapter, we examine how such attitudes combined with vague diagnostic criteria for BPD may have detrimental effects on patients' sense of moral agency.[1] Focusing on anger and BPD, we take seriously and expand on Nancy Potter's (2009) worry that clinicians "run the risk of assuming that

[1] We use "patient(s)" because we focus on anger assessments in a clinical setting, and we believe that in this setting there exist very real power differentials that may be obscured by insistent use of terms such as "client" or "service user" (Leaker, 2002; Sadler, 2005).

excessive anger is so much a part of a patient's character that she is unable ever to be reasonably angry. A patient's sense of herself as an adequate reasoner and moral agent is at stake here [. . .]" (p. 45).

First, we provide a brief overview of anger in the context of BPD (Section 18.2). Specifically, we look at the "inappropriate anger criterion" and highlight different philosophical accounts of the nature of anger and what makes it (in)appropriate. We suggest that the openness of the criterion heightens the risk of the situation described by Potter wherein BPD anger is assumed to be unreasonable or excessive in a way that disrespects patients' moral standing and agency. Throughout the chapter we use "BPD anger" as a shorthand for anger experienced, expressed, and assessed in a context where the angry person is diagnosed with BPD. Thus, BPD anger may or may not be the kind of anger picked out by the inappropriate anger criterion (whatever kind of anger that might be), it may be both appropriate and inappropriate, prudent or imprudent, fitting or unfitting.

Next, we tentatively analyze this as a case of testimonial injustice (Section 18.3). This is a form of epistemic injustice wherein negative prejudices about a speaker's identity lead hearers to deflate the speaker's credibility. In the case of BPD anger, we suggest that negative BPD-related stereotypes may result in clinicians underestimating the credibility of what is communicated through and by BPD anger. Yet, solely analyzing this as a case of testimonial injustice would overlook the fact that what is dismissed is not just some evaluation or appreciation of moral offense, but also the very experience of anger, its "affective force" (Whitney, 2018).

Hence, we propose analyzing this as a case of "affective injustice," broadly defined as "a wrong done to someone specifically in their capacity as an affective being" (Archer & Matheson, 2022, p. 8) (Section 18.4). Drawing on work by Srinivasan (2018) and Whitney (2018), we sketch how patients diagnosed with BPD can be subject to affective injustice in virtue of how their anger is dismissed. Finally, we suggest that persistent exposure to this kind of injustice can undermine patients' moral agency in case they internalize the disrespectful idea that they are unable to experience justified anger in response to moral offense.

18.2 Borderline Anger

There are nine diagnostic criteria for the DSM-5-TR Axis II diagnosis of borderline personality disorder (BPD), one of which refers to the display of "Inappropriate, intense anger or difficulty controlling anger (e.g., frequent displays of temper, constant anger, recurrent physical fights)" (APA, 2022). According to this criterion, such anger may manifest itself in "extreme sarcasm, enduring bitterness, or verbal outbursts" in response to perceived neglect, withholding, lack of care, or abandonment of a person close to the patient such as a lover, family member, or caregiver (APA, 2022).[2]

To determine whether this criterion is satisfied in a particular case, one must determine, for example, when physical fights and verbal outbursts are recurring and when eliciting conditions or prompting events (e.g., that a caregiver is seen as withholding) are instantiated. These are difficult questions that leave a lot of room for interpretation. Not only would it be hard to tell, say, if a caregiver is withholding if we had a precise notion of being withholding, we hardly *do* have a precise notion of being withholding. Moreover, is it, according to the criterion, the intensity of the anger in response to neglect (the caregiver is somewhat neglectful, but the strong anger is disproportionate to the low degree of neglect), the expressions of the anger (through "verbal outbursts"), and/or the anger itself (the patient misperceives the caregiver as neglectful) that is inappropriate? Is it something else? Even if we settle the question of whether to emphasize intensity, eliciting conditions, or expression in assessments of anger's appropriateness, further questions arise about thresholds for and characteristics of appropriate intensity, eliciting conditions, and expressions.

We will not attempt to settle any of these questions here. Instead, our aim is to illustrate the openness of the criterion by providing a brief sketch of varied philosophical approaches to defining and assessing anger, none of which are excluded by the criterion. This can make way for heterogeneous and potentially harmful evaluations wherein BPD anger is "cast as pathological too quickly in clinical settings" (Potter, 2009, p. 156). Although our focus is the inappropriate anger *diagnostic* criterion, we take our argument to apply beyond the diagnostic process because such criteria influence how diagnoses and specific patient groups are viewed. Thus, although not active in the business of diagnosing, clinicians (perhaps, especially those specialized in areas other than PDs) will still encounter patients with a BPD diagnosis knowing that they have been found to meet a minimum of five diagnostic criteria, one of which may be the inappropriate anger criterion.

18.2.1 A Note on Anger

Anger is an emotional experience with cognitive, physiological, expressive, and experiential components stimulated by or in reaction to something in the world. Anger typically involves unpleasant bodily sensations such as an increased heart rate, one's face flushing, or teeth clamping together (Linehan,

[2] There are a total of nine criteria for BPD whereof a minimum of five must be met for a diagnosis to be made. Although we focus on the inappropriate anger, our arguments may be relevant to other criteria relating to affect such as "Affective instability due to a marked reactivity of mood" and "Chronic feelings of emptiness" (APA, 2022).

2015), in response to some form of obstruction, offense, unfairness, or injury – often labeled as the formal object of anger (Brady, 2013; Osler, 2023).[3] Following Potter (2009), we focus on a type of anger – moral anger – the formal object of which is *moral* offense, violation, or transgression (Cherry, 2022; Srinivasan, 2018).[4] So, when we refer to anger and BPD anger, we intend for this to be understood as moral anger.

There is an evaluative component implicit in the formal object of moral anger. Thus, it is a "reactive assessment" or appreciation of something as morally offensive or unfair (Potter, 2009, p. 36; Srinivasan, 2018). The nature of this assessment or appreciation is a topic of ongoing philosophical discussion. Some argue that emotions' evaluative content amounts to beliefs or judgments distinguishable from their experiential components (Marks, 1982; Nussbaum, 2004, 2015; Solomon, 1976), whereas others favor the view that the phenomenology or affective aspects of emotions cannot be distinguished from their intentionality in this way. For example, embodied accounts of emotions as "felt evaluations" (Helm, 2020), "felt recognitions" (Furtak, 2018), or "evaluative presentations" (D'Arms & Jacobson, 2000) describe the phenomenology and intentionality of emotions as inseparable: the affective nature of emotions is thought to be part of their evaluative character.[5] Although Potter seemingly aligns herself with the view that anger comprises belief or judgment in claiming that it involves "perception, belief, and interpretation" (2009, p. 37), we want to avoid making this claim here. Rather, we intend to show that even if one holds that the evaluation implicit in moral anger is inseparable from its phenomenal content and may at best be described as quasi-judgmental (D'Arms & Jacobson, 2000), one can still entertain Potter's claim. One need only accept that the evaluative content of moral anger can be crucial to moral reasoning and agency.

18.2.2 What Makes Anger (In)appropriate?

With this brief outline of anger in mind, let us look at possible interpretations of the inappropriate anger criterion for BPD. We provide a rough sketch of two prominent philosophical accounts of how to assess emotions such as anger – prudential and fittingness accounts – neither of which are excluded or required

[3] Comparatively, fear tends to involve a sensation of a pit in the gut or hearing one's heartbeat and its formal object is a dangerous thing.

[4] We are sympathetic to the view that anger need not always be a reaction to moral transgression. You might be angry at yourself for forgetting to bring water or at your flatmate for not closing the fridge properly. These cases involve obstruction or frustration of a goal or expectation leading to an emotional reaction we tend to describe as anger. What is blocked or obstructed, however, is not of particular moral relevance, so we are not dealing with moral offense.

[5] Furtak, for example, argues that emotions' evaluative content is "made available to us *in* and *through* the visceral feelings of being shaken with fear" or being in the grip of anger (2018, pp. 76–77; emphasis in original).

by the criterion. Consequently, they may or may not be employed by clinicians in their assessments of whether a person experiences "[i]nappropriate, intense anger or difficulty controlling anger" (APA, 2022).

First, Potter states that "many clinicians posit BPD anger as a regression to primitive" defense mechanisms such as acting out, projection, or denial (2009, p. 38). Despite their developmental utility, these defenses are primitive because they are thought to be pathological responses to past wounds impeding "mature psychological health" (Potter, 2009, p. 42). Primitive defenses are, by definition, unreasonable. Looking to the inappropriate anger criterion, one can find vindication of this approach in examples of "acting out" behaviors like "verbal outbursts," "extreme sarcasm," and "recurrent physical fights" (APA, 2022).[6] Implicit in the primitive defenses approach is a judgment that anger is bad for the angry person. In short, it is imprudent. At the core of prudential approaches to anger evaluation is the question of whether anger is good or bad for the bearer of anger. From this perspective anger at a caregiver seemingly failing to provide adequate care could be inappropriate if it makes the caregiver more withholding or the patient experience a negative feeling of "being evil" (even in cases where the caregiver has indeed withheld care in a morally wrongful way; APA, 2022). The anger can be counterproductive to building a positive sense of self or maintaining the caring relationship on which the patient may depend for help and recognition. Notably, prudence is relative to personal goals and interests, and these can vary significantly from person to person. Moreover, whether an emotional experience and expression thereof is prudent or not may be largely contingent on how others respond to it.

A second influential philosophical understanding of the appropriateness of anger emphasizes the "fit" between emotion and the world. Fittingness accounts argue that even if an emotion is imprudent, it can still get something "right" about or "fit" the world in a manner analogous to how true belief fits the world (D'Arms & Jacobson, 2000; Srinivasan, 2018). Assessing emotional fittingness or aptness requires examining whether the evaluative content of the emotion accurately captures the features of its object, that to which it is a reaction. For example, because envy represents something as enviable, envy is a fitting emotional response to the enviable. As the formal object of BPD anger is moral offense, fittingness accounts would take such anger to be appropriate only in cases where something really is morally offensive. If a caregiver's failure to provide care constitutes a moral offense, then anger

6 Relatedly, "splitting" – the tendency to view self and others as either all good or all bad – is often described by psychodynamic thinkers as a primitive defense mechanism characteristic of borderline personality disorder and may also be relevant to anger assessments, for example when intense anger is linked with an overly rigid representation of something as all bad (Yeomans & Delaney, 2018; Linehan, 1993).

would be appropriate, even if it may be prudentially bad for the care recipient to express or even experience such anger.

Imagine a patient who experiences anger in response to the fact that a therapist will not take them on as a client. The patient thinks that this decision rests on feelings of animosity toward or negative prejudices about patients diagnosed with BPD. Yet, the therapist rejected the patient due to a lack of capacity to take on new clients, and the patient's anger is grounded in false belief, a faulty representation of the facts of the matter.[7] Consequently, the anger is inappropriate on a fittingness picture: rejection due to lack of capacity is not morally offensive. Were it, on the other hand, the case that therapist rejected the patient because of negative prejudices about their diagnosis, then the therapist's decision seems to rest on morally dubious, perhaps even morally offensive, reasons. Because this approach emphasizes fit between world and affect, seemingly unfitting BPD anger may also be described as reality distortions. These distortions including unfitting anger might even be thought to result from an underlying BPD-related defect in the relevant person's sense of reality. On this picture, the unfitting BPD anger is framed as a result of an underlying pathological defect in reality testing rather than one-off faulty representations of the world (more on this in Section 18.4). Although we have focused on appropriateness as it relates to the experience of anger, prudential and fittingness considerations apply to emotional intensity and expression as well. For example, expressions of anger in the form of verbal outbursts or physical altercations can be imprudent and a particularly intense experience of anger can fail to fit, for instance to be disproportional to, the severity of the offense to which it is a reaction.[8]

The fact that the inappropriate anger criterion for BPD is open to different interpretations and heterogeneous clinical application may heighten the risk identified by Potter of undue dismissal of BPD anger as pathological and unreasonable. Research on stereotyping in healthcare and other types of frontline work suggests that high levels of uncertainty and lack of informational clarity can increase use of stereotyping in, for example, clinical encounters (Assouline et al., 2022).[9] Hence, the vagueness of the criterion can increase the risk that clinical assessments of BPD anger are guided by the kind of negative stereotypes and attitudes mentioned in the introduction. In the next section, we show how this can lead to undue dismissal of BPD anger as inappropriate by tentatively analyzing the situation as one of epistemic

[7] We leave it open whether the anger itself involves a false belief or is a response to such a belief.

[8] Inversely, unfitting exaggerated expressions of anger not reflecting the experience of anger can in some cases be productive. Relatedly, repressing and failing to express anger can be counterproductive to personal health, for example, increasing stress (Cherry, 2021).

[9] For a more detailed overview of public administration research on stereotyping, ambiguity, and the inappropriate anger criterion, see Oredsson (2023).

injustice – a distinct form of injustice wherein a person is wronged in their capacity as a knower.

18.3 Testimonial Injustice

In the past decade, a growing literature has employed the notion of testimonial injustice to analyze the wrongfulness of dismissing certain forms of patient testimony in healthcare including in psychiatry (Byrne, 2020; Gosselin, 2019; Carel & Kidd, 2014; Scrutton, 2017). Focusing on the relationship between social injustice and knowledge, Fricker (2007) describes epistemic injustice as the phenomenon whereby unjust social structures are enacted through and reproduced by our knowledge practices in ways that undermine some people's social position as knowers. This can happen when efforts to relay knowledge are halted due to prejudices about a person's social identity held by would-be hearers, or when a gap in "collective interpretive resources" damages people's (most often marginalized groups') chances of making sense of and communicating important aspects of their social experiences and life under oppression (2007, p. 1). The former kind is known as testimonial injustice, the latter is hermeneutical injustice. Our focus is testimonial injustice as this has been the dominant line in philosophical work on patient testimony.

A (if not *the*) central case of testimonial injustice according to Fricker (2007) is a scene in Harper Lee's novel *To kill a mockingbird* from 1960. Set in 1930s Alabama, the scene features a black man, Tom Robinson, on trial for the rape of a white girl, Mayella Ewell. Tom has been falsely accused: in court we are presented with overwhelming evidence for his innocence. When questioned about making a stop at the Ewell residence, Tom replies that he stopped to help Mayella with her chores because he felt sorry for her. Yet, against the backdrop of the widespread white supremacist beliefs characteristic of 1930s Alabama, the all-white jury cannot make sense of Tom's expression of sympathy toward Mayella. Moreover, the "idea that the black man is to be epistemically trusted, and the white girl distrusted is virtually a psychological impossibility" (Fricker, 2007, p. 25). As a result, Tom's true testimony is deemed unreliable by the jury. This results in a credibility deficit: his testimony is seen as less credible than what is the case.

The fact that racist prejudices drive this assessment is vital. This is where social power comes into the picture. Credibility deficits in central cases of testimonial injustice are results of negative prejudices about speakers' social identities, prejudices influenced by wider structures of social inequality and oppression. Thus, testimonial injustice can be thought of as involving an identity-prejudicial credibility deficit, where the identity prejudices at stake are negative and systematic, tracking "the subject through different dimensions of social activity" (Fricker, 2007, p. 27).

18.3.1 Is This a Case of Testimonial Injustice?

For our case – undue dismissal of BPD anger as inappropriate when it is not – to be one of testimonial injustice it must satisfy two conditions: (i) there should be a credibility deficit, and (ii) negative prejudices about patients' identities must, at least in part, shape assessments of their anger testimony in ways resulting in said credibility deficit. Below we suggest that the case satisfies both conditions. Nevertheless, analyzing this solely as an example of testimonial injustice would fail to capture something important about the kind of wrong at play. Namely, the patients are not only wronged as knowers, but also as affective beings.

One might wonder whether patients diagnosed with BPD are subject to the kind of negative and systematic prejudices described above qua their diagnosis at all. Writing specifically on epistemic injustice in psychiatry, Knox introduces the term "psychopathologized" to describe a social group "united by the experience of being seen and treated as having a psychopathology" (2022, p. 256). Members of this group may be subject to involuntary treatment and social stigmatization by virtue of being psychopathologized of their group membership. Accordingly, Knox argues that the psychopathologized share experiences that those outside the group do not; the psychopathologized "constitute a marginalized group with an epistemic standpoint similar to other groups discussed by standpoint epistemologists" and others concerned with epistemic injustice (2022, p. 256). As BPD is a psychiatric diagnosis, patients with BPD are indeed members of this social group and likely face the kind of first-order injustice underlying epistemic injustice in virtue of their diagnosis.

Moreover, although patients with a BPD diagnosis are subject to a host of harmful prejudices by virtue of being psychopathologized, we might still ask whether they are the right sort of stereotypes or prejudices, the sort that shape credibility assessments. We believe so. First, there are various prejudices about not thinking clearly or being in one's "right mind" generally associated with being psychopathologized and mental illness (namely, the diagnostic criterion discussed above). These have an obvious bearing on judgments of epistemic capabilities. Second, and specific to the case of BPD anger, are the stereotypes mentioned in the introduction, that is that patients diagnosed with BPD are manipulative and attention-seeking (Bodner et al., 2015; Gallop et al., 1983; Markham & Trower, 2003).[10] If you are viewed as a manipulative person, it

[10] Although sample sizes in these studies are generally low, anecdotal evidence from researchers and clinicians (Brodsky, 2018; Pickard, 2011; Stanley & Singh, 2018) as well as carers and

becomes hard to be seen as a credible testifier. For example, lying and deceiving are often described as integral to manipulation (Potter, 2006). If you are thought to lie and deceive people for your own gains (e.g., to get attention), then people are unlikely to view your testimony as credible and your expressions of emotion as genuine. Moreover, in the case of BPD anger, being thought of as especially violent or antagonistic will likely make people more willing to dismiss your anger as unreasonable, pathological, and a result of some character defect (or disorder) than a response to an external, morally offensive situation. We think it reasonable, then, to conclude that in our case there are indeed stereotypes – whether BPD-specific or about psychopathology more generally – at play that can sway credibility assessments in a way that leads clinicians to assign less credibility than what is due.

18.3.2 Emotional Experience

Ending our analysis here, however, would fail to discern important nuances of the case. Namely, if we describe such dismissals of BPD as (only) involving an *epistemic* wrong, we may lose sight of another wrong to which patients are subjected, a distinctly affective wrong.

As mentioned in Section 18.2.1, there is ongoing philosophical debate about how to make sense of the intentional and evaluative components of emotions. Brady describes emotions as intentional not just because they are about something in the world – drawing our attention to an object or event – but also because they alert "us to *the way in which* some object or event is important or significant" to us (2013, p. 27; emphasis in original). But what are we to make of this disclosure or appreciation of value or disvalue? Is it, perhaps, a form of perception of affective or normative qualities? Does anger necessarily involve a *belief* that something is offensive? Or does such belief occur immediately prior to or after the experience of anger, where the appreciation of something as morally offensive involved in anger is something else, perhaps best described as quasi-judgmental and/or quasi-perceptual (D'Arms & Jacobson, 2000)?[11]

Although we are unsure of how best to answer these questions, we believe that analyzing BPD anger only as a claim to knowledge would misrepresent such anger and emotions as more reflective and detached than is the case. Think (again) of the increased heart rate and teeth clenching associated with anger; the cold sweat, dizziness, and numbness associated with intense fear; the butterflies and warm sensation associated with happiness. These are

patients themselves (Lamont & Dickens, 2021; Tusiani-Eng & Tusiani, 2018) support the hypothesis that negative BPD-related stereotypes are widespread in healthcare and influence clinical encounters.

[11] For an in-depth exploration of these and related questions see Goldie (2000), Helm (2001), Russell (2003), and Tappolet (2016).

physiological elements central to emotions over which we may have limited to no control. Comparatively, believing that tomorrow is Thursday or that water is H_2O does not usually involve such physiological experiences: it is perfectly possible to believe, and claiming to know that Thomas Kuhn (1962) wrote *The structure of scientific revolutions* without experiencing cold sweats, crying, or butterflies.

What is dismissed in cases where BPD anger is categorized as an unreasonable primitive defense mechanism is not just the moral valuation of something as morally offensive, it is also the *experience* of something as morally offensive. The increased heart rate, the flushed face, and the clenched teeth, these are part of the anger. Accordingly, part of dismissing BPD anger as unreasonable or inappropriate involves the dismissal of such phenomena as well. What is dismissed is not (just) belief or valuation, but "affective force" and experience (Whitney, 2018). Analysis of undue dismissal of BPD anger simply as testimonial injustice would not pay due attention to this. What is at stake is not just patients' standing as (moral) knowers, but their status and experiences as affective beings.

In the next section, we turn to the framework of "affective injustice" to provide a preliminary analysis of how the dismissal of BPD anger described by Potter can involve a distinctly affective – as opposed to epistemic – wrong. This form of injustice includes disrespect of patients' standing as affective and moral beings. Further, in cases where patients internalize such disrespect it may undermine their moral agency.

18.4 Affective Injustice and Moral Agency

Drawing on Fricker's (2007) definition of epistemic injustice, Archer and Matheson define affective injustice as "a wrong done to someone specifically in their capacity as an affective being" (2022, p. 8). There are several ways in which this wrong may be enacted, several kinds of affective injustice. Srinivasan (2018), for example, describes affective injustice as a normative conflict encountered by racialized (or otherwise marginalized) people between their apt anger at racism (or other forms of oppression) and wanting to better their situation. When their anti-racist anger is dismissed as aggressive and counterproductive to constructive debate, racialized people must engage in a psychically taxing process of emotion suppression if their experiences of racism are to be taken seriously (Archer & Mills, 2019; Plunkett, 2021). Crucially, the anger's imprudence is contingent upon socially unjust structures: it is counterproductive "because the anger of victims of systematic injustice is treated as sufficient reason to further ignore, marginalise, or oppress them" (Srinivasan, 2018, p. 135, fn. 44). Drawing inspiration from Young's (1990) "five faces" of oppression, Whitney (2018) describes distinctly affective forms of marginalization, exploitation, and violence as variations of affective injustice. This account is supplemented by Archer and Matheson (2022), who characterize what they call "emotional imperialism" as another form of affective injustice. This is the phenomenon whereby a powerful group imposes their cultural and social affect norms on a less-powerful group "whilst at the same time marking out the other culture's emotional norms and standards as deviant and inferior" (2022, p. 11). It is beyond the scope of this paper to provide a detailed account of these different forms of affective injustice. Instead, we focus on Whitney's (2018) notion of affective marginalization and the normative conflict characterized by Srinivasan (2018) as affective injustice. We do this because these phenomena involve a harmful localization of anger's cause or reason within the angry individual that we believe takes place in the dismissals of BPD anger with which we are concerned.

18.4.1 Borderline Anger and Its Reasons

Like Srinivasan (2018), Whitney (2018) focuses on anger in the context of oppression – racist, colonial, and sexist. On her account, affective injustice "damages the weight afforded to one's feelings" (2018, p. 495). In the case of affective marginalization – one kind of affective injustice – the wronged person's anger is reduced to "mere" affect in a way that disables its intentionality. Instead of being treated as intentionally engaged with the external world, the affectively marginalized person's anger is seen as a reflection of their (inferior) character such as their emotional instability or sensibility. Thus, dismissing women's anger as a result of their being "hysterical" or "shrill" locates the reasons for the anger within the individual in a way that involves "expulsion from participation in affect circulation that depletes affective agency, influence, or authority" (Whitney, 2018, p. 497; Cherry, 2018; Frye, 1983). When anger is characterized as a product of a person's character in this way, that person is excluded from the community of people whose emotions involve an appreciation (apt or not) of the (dis)value of external states of affairs. In the case of affective injustice, this form of intentionality-disabling refusal of uptake is intricately linked with wider unjust social structures.

These are not one-off occurrences but, rather, reflective of widespread ideas about the inferior character of members of marginalized groups. This marks an important point of convergence between Srinivasan's (2018) and Whitney's (2018) accounts of affective injustice: both are concerned with the refusal to acknowledge that the anger in question may be an apt response to socially unjust conditions or oppression. Whereas Whitney explicitly focuses on dismissals grounded in demeaning beliefs and prejudices about the emotionality of marginalized people, Srinivasan highlights the fact that the prudential focus of counterproductivity critiques against anti-racist anger "shifts us from the space of intrinsic reason to the space of instrumental reason, thereby obscuring the possibility that the agent's anger is apt" (2018, p. 128). Whereas intrinsic, that is, formal objective-responsive, reasons for anger involve, for example, moral violation, instrumental and circumstances-responsive reasons for anger may be anger for pleasure's sake (in case you derive pleasure for anger) or anger as a means of getting attention.[12] Srinivasan (2018) also acknowledges the systematic framing of marginalized people's anger as a product of inferior character, describing it as part of the socially contingent structures that "make" this anger counterproductive (Cherry, 2018, 2021). Expressions of anti-racist anger can be seen or framed as confirmation of the emotional instability of the angry person, an instability conceived as counter to "rational" and respectful debate and conversation about racism.

In both instances explanation for the individual's anger is sought not by looking at that to which the anger is a response. Consequently, the appreciation of (dis)value – of moral offense – involved in and communicated through anger remains unacknowledged. We believe that in the case described by Potter (2009) something very similar is going on: when BPD anger is assumed to be a pathological primitive defense mechanism, the possibility that this anger may be a reasonable, fitting, or apt response to moral offense is obscured. Focus is shifted from the object of the anger to the mental and emotional instability of the patient. The "failure to give uptake to the patient's sense that a norm or moral right has been violated" (Potter, 2009, p. 41) moves attention away from external reasons onto the angry person's character or sanity in much the same way as in Srinivasan's (2018) and Whitney's (2018) accounts of affective injustice. In fact, the very expression of the features associated with BPD may be seen as confirmation of pathology and, thus, further reason not to give uptake to the evaluative content of and injury underlying said anger.[13] Consequently, the undue dismissal of BPD anger described by Potter can be understood as a case of affective injustice wronging patients as affective beings.[14]

18.4.2 Moral Agency

Let us turn, now, to the latter part of Potter's worry, namely that what is at stake is the "patient's sense of herself as an adequate reasoner and moral agent" (2009, p. 45). If we were to formulate the undue dismissal of BPD anger as

[12] Thus, intrinsic and instrumental reasons for anger maps onto fittingness (or aptness) and prudential accounts of the appropriateness of anger.

[13] Failing to give uptake to patients' anger or being too quick to attribute "hostile intent" may also generate further anger and create an invalidating and potentially retraumatizing therapeutic environment (Linehan, 1993; Potter, 2009).

[14] The negative stereotyping of the psychopathologized more widely and patients with a BPD diagnosis in particular may encourage such dismissals, and the openness of the inappropriate anger criterion is likely to increase the risk of such stereotypical anger assessments.

a case of testimonial injustice and accept that said anger involves moral belief, then the link would be straightforward: dismissing BPD anger as always unreasonable would mean dismissing the possibility that patients diagnosed with BPD can engage in sound moral reasoning or be wronged. Thus far, however, we have resisted this picture (at least when seen as the complete picture) and steered clear of the claim that BPD anger necessarily involves moral belief. Instead, we have described the case as one of affective injustice directed at anger that involves disclosure or appreciation (perception- or belief-like) of something as morally offensive. As a result, we need to do a bit more work to show how this case of affective injustice can negatively influence patients' sense of themselves as adequate moral reasoners and agents.

First, affective injustice in the case of BPD anger involves a disrespect for patients' standing as affective *as well as* moral agents. Part of what it means to be wronged as an affective being is to have your ability to appreciate the value of things through affective experience be disrespected. Kauppinen, for example, argues that to "treat your anger as a symptom of something that's wrong with you" would be to disrespect you as a moral agent (2018, p. 37). In the case of BPD anger – the formal object of which is moral offense – affective injustice involves disrespect of patients' ability to affectively appreciate and register moral (dis)value. Furthermore, when the anger is a response to moral offense done to patients themselves, we are also dealing with a failure to acknowledge the patients' standing as moral agents deserving of respect. In fact, species of anger such as resentment and indignation have long been described as reactive attitudes central to moral agency, self-respect, and holding others morally responsible for their actions (Murphy, 1982; Strawson, 1962). Thus, the person who assumes that BPD anger is always or nearly always unreasonable as opposed to a possibly fitting response to moral offense fails to acknowledge and respect "the patient as a sometimes-reasonable moral agent" (Potter, 2009, p. 43).

Second, repeated exposure to this kind of affective injustice can lead patients to internalize this disrespect to a degree that undermines their moral reasoning and agency. Imagine a person whose anger is repeatedly dismissed as dysfunctional, inappropriate, or pathological. Over time they begin to believe that their anger is in fact an inappropriate and pathological defense mechanism (even when it is a fitting response to moral offense). Wanting to be a "good patient" and to "get better," they set out to restrain their anger, to engage in some serious emotion regulation – "processes by which individuals influence which emotions they have, when they have them, and how they experience and express these emotions" (Gross, 1998, p. 275). This could bring about a situation wherein the patient learns and begins to "explain away all insults [and moral offenses] as benign and unimportant," as unworthy of an angry reaction (Potter, 2009, p. 38). Consequently, the patient may lose sight of her own moral worth.

Murphy, for example, argues that "a failure to resent moral injuries done to me is a failure to care about the moral value incarnate in my own moral personality" (Murphy, 1982, p. 505; as quoted in Potter, 2009, p. 37). Further, as a reactive attitude, experiencing and expressing moral anger may be necessary to assert not only our own moral worth and responsibility, but also that of others (Menges, 2016; Strawson, 1962; cf. Pettigrove & Tanaka, 2014).

Finally, there is a line of scholarship that links emotions such as moral anger intricately to moral reasoning while stopping short of describing belief as a constitutive component of such anger. For example, one might think that emotions play a crucial motivational role in moral reasoning, that emotions can act as moral cues. Emotions capture and direct our attention in ways that "motivate search for reasons that could justify our emotional responses" (Silva, 2021, p. 668; Brady, 2013). So, our anger can lead us to reflect on our own moral commitments and values as well as the moral status of specific situations or actions, for instance, a loved one not offering the care we expect or a therapist refusing to work with us. Alternatively, one could take the stance that emotions can have direct justificatory force, that they provide defeasible justification for evaluative and moral beliefs (Silva, 2021).[15] Here an even closer connection is drawn between emotions and moral belief: the very experience of anger can be a justificatory (yet defeasible) reason for the belief that an action is morally offensiveness. On both accounts, the sort of distrust of BPD anger brought about by repeated dismissal of it as pathological, dysfunctional, or inappropriate is likely to have grave consequences to patients' sense of themselves as moral reasoners and agents.

18.5 Conclusion

Our point of departure in this chapter was a brief examination of how negative attitudes toward people with a BPD diagnosis combined with vague diagnostic criteria for BPD can result in an unjustifiably dismissive response to their emotions – for example, most importantly their anger – due to how this emotion is mentioned in the diagnostic criteria. We submitted that such dismissal could involve epistemic injustice, namely, testimonial injustice. Yet, we also noted that an analysis of the dismissal of BPD anger described by Potter (2009), which is restricted to the concept of epistemic injustice, provides only a limited insight into the affective and moral nature of the case. This is because such situations might also involve injustice to patients diagnosed with BPD qua their affective standing and that in turn might result in an erosion of their sense of moral agency. When BPD anger is dismissed as merely symptomatic of an underlying pathology and not fitting given the way they are being treated,

[15] Hutton (2022) goes so far as to argue that moral experience – the basis for moral knowledge – consists of emotion.

people diagnosed with BPD might adopt an objectifying stance toward themselves and embark on internal anger management, resulting in distrust of their own moral experiences, standing, and agency.

References

American Psychiatric Association. (2022). Personality disorders. In *Diagnostic and statistical manual of mental disorders* (5th ed., text rev.). American Psychiatric Association.

Archer, A., & Matheson, B. (2022). Commemoration and emotional imperialism. *Journal of Applied Philosophy, 39*, 761–777. https://doi.org/10.1111/japp.12428.

Archer, A., & Mills, G. (2019). Anger, affective injustice, and emotion regulation. *Philosophical Topics*, *47*(2), 75–94.

Assouline, M., Gilad, S., & Ben-Nun Bloom, P. (2022). Discrimination of minority welfare claimants in the real world: The effect of implicit prejudice. *Journal of Public Administration Research and Theory, 32*(1), 75–96.

Bodner, E., Cohen-Fridel, S., Mashiah, M., Segal, M., Grinshpoon, A., Fischel, T., & Iancu, I. (2015). The attitudes of psychiatric hospital staff toward hospitalization and treatment of patients with borderline personality disorder. *BMC Psychiatry, 15*(2). https://doi.org/10.1186/s12888-014-0380-y.

Brady, M. S. (2013). *Emotional insight: The epistemic role of emotional experience.* Oxford University Press.

Brodsky, B. S. (2018). Meeting the clinical challenges of managing borderline personality disorder. In B. Stanley & A. S. New (eds.), *Borderline personality disorder* (pp. 363–376). Oxford University Press.

Byrne, E. A. (2020). Striking the balance with epistemic injustice in healthcare: The case of chronic fatigue syndrome/myalgic encephalomyelitis. *Medicine, Health Care and Philosophy, 23*, 371–379. https://doi.org/10.1007/s11019-020-09945-4.

Carel, H. H., & Kidd, I. J. (2014). Epistemic injustice in healthcare: A philosophical analysis. *Medicine, Health Care and Philosophy, 17*(4), 529–540.

Cherry, M. (2018). The errors and limitations of our "anger-evaluating" ways. In M. Cherry and O. Flanagan (eds.), *The moral psychology of anger* (pp. 49–65). Rowman and Littlefield International Ltd.

Cherry, M. (2021). *The case for rage: Why anger is essential to anti-racist struggle.* Oxford University Press.

Cherry, M. (2022). Political anger. *Philosophy Compass*, *17*(2), e12811.

D'Arms, J., & Jacobson, D. (2000). The moralistic fallacy: On the "appropriateness" of emotions. *Philosophy and Phenomenological Research*, *61*(1), 65–90.

Fricker, M. (2007). *Epistemic injustice. Power & the ethics of knowing.* Oxford University Press.

Frye, M. (1983). *The politics of reality: Essays in feminist theory.* Crossing Press.

Furtak, R. (2018). *Knowing emotions: Truthfulness and recognition in affective experience*. Oxford University Press.

Gallop, R., Lancee, W. J., & Garfinkel, P. (1989). How nursing staff respond to the label "borderline personality disorder". *Hospital Community Psychiatry, 40*, 815–819.

Goldie, P. (2000). *The emotions: A philosophical exploration*. Clarendon Press.

Gosselin, A. (2019). "Clinician knows best"? Injustices in the medicalization of mental illness. *Feminist Philosophy Quarterly*, *5*(2), Article 2.

Gross, J. J. (1998). The emerging field of emotion regulation: An integrative review. *Review of General Psychology*, *2*(3), 271.

Helm, B. W. (2001). *Emotional reason: Deliberation, motivation, and the nature of value*. Cambridge University Press.

Helm, B. W. (2020). Affective intentionality and the reactive attitudes. In T. Szanto & H. Landweer (eds.), *The Routledge handbook of phenomenology of emotion*. Routledge.

Hutton, J. (2022). Moral experience: Perception or emotion? *Ethics*, *132*(3), 570–597. https://doi.org/10.1086/718079.

Kauppinen, A. (2018). Valuing anger. In M. Cherry & O. Flanagan (eds.), *The moral psychology of anger* (pp. 31–48). Rowman and Littlefield International Ltd.

Kidd, I. J., & Carel, H. (2017). Epistemic injustice and illness. *Journal of Applied Philosophy*, *34*(2), 172–190. https://doi.org/10.1111/japp.12172.

Knox, B. (2022). Exclusion of the psychopathologized and hermeneutical ignorance threaten objectivity. *Philosophy, Psychiatry, & Psychology*, *29*(4), 253–266.

Kuhn, T. S. (1962). *The structure of scientific Revolutions*. University of Chicago Press.

Lamont, E., & Dickens, G. L. (2021). Mental health services, care provision, and professional support for people diagnosed with borderline personality disorder: Systematic review of service-user, family, and carer perspectives. *Journal of Mental Health*, *30*(5), 619–633. https://doi.org/10.1080/09638237.2019.1608923.

Leaker, C. (2002). Speaking across the border: A patient assessment. In J. Z. Sadler (ed.), *Descriptions and prescriptions: Values, mental disorders, and the DSMs* (pp. 229–250). Johns Hopkins University Press.

Lee, H. (1960). *To kill a mockingbird*. William Heinemann.

Linehan, M. (1993). *Cognitive-behavioral treatment of borderline personality disorder*. The Guilford Press.

Linehan, M. (2015). *DBT skills training handouts and worksheets*, 2nd ed. The Guilford Press.

Markham, D., & Trower, P. (2003). The effects of the psychiatric label 'borderline personality disorder' on nursing staff's perceptions and causal attributions for challenging behaviors. *British Journal of Clinical Psychology*, *42*(3), 243–256.

Marks, J. (1982). A theory of emotions. *Philosophical Studies*, *42*, 227–242.

Menges, L. (2016). The emotion account of blame. *Philosophical Studies*, *174*(1), 257–273.

Murphy, J. (1982). Forgiveness and resentment. *Midwest Studies in Philosophy*, *7*(1), 503–516.

New, A. S., & Triebwasser, J. (2018). A history of borderline personality disorder. In B. Stanley & A. S. New (eds.), *Borderline personality disorder* (pp. 1–16). Oxford University Press.

Nussbaum, M. (2004). Emotions as judgments of value and importance. In R. C. Solomon (ed.), *Thinking about feeling: Contemporary philosophers on emotions* (pp. 183–199). Oxford University Press.

Nussbaum, M. (2015). Transitional anger. *Journal of the American Philosophical Association*, *1*(1), 41–56. https://doi.org/10.1017/apa.2014.19.

Oredsson, A. F. (2023). Women "out of order": Inappropriate anger and gender bias in the diagnosis of borderline personality disorder. *Journal of Psychosocial Studies*, *16* (2), 149–162. https://doi.org/10.1332/147867323X16863891304659.

Osler, L. (2023). WTF?! Covid-19, indignation, and the internet. *Phenomenology and the Cognitive Sciences*, *22*, 1215–1234. https://doi.org/10.1007/s11097-023-09889-z.

Pettigrove, G., & Tanaka, K. (2014). Anger and moral judgment. *Australasian Journal of Philosophy*, *92*(2), 269–286. https://doi.org/10.1080/00048402.2013.795990.

Pickard, H. (2011). Responsibility without blame: Empathy and the effective treatment of personality disorder. *Philosophy, Psychiatry & Psychology*, *18*(3), 209–223.

Plunkett, D. (2021). Debate: Anger, fitting attitudes, and Srinivasan's category of "affective injustice". *The Journal of Political Philosophy*, *29*(1), 117–131.

Potter, N. N. (2006). What is manipulative behavior, anyway? *Journal of Personality Disorders*, *20*(2), 139–156.

Potter, N. N. (2009). *Mapping the edges and the in-between: A critical analysis of borderline personality disorder*. Oxford University Press.

Russell, J. A. (2003). Core affect and the psychological construction of emotion. *Psychological Review*, *110*(1), 145–172.

Sadler, J. Z. (2005). *Values and psychiatric diagnosis*. Oxford University Press.

Sansone, R. A., & Sansone, L. A. (2013). Responses of mental health clinicians to patients with borderline personality disorder. *Innovations in Clinical Neuroscience*, *10*(5–6), 39–43.

Scrutton, A. P. (2017). Epistemic injustice and mental illness. In I. J. Kidd, J. Medina, & G. Pohlhaus (eds.), *The Routledge handbook of epistemic injustice*. Routledge.

Silva, L. (2021). The epistemic role of outlaw emotions. *Ergo*, *7*(23), 664–691.

Solomon, R. C. (1976). *The passions: The myth and nature of human emotion*. Anchor Press.

Srinivasan, A. (2018). The aptness of anger. *The Journal of Political Philosophy*, *26*(2), 123–144.

Stanley, B., & Singh, T. (2018). Diagnosis of borderline personality disorder. In B. Stanley, & A. S. New (eds.), *Borderline personality disorder* (pp. 17–34). Oxford University Press.

Strawson, P. F. (1962). Freedom and resentment. *Proceedings of the British Academy*, *48*, 1–25.

Sulzer, S. H. (2015). Does "difficult patient" status contribute to de facto demedicalization? The case of borderline personality disorder. *Social Science & Medicine*, *142*, 82–89.

Tappolet, C. (2016). *Emotions, values, and agency*. Oxford University Press.

Tusiani-Eng, P., & Tusiani, B. (2018). Borderline personality disorder and advocacy: Individuals and family members speaking out for change. In B. Stanley, & A. S. New (eds.), *Borderline personality disorder* (pp. 421–436). Oxford University Press.

Whitney, S. (2018). Affective intentionality and affective injustice: Merleau-Ponty and Fanon on the body schema as a theory of affect. *The Southern Journal of Philosophy*, *56*(4), 488–515.

Yeomans, F. E., & Delaeny, J. C. (2018). Transference-focused psychotherapy: A psychodynamic treatment of personality disorders. In B. Stanley, & A. S. New (eds.), *Borderline personality disorder* (pp. 271–288). Oxford University Press.

Young, I. M. (1990). *Justice and the politics of difference*. Princeton University Press.

Part V

Perspectives on Borderline and Narcissistic Personality

19 How and Why Emptiness Manifests in Everyday Life

Borderline Personality Disorder and Beyond

Nancy Nyquist Potter

This chapter explores the criterion of emptiness found in borderline personality disorder (BPD). In Section 19.1, I address why it is important to study the concept and experience of emptiness. In Sections 19.1.1 and 19.1.2, I examine the question of what emptiness is and discuss prevailing theories of how it develops. I point out that feelings of emptiness are also found in other clinical diagnoses. In Section 19.2, I discuss emptiness in everyday life. Sections 19.2.1 and 19.2.2 turn to the question of whether emptiness is inherently negative, with the idea that mindfulness meditation can address emptiness both within the clinic and beyond. I argue that learning how to conceptualize and experience emptiness differently can be healing.

The *Diagnostic and statistical manual of mental disorders* (DSM; American Psychiatric Association, 2013, 5th ed.) states that "Borderline personality disorder (BPD) is a pervasive pattern of instability in interpersonal relationships, self-image, and affects, and marked impulsivity, beginning by early adulthood and present in a variety of contexts" (DSM-5: 663). Although I focus here on one criterion, the presence of just one criterion or symptom is not sufficient to make a diagnosis of BPD; the psychiatrist must identify at least five of the nine criteria to give a person this diagnosis. The criteria for diagnosis of BPD found in the DSM are as follows:

1. Frantic efforts to avoid real or imagined abandonment.
2. A pattern of unstable and intense interpersonal relationships characterized by alternating between extremes of idealization and devaluation.
3. Identity disturbance: markedly and persistently unstable self-image or sense of self.
4. Impulsivity in at least two areas that are potentially self-damaging (e.g., spending, sex, substance abuse, reckless driving, binge eating.
5. Recurrent suicidal behavior, gestures, or threats, or self-mutilating behavior.

6. Affective instability due to a marked reactivity of mood (intense episodic dysphoria, irritability, or anxiety usually lasting a few hours and only rarely more than a few days).
7. Chronic feelings of emptiness.
8. Inappropriate, intense anger or difficulty controlling anger (e.g., frequent displays of temper, constant anger, recurrent physical fights).
9. Transient, stress-related paranoid ideation or severe dissociative symptoms. (DSM-5: 663)[1]

It may be thought that personality disorders are intractable given that they are or seem to be an unchangeable part of a person's personality. However, such a view seems to be false when we assess current research. It is more often found that people diagnosed with BPD can recover over time (Korner et al., 2008: 378; Zanarini, 2018).

19.1 Why Study Emptiness?

Chronic emptiness is reported in approximately 70% of service-users diagnosed with BPD (Klonsky, 2008: 419). Studies show that emptiness in those diagnosed with BPD is virtually always experienced as negative – uncomfortable, unpleasant, and often terrifying. In fact, feelings of emptiness can present high risks; in particular, it overlaps with hopelessness, and hopelessness is a predictor of suicide (Klonsky, 2008; see also Wilson et al., 2021). Kiera Van Gelder's (2010) memoir on recovery from BPD is a powerful reminder of just how much suffering, terror, and despair a person with the symptoms listed in the DSM experience in their everyday lives. As Marsha Linehan (1993a: 107) writes, "The lives of suicidal, borderline individuals are unbearable as they are currently being lived." The serious risk factors and intensity of suffering reported by so many service-users diagnosed with this personality disorder itself are reasons for probing this criterion. Second, it is the least researched of the nine criteria, and most research shows vague boundaries and overlap between concepts (Miller et al., 2020). As noted, hopelessness and emptiness often overlap, but also loneliness, isolation, depression, and boredom.

A third reason to study the concept of emptiness is likely related to the first two points: it is the longest of symptoms to show remission after clinical treatment. That is, it appears to be the most intractable of the criteria. On the other hand, treatment for chronic feelings of emptiness often is not targeted. Thus, slow remission may be due to not targeting treatment accordingly, and the fact that the concept of emptiness is unclear may contribute to an interplay between all three of these issues in the seventh criterion.

[1] I have discussed many of these criteria in Potter (2009).

Finally, feelings of emptiness are neither specific to people diagnosed with BPD nor exclusive to psychopathology. There are reasons to believe that emptiness is experienced by most people at some times (see Section 19.2).

19.1.1 What Is Emptiness?

It is crucial that we listen well to service-users' voices about their own experiences of emptiness (Potter, 2019). This applies to people diagnosed with BPD as well as those with other diagnoses. Service-users seem to be in agreement that experiences of emptiness and disconnection are negatively valanced (D'Agostino, 2020). These feelings of emptiness play a central role in the person's fear, despair, and intolerable suffering.

Qualitative studies cite words and phrases people diagnosed with BPD use to describe what emptiness feels like for them: deadness, nothingness, a void, feeling swallowed, a sense of vagueness, a feeling of internal absence, aloneness, isolation, numbness, purposeless, and hollowness (Price et al., 2020; Miller et al 2020, 2021). Discursively, one person describes their experience of emptiness as "not living a life of fulfillment . . . there's something missing, I'm not living the life that I want to live . . . why . . . why, what am I doing right now, like why . . . What am I doing with my life that is fulfilling me right now?" (Miller et al., 2021: 4).

When asked if they could give a metaphor that describes how they experience emptiness, one person says, "It's like wind inside a tin can . . . like you're the tin can." Another says "Um, I suppose like just a depressing, empty swimming pool. Like a concrete swimming pool with, like, a little bit of water and lots of mould . . . Yeah. Like not one that people skate in." Another says, "It's just your kind of very robotic and very, like – there is no meaning or purpose, I guess, would be my definition of it" (Miller et al., 2021: 4).

Elsner et al.'s (2018) list below also illustrates first-person descriptions of how emptiness feels to them:

"Verbatim descriptions of experiences of chronic emptiness

'It feels like there's a hole inside me from the front of me right through to my back'
'Hopelessness and existential nihilism'
'A sense of purposelessness'
'I feel hollow – a true emptiness, a void, where my heart is'
'There's always something missing – I'm looking for something that's not there'
'I get heartaches'
'It's like a pit or a big black cloud'
'I'm on automatic pilot'
'I feel hollow, like a shell'
'Constant despair'
'Like an egg shell without a yolk in it'
'I feel like I'm missing lots of things that other people have'

'It's like I have an empty brain'
'An existential angst, with no purpose or meaning'" (Elsner et al., 2018: 89)

One can understand from these comments how disturbing and painful feelings of emptiness can be. Service-users' voices describe suffering through their attempts to describe this internal experience of a void, a hole, a hollow feeling. Although there is no unifying concept of emptiness that holds together the various responses to questions of what emptiness is, Miller et al.'s (2021) qualitative approach and Elsner et al.'s (2018) research paint a picture of deep suffering that may lead to self-harm, suicide attempts and completions, and other desperate measures to escape this misery.

To summarize so far, there is no clear construct of what emptiness is. On the other hand, Sani and Herron offer a definition of it:

> A feeling that one is going through life mechanically, devoid of emotions and purpose, and therefore is empty inside, with emptiness often being bodily felt in the form of a discomfort in the chest. This is coupled with feelings that one is disconnected from others, in some way invisible to others, and unable to contribute to a world that remains the same, but from which one is distant and detached. (Herron & Sani, 2022: 192)

These researchers emphasize that this is an ideal type or prototype. It is more descriptive than many people would accept as a definition or ideal measure. This step, however, is an important one to offer because it serves as a working definition for providing more clarity.

What does seem to be clear is that people who experience it have some difficulty articulating just what it feels like, and a wide variety of terms is used when asked. The criterion is not adequately researched and queried. Yet people diagnosed with BPD suffer immensely from feelings and experiences called "emptiness."

19.1.2 Why Do Feelings of Emptiness Develop?

It is currently unclear why people diagnosed with BPD develop feelings of emptiness. In part, this absence is due to a relative lack of research compared with the other criteria for BPD. In this section, I call attention to primary theories of its etiology.

Stone (2024) identifies two models that currently are drawn upon to hypothesize causes of the development of BPD and emptiness. One is the Tripartite Model of the Development of BPD; the second is the Biosocial Development Model of BPD. The tripartite model "consists of loosely defined traumatic childhoods, a vulnerable or hyperbolic temperament, and an event or series of events that trigger the onset of BPD" (Stone, 2024: 4). Mary Zanarini and Frances Frankenburg (1994), who developed this model, suggest that the three factors in their model are necessary but not sufficient for the development of

BPD or its symptoms (Stone, 2024: 4). Some research now examines genetic contributions to the etiology of BPD, but Stone suggests that more needs to be done in this area.

The second model is the biosocial model, developed by Marsha Linehan (Stone, 2024). The biosocial theory of the development of psychopathology highlights the interactions between biology-genetics, personality, and stressful events. These interactions are key factors in creating vulnerability (Pollack, 2001). Linehan holds that vulnerability is a tendency to be readily and strongly reactive and to have difficulty returning to a more balanced state (Stone, 2024). Linehan proposes that a poor fit between environmental opportunities in the child's life and the capacities of the child creates an invalidating environment that creates conditions for the development of BPD. Her assessment of the biosocial model is that BPD is primarily a disorder of the emotion regulation system (Linehan, 1993a: 43). Many service-users who are diagnosed with BPD tend to try to inhibit emotional responses which, in turn, may contribute to a lack of sense of identity. The numbness that appears to arise from emotional inhibiting is often experienced as emptiness (Linehan, 1993a: 61). Identity disturbance is another significant symptom of BPD. As I understand it, emotional dysregulation and identity disturbance are in part caused by invalidation experienced at an early age and that they interact to heighten each individual symptom, possibly resulting in a vicious cycle and, more pertinently, in feelings of emptiness.

It seems reasonable to accept the current research building on the biosocial model; that is, the evidence that adverse childhood experiences such as poverty; parental drug abuse; physical, sexual, and emotional abuse; and intrauterine events may interact with a person's genetic makeup and temperament to influence brain development has more standing for good reasons (Leichsenring et al., 2023: 673). As Korner et al. (2008) note, service-users with BPD have an inner world where negative emotional beliefs and patterns are set down early in life in the context of difficulties with having relationships with others (377).[2] Studies on the role of genetics in the development of BPD symptoms highlight the many factors that can lead to the development of often-devastating experienced of BPD symptoms.

[2] I stress the following: both models consider childhood trauma as one of the mechanisms that likely are causally related to feelings of emptiness. As Wilson et al. state, it appears that individuals diagnosed with BPD are 13 times more likely to report childhood adversity than non-clinical controls (Wilson et al., 2021: 132). "Nonetheless, childhood maltreatment is currently considered to be neither causative nor specific to BPD. Indeed, 80% of subjects with a history of sexual abuse do not fulfil criteria for the disorder and longitudinal follow-up studies of abused children showed high rates of resilience" (Wilson et al., 2021: 132). These statistics deserve attention in that they remind us that no one causal path (or combination of paths), as of now, can determine whether a person may develop symptoms of BPD.

A third model, a psychodynamic one, also has traction in understanding the etiology of BPD. On this model, two of the criteria for BPD diagnosis (chronic feelings of emptiness and frantic efforts to avoid abandonment) can be grouped together into the concepts of "solitude and emptiness" (Pazzagli & Monti, 2000). Pazzagli and Monti explain that a person struggling with experiences of emptiness simultaneously may feel unable to tolerate solitude. In such cases, people try to find ways to fill this internal feeling of emptiness.

> The solitude of the BPD patient is actually an intolerance of true solitude, the solitude of being able to be alone. It is a solitude dominated by emptiness: a void in the outside world, made up of inadequate objects, sporadic, stormy, and superficial relationships prone to sudden break-ups, and a void in the inner world, always subject to the threat of rupturing and the loss of limits. (Didonna & Gonzalez, 2009: 135)

Others, too, have found that chronic emptiness and identity disturbance show a stronger relation to one another than to other BPD symptoms (Martin & Levy, 2022). "Individuals with BPD are believed to experience feelings of emptiness in response to the various instabilities present in their lives, to include instability in identity, mood, interpersonal and romantic relationships, and behavior" (8).[3] These findings seem relevant to the biosocial model as well.

To varying degrees, each model suggests that chronic feelings of emptiness reflect emotional dysregulation intertwined with identity disturbance. Emptiness is sometimes understood as an attempt to suppress intense emotions, which can lead to a rather undeveloped sense of self. In psychodynamic models, attachment theory explains experiences of chronic emptiness as the result of insecure attachments with parental figures – hence efforts to avoid abandonment. Others explain the etiology of emptiness arising from a person not knowing their own experiences and having experienced invalidation from parental figures. "Specifically, emptiness is a consequence of the absence of the psychological self – the secondary representation of self which allows an understanding of one's own internal world, and the world seen through the eyes of others" (Miller et al., 2020: 2).

Despite the theorizing on causes of emptiness in those diagnosed with BPD or developing symptoms of it, "it is not typically accounted for in aetiological models of BPD" (Miller et al., 2020: 2). It matters which models of BPD etiology are drawn upon to investigate further characteristics that work together to produce BPD symptoms. This is especially the case with ones that study feelings of emptiness. The choice of models, of which I have described only three, matters because models help us focus on what treatment options might best serve the service-user and what sorts of early interventions are necessary to ameliorate the

[3] For more literature on the etiology of BPD or emptiness, see Juraś-Darowny et al. (2023), Pazzagli & Monti (2020), Wilson et al., (2021), Winsper (2018), Korner et al. (2008), Livesley (2008), and Levy (2005).

development of BPD. Because experiences of emptiness seem quite intractable, because they seem more likely than any other BPD symptom to lead to self-harm and suicidality, and because they significantly contribute to intense suffering, it is necessary that causal explanations continue to be studied and honed in order to decrease the likelihood of development of people who are identified with BPD. In addition, as I have noted, definitions of emptiness are messy and unclear; hence, it is not clear which aspects of emptiness should be emphasized in treatment methods (Elsner et al., 2018: 90; see also Section 19.1).

19.2 Emptiness as Transdiagnostic

One reason for lack of clarity about what emptiness is and why some people develop the characteristics associated with this criterion might be found in its expectation that experiences of emptiness are specific to BPD. However, some recent research indicates that feelings of emptiness are common in the broader clinical population, suggesting that emptiness should be thought of as transdiagnostic rather than pathology-specific experience. As D'Agostino et al. (2020) say that it is not only people with BPD who may experience emptiness, but also some of those with other mental diagnoses as well. (See also Klonsky, 2008: 419; Konjusha et al., 2021.) A transdiagnostic model may group factors such as depression, generalized anxiety disorder, and social anxiety disorder that are in the internalizing domain (Rodriguez-Seijas et al., 2015: 428). Transdiagnostic features, then, represent core dispositional characteristics that saturate common disorders as well as normal-range personality traits. Research suggests that emptiness is a relatively narrow symptom most strongly related to constructs in the broad internalizing domain of psychopathology, whereas aggression and impulsivity are more strongly associated with externalizing constructs than with internalizing ones such as emptiness (Price et al., 2020: 2).

19.2.1 Emptiness in Everyday Life

People diagnosed with BPD report feelings of emptiness. People with other diagnoses also report such feelings (D'Agostino et al., 2020; Konjusha et al., 2021). In fact, feelings of emptiness may be more common than is recognized. As Sani and Herron report, their research findings suggest that times of feeling empty are far more widespread than previously believed. Feelings of emptiness can be experienced by anyone, regardless of their mental health history (Sani & Herron, 2021). In their research, Sani and Herron found that half of participants had never struggled with a mental health difficulty – showing us that emptiness is not only experienced by people who carry a diagnosis of BPD, but that it can be experienced by people with and without mental health problems (Sani &

Herron, 2021: 193–194). Similarly, Didonna and Gonzales (2009) found that experiences of emptiness seem "to be a universal human experience and might not always seem directly linked to a pathology. Each of us occasionally can experience feelings of emptiness even when we are not currently struggling with a mental illness" (2009: 25). People might feel empty when they retire, are between jobs, hate the job they have, don't have a child, people whose children have been placed in care, whose children are grown to adulthood and move away, or whose communities are internally displaced or forced into migration.

It is important to consider that the economic and social context in which many parts of the world work, play, and live their lives may also contribute to emptiness in people without mental illnesses (see Alvesson, 2013; Biebricher & Johnson, 2012). In capitalist economies, the disappointments in life and with our personal shortcomings are trumpeted as things able to be overcome through consumption. Fantasies of success, acquisition, production (of policies, ethics standards, graduates, and so on) drive people toward more and higher aims, only to find that even higher striving is necessary for satisfaction. Such values, aims, and goals tell us what sort of person we should be and how to judge ourselves and others. A cycle of goal-setting, consuming, and achieving may be valued as the norm for living a good life, but in between the aiming-toward is dissatisfaction, disappointment, and even despair. Many people live and work in environments where they periodically feel the pointlessness and meaninglessness of constant striving, where satisfaction is short-lived. As Michael Friedman (2022) says, "Sometimes, we feel empty not because there is something 'wrong' with us per se but because there is something 'right' with us. We are truly not connecting with the environment around us because that environment is somehow toxic and not consistent with our purpose and our life goals."

In this case, emptiness may signify an openness – a willingness to experience new and positive connections. This way of thinking about emptiness offers us a way to deeply connect with ourselves and the world around us. Our hollow or empty feeling would be understood as an opportunity rather than a disconnect (Friedman, 2022). Section 19.3 turns to Buddhist meditation as a pathway to such an opportunity for those diagnosed with BPD and others, including those not currently carrying a diagnosis of any mental illness.

19.2.2 Beyond Western Conceptions of Emptiness

Cultural differences such as values, beliefs, social norms for behavior, and socioeconomic factors may alter how people conceptualize the term "emptiness" – raising additional questions about what it is, how it is experienced, and how others who hear someone who talks about feelings of emptiness respond to such descriptions of anguish and suffering.

Indirect evidence suggests that BPD is socially sensitive, occurs in specific social contexts, and is more likely to develop when social cohesion and social capital are compromised. Patients with a BPD diagnosis might therefore be considered, at least in some ways, as casualties of modernity and the rise of individualistic values (Paris & Lis, 2013).

Context and culture are important to investigate to see to what extent emptiness is experienced differently or even whether emptiness means similar things to what is reported in Western cultures. Such research is important to expand because it raises the possibility of understanding when emptiness is a pathology, how to develop a construct of emptiness that includes dimensions of Western ideas as well as emptiness as discussed in some other cultures – without collapsing understandings in Western culture into multiculturalism; that approach tends to retain Western dominance in science and psychology. Still, it is important to appreciate the need loosely to attend to the construct of emptiness ranging from Northern/Western cultures to Southern and Eastern cultures so that we can more deeply understand the complexity of feelings and experiences of it. This work likely will not give us necessary and sufficient conditions for this thing called "emptiness," but it may help direct treatment options that are culturally sensitive (see Chung et al., 2020; Williams et al., 2021; Tao et al., 2022; Lesham, 2013).[4]

[4] The fact as of now is that there is very little literature on emptiness as a cross-cultural phenomenon. I call attention to a few research projects that are either cross-cultural or non-Western.

Chung et al. (2020) researched older people who live in long-term care facilities (LTCF) in two cultures, western China (Hong Kong) and Sweden, to see to what degree their feelings and experiences of aging in such facilities are more similar or different. Older people who move into LTCF are faced not only with losses associated with aging but also with loss of a network, meaningful roles and projects, and some basic freedoms they formerly held. Many people in this situation report sadness, emptiness, and what the authors call existential loneliness (EL). This kind of loneliness seems to be different from more prevalent loneliness studied. Existential loneliness is "the intolerable emptiness and lack of meaningful existence resulted from the losses they have experienced" (Chung et al., 2020: 1–2). A central difference found between Western cultures and Chinese/Swedish ones is in how they *experience* EL. In general, both Chinese and Swedish older adults in this study described their EL experience as "overcoming" rather than "being trapped" as is reported in studies of Western cultures. Chung et al.'s study found that people who moved into LTCF experienced EL in their feelings of losing control of their lives, absence of being understood, isolation, and difficulty finding meaning and purpose in their lives (Chung et al., 2020: 9).

In research on Canadian women, Williams et al. (2021) focused on First Nations, Métis, and Inuit (FNMI) women's experiences and effects of intimate partner violence (IPV). The context with respect to FNMI women is that of continuing colonization of FNMI women who have less assistance in escaping IPV, less access to safety and the concern of health care providers and the government, less financial support necessary to stay away from a violent partner instead of returning for practical reasons. A crucial aspect of most of their experiences includes trauma from being placed in residential schools where many were abused, shamed, forced to try to assimilate by forbidding use of their languages and cultural values and beliefs. The blockades to escaping IPV compound their anguish and despair coupled with ongoing colonization and experiences of placement in violent and alienating schools that continue to cause immense

19.3 Meditation and Emptiness

There is no question that most people diagnosed with BPD experience tremendous suffering, some to the point of attempting or completing suicide or engaging in self-harm. Feelings of emptiness are one aspect of that suffering. Research suggests that emptiness is virtually always a painful, even terrifying experience, with strong negative emotions and potentially destructive behaviors accompanying it. However, this is not a necessary truth about emptiness. In this section, I turn to mindfulness meditation to shift toward an idea of emptiness that is positive and freeing. Mindfulness, or insight meditation, may offer a path of recovery for some people diagnosed with BPD.

Linehan (1993a) developed a treatment for those struggling with symptoms of BPD called dialectical behavioral therapy (DBT). This treatment has been found to be highly successful for many people (Barnicot & Crawford, 2019; Bohus et al., 2000; Lynch et al., 2007; Schmidt et al., 2021). Dialectical behavioral therapy focuses on helping people diagnosed with BPD to become aware that their core beliefs about themselves and the world are not the only truths they hold. For example, a person who firmly believes they will always want to die may come to recognize experiences where they did not want to die. Holding both to be true while being aware that that belief is contradictory can gradually shift their beliefs toward a new way of being in the world. Change is an aim in the long-term treatment with DBT but it must be preceded by acceptance of current feelings and beliefs, moving toward a synthesis of the two contradictory beliefs or feelings. As Linehan says, "in most descriptions of BPD, the emphasis is on identifying the pathology that sets the individual apart

harm. Qualitative studies that Williams et al. reviewed show that a major theme within FNMI women is the feeling of emptiness. One woman says: "There is such a void, when you come out of that place [residential schools, displacement to reserves, and violence in their lives], there is such a void. There is such a cloud of emptiness and you need to fill it and for me I filled it with food and work . . . That whole emptiness . . . your spirit being removed" (Williams et al., 2021: 1004). This description of emptiness resonates with Western research on first-person descriptions of what emptiness feels like.

In China, many symptoms of mental problems have emerged during the Covid pandemic, such as panic, tension, melancholy, and helplessness, but emptiness is not one of them (Tao et al., 2022: 1). Instead, emptiness is considered a healing state. An English way of characterizing emptiness in Chinese philosophy is that it is a neutral, non-positive, and non-negative state of existence instead of a state of action. People who are struggling with mental distress are encouraged to put those feelings into an emptiness state; emptiness, then, is an area of inner experience whence their distress will no longer exist (Tao et al., 2022: 1–2).

An interesting analysis of Israeli/Palestinian relations is found in Lesham (2013). He focuses on emptiness in Palestine in terms of geography and spatial relationships on land as an effect of wars. Emptiness does not seem to refer to personal or interpersonal phenomena but instead to refer to economic and power issues between Israel and Palestine. It would be interesting empirically to investigate whether there is any relationship between spatial emptiness and emptiness as an internal experience of people and, if so, to analysis similarities and differences in culturally inflected more individualized experiences of emptiness.

from others. Treatment is then designed to ferret out the pathology and *create conditions for change*. A dialectical perspective, however, suggests that within dysfunction there is also function; that within distortion there is accuracy; and that within destruction one can find construction" (1993a: 32; emphasis added).

Linehan's treatment, therefore, doesn't primarily focus on service-users' acceptance of painful emotional states and problematic environmental events. Robins, Schmidt, and Linehan (2004) explain that focusing exclusively on change or on acceptance may result in the patient feeling invalidated (31). In therapy, patient and clinician need to find a way to simultaneously hold acceptance and change. This can lead to a synthesis that, when found, can engender both new patient change and acceptance of new perspectives of themselves, others, and the world.[5]

The dialectical approach is relevant to this section of the chapter in that it is partly grounded in Buddhist practices. Skills training for the people diagnosed with BPD or experiencing some of the symptoms along those lines aims to increase four central behaviors: interpersonal skills, emotion regulation skills, distress tolerance, and core mindfulness skills including "observing, describing, participating, taking a nonjudgmental stance, focusing on one thing in the moment, [and] being effective" (Linehan, 1993a: 144; Linehan, 1993b). Mindfulness involves developing a capacity for awareness that people can bring into their everyday lives (Linehan, 1993a: 144).

Dialectical behavioral therapy is quite effective in helping people diagnosed with BPD or who experience some of the symptoms to manage their lives more constructively. For some people, Buddhist meditation may be a next step in a recovery process. One reason is that it is a powerful way to promote well-being and healing. From a Buddhist perspective, emptiness does not mean nothingness. Thich Nat Hanh explains that it means we are open to the experience of emptying ourselves of the idea of a permanent, separate self (2017). When we hold dualistic ontological and existential beliefs, we concretize our

[5] Dialectics, like other dialectical methods, relies on a contradictory process between opposing sides. In Hegel's epistemology, "the 'opposing sides' are different definitions of consciousness and of the object that consciousness is aware of or claims to know. As in Plato's dialogues, a contradictory process between 'opposing sides' in Hegel's dialectics leads to a linear evolution or development from less sophisticated definitions or views to more sophisticated ones later" (*Stanford encyclopedia of philosophy*). "The first moment – the moment of the understanding – is the moment of fixity, in which concepts or forms have a seemingly stable definition or determination (EL §80). The second moment – the '*dialectical*' (EL §§79, 81) or '*negatively rational*' (EL §79) moment – is the moment of instability. In this moment, a one-sidedness or restrictedness (EL Remark to §81) in the determination from the moment of understanding comes to the fore, and the determination that was fixed in the first moment passes into its opposite (EL §81) . . . The dialectical moment thus involves a process of *self*-sublation, or a process in which the determination from the moment of understanding sublates *itself*, or both cancels and preserves *itself*, as it pushes on to or passes into its opposite." The third moment "grasps the unity of the opposition between the first two determinations" (*Stanford encyclopedia of philosophy*, emphasis in original). This step is often called" synthesis."

selfhood, which can keep us stuck in narrow and painful responses. When we are ontologically committed to such beliefs, we take a Western metaphysics of the self as given, which can trap us in narrow and painful experiences and responses. If we can move away from rigid beliefs about an inherently and independently existing "I," we have less "self" for unskillful stories about who we "truly" are. We needn't be snagged by attaching how things are, at the present moment, to a "self" and then assume that the core self has been, is, and always will be that way. For example, when a person says "I'm feeling bitter" or "I'm feeling lonely," they do not need to make this a fact about their self. We can learn how not to turn such experiences into "I am a bitter and lonely person." This is not primarily a philosophical shift but an experiential one – although it may engage the person in knotty questions or shifts about metaphysical beliefs. (See Section 19.4.)

Without a rigid belief in an inherently and independently existing "I," there is a reduced locus of self upon which conceptual and emotional baggage can accrue. Instead of repeating "I'm a screw-up" or "I am destined to stay depressed, needy, and suicidal for my whole life," Buddhist meditation helps people let go of attachment to a core self that some are reluctant to question because they see particular qualities of themselves that they experience as their identity. Without learning to let go of an attachment to a metaphysics of selfhood, emptiness feels like an aversive experience (see Van Gordon et al., 2021).

Kiera van Gelder, a person diagnosed with BPD, went through DBT skill development and then turned to Buddhist meditation. She writes that this kind of meditation has commonalities with DBT treatment, but that Buddhist meditation "involves a much more sustained effort . . . Thirty seconds of pure awareness is a long time, especially after a lifetime of escaping yourself at all costs" (2010, 164–165). Another similarity is that, as in DBT, people need a guiding teacher and a support community in their meditation practice (182). The effort involved may present serious challenges to those who would start practicing Buddhist meditation.

19.4 Conclusion

One core concept in DBT treatment for those diagnosed with BPD is that of mindfulness, a skill and practice derived from Buddhist meditation and other forms of insight meditation. Although DBT and Buddhist mindfulness practice are not the same, they are, in some ways, quite similar in that DBT draws on ideas from Buddhist practices when working on skill building with people diagnosed with BPD.

Still, the enthusiasm of many clinicians to endorse the treatment of mindfulness as a way to recover from BPD has raised concerns that enthusiasts neglect potential worries of advocating for this treatment. Ratnayake and Merry (2018) argue that a Buddhist meditation program is metaphysically loaded in that it conflicts with a metaphysics that is widely accepted – specifically, that the doctrine of no-self in Buddhist meditation is at odds with commonplace understandings of the self in Western cultures (568). Because of the current embrace of mindfulness as a treatment method, contemporary psychology is replete with a controversial conceptualization of mental states as "somehow separate from, or unrelated to, the self" (569). Thus, doing mindfulness exercises may create an epistemic dissonance that may not only not be helpful but, in fact, may be harmful to some service-users.[6] Ratnayake and Merry do point out that many other treatment plans have negative aspects to them and that clinicians and their service-users need to weigh the benefits and possible costs after informed consent. Certainly, like any other treatment for BPD such as CBT or DBT, mindfulness may not be appropriate for some people or may not offer the degree of healing that one might wish for. Experiencing emptiness through Buddhist meditation is also quite difficult and frustrating, at least to some in the beginning. But it is possible and even worthwhile to shift from interpreting experience as devastating to interpreting it as a move toward a life worth living.

Another criticism of my argument is that some people may see emptiness experienced by people diagnosed with BPD and emptiness in Buddhist meditation practices as different in kind. It is true that "the concept of emptiness in Eastern psychology and culture is, in some ways, unrelated to that of the West, especially considering the negative value that is commonly ascribed to it in the West. An analysis of the classical texts of Taoism or Chinese Buddhism seems enough to draw the conclusion that the Christian–Western concepts are basically opposite of those illustrated in Eastern thought" (Didonna & Gonzalez, 2009: 132). That said, I reserve judgment until research is undertaken with people diagnosed with BPD and experiencing emptiness engage in Buddhist meditation. Some might wonder why people who experience painful and debilitating feelings of emptiness should study and practice emptiness from a Buddhist perspective. I suggest that, even if Western and Eastern thought are radically different, they are not, in my view, incommensurable.

I have argued that Buddhist meditation offers one direction for healing from experiences of emptiness associated with BPD. In fact, there is evidence that neural pathways are changed over time when a person practices meditation.

[6] The authors raise concerns that mindfulness exercises often collide with our common values and beliefs about the self and other metaphysical commitments. However, they seem not to question whether holding on to "commonsense" beliefs is aways desirable in the longer term. Although epistemic conflict may be uncomfortable, it is often unavoidable in everyday life. In fact, the move to synthesis in DBT can also create epistemic discomfort in service-users. Even so, DBT does have a good track record for recovery.

Treadway and Lazar report that meditation has both state and trait effects. State-like changes occur when a person is actively meditating. Trait-like effects, however, occur gradually as a result of sustained meditation and persist through the day. Trait-like effects are believed to come about from "stable, long-term transformations in brain activity and structure" (Treadway & Lazar, 2009: 45–46; see also Allen et al., 2012; Gibson, 2019; Scherpiet et al., 2015).

These studies support claims reported by experienced meditators about the effects of their practice: regular meditation practice does appear to increase an individual's capacity for attention and to decrease habits that cause suffering. These neurological and experiential effects may contribute to clinical benefits that develop from meditation practices (Treadway & Lazar, 2009: 48). Over time, Buddhist meditation changes feelings of emptiness and offers healing qualities that are associated with changes in brain patterns, such as increased time living in the present moment, increased positive affect; reduced stress activity in the brain; and enhanced cognitive capabilities (53–54).

It seems to follow from this analysis that one focus for healing from feelings of emptiness, meaninglessness, and disconnection needs to be on helping people effectively to learn to live with difficult stimuli, to learn to find equanimity, and to learn to live with change. Healing can take traditional forms of clinical treatment, cognitive behavioral therapy, DBT, or might include Buddhist mindfulness meditation. They can be done in conjunction with one another or not. Whatever treatment is considered, it should aim for fitness with the person's needs and current state and, most importantly, it should aim for reducing suffering and preventing suicides. Of course, emptiness is just one of the criteria that may indicate the development of BPD, but as it is much less a target of research and is a central effect of some very strong painful and difficult feelings, it calls for more investigation.

References

Allen, M., Dietz, M., Blair, K. S., van Beek, M., Rees, G., Vestergaard-Poulsen, P., Lutz, A. & Roepstorff, A. (2012). Cognitive-affective neural plasticity following active-controlled mindfulness intervention. *Journal of Neuroscience*, *32*(44), 15601–15610.

Alvesson, M. (2013). *The triumph of emptiness: Consumption, higher education, and work organization*. Oxford University Press.

American Psychiatric Association. (2013). *Diagnostic and statistical manual of mental disorders* (5th ed.). American Psychiatric Association.

Barnicot, K., & Crawford, M. (2019). Dialectical behaviour therapy *v.* mentalisation-based therapy for borderline personality disorder. *Psychological Medicine*, *49*(12), 2060–2068.

Biebricher, T., & Johnson, E. (2012). What's wrong with neoliberalism? *New Political Science*, *34*(2), 202–211. https://doi.org/10.1080/07393148.2012.676398.

Bohus, M., Haaf, B., Stiglmayr, C., Pohl. U., Böhme, R., & Linehan, M. (2000). Evaluation of inpatient dialectical-behavioral therapy for borderline personality disorder – A prospective study. *Behaviour Research and Therapy*, *38*, 875–887.

Chung, B., Olofsson, J., Wong, K., & Rämgård, M. (2020). Overcoming existential loneliness: A cross-cultural study. *BioMedCentral Geriatrics*, *20*(347), 1–12.

D'Agostino, A., Pepi, R., Monti, M., & Starcevic, V. (2020). The feeling of emptiness: A review of a complex subjective experience. *Harvard Review of Psychiatry*, *8*(5), 287–295.

Didonna, F., & Gonzalez, Y. R. (2009). Mindfulness and feelings of emptiness. In F. Didonna (ed.), *Clinical handbook of mindfulness* (pp. 125–151). Springer.

Elsner, D., Broadbear, D., & Rao, S. (2018). What is the clinical significance of chronic emptiness in borderline personality disorder? *Australasian Psychiatry*, *26*(1), 88–91.

Friedman, M. (2022). Why we feel empty and how we can cope with emptiness. *Psychology Today*, July 5. www.psychologytoday.com/gb/blog/brick-brick/202207/why-we-feel-empty.

Gibson, J. (2019). Mindfulness, interoception, and the body: A contemporary perspective. *Frontiers in Psychology*, *12*, 1845–1848. https://doi.org/10.1007/s12671-020-01586-1.

Gunderson, J. G., Herpertz, S. C., Skodol, A. E., Torgersen, S., & Zanarini, M. C. (2018). Borderline personality disorder. *Nature Reviews Disease Primers*, *4*(1), 1–20.

Hanh, T. N. (2017). *The art of living*. Penguin Random House.

Herron, S. J. & Sani, F. (2022). Understanding the typical presentation of emptiness: A study of lived-experience. *Journal of Mental Health*, *31*(2), 188–195. https://doi.org/10.1080/09638237.2021.1922645.

Juraś-Darowny, M., Strzelecki, D., & Talarowska, M. (2023). Borderline personality – From psychoanalysis to epigenetics. Biological basis of attachment. *Psychiatria Polska*: 1–15.

Klonsky, E. (2008). What is emptiness? Clarifying the 7th criterion for borderline personality disorder. *Journal of Personality Disorders*, *22*(4), 418–426.

Konjusha, A., Hopwood, C., Price, A., Masuhr, O., & Zimmermann, J. (2021). Investigating the transdiagnostic value of subjective emptiness. *Journal of Personality Disorders*, *35* (5), 788–800.

Korner, A., Gerull, F., Meares, R., & Stevenson, J. (2008). The nothing that is something: Core dysphoria as the central feature of borderline personality disorder: Implications for treatment. *American Journal of Psychotherapy*, *62*(4), 377–394.

Leichsenring, F., Heim, N., Leweke, F., Spitzer, C., Steinert, C., & Kernberg, O. (2023). Borderline personality disorder: A review. *Journal of the American Medical Association*, *329*(8), 670–679. https://doi.org/10.1001/jama.2023.0589.

Lesham, N. (2013). Repopulating the emptiness: a spatial critique of ruination in Israel/Palestine. *Environment and Planning D: Society and Space*, *31*, 522–537.

Levy, K. (2005). The implications of attachment theory and research for understanding borderline personality disorder *Development and Psychopathology*, *17*, 959–986. https://doi.org/10.10170S0954579405050455.

Linehan, M. (1993a). *Cognitive-behavioral treatment of borderline personality disorder*. Guilford Press.

Linehan, M. (1993b). *Skills training manual for treating borderline personality disorder*. Guilford Press.

Livesley, J. (2008). Toward a genetically-informed model of borderline personality disorder. *Journal of Personality Disorders*, *22*(1), 42–71.

Lynch, T., Trost, W., Salsman, N., & Linehan, M. (2007). Dialectical behavior therapy for borderline personality disorder. *Annual Review of Clinical Psychology*, *3*, 181–205.

Martin, J., & Levy, K. (2022). Chronic feelings of emptiness in a large undergraduate sample: Starting to fill the void. *Personal Mental Health*, *16*(3), 190–203.

Miller, C., Townsend, M., Day, N., & Grenyer, B. (2020). Measuring the shadows: A systematic review of chronic emptiness in borderline personality disorder. *PLoS One*, *15*(7), e0233970. https://doi.org/10.1371/journal.pone.0233970.

Miller, C., Townsend, M., & Grenyer, B. (2021). Understanding chronic feelings of emptiness in borderline personality disorder: A qualitative study. *Borderline Personality Disorder and Emotion Dysregulation*, *8*(24), 1–9. https://doi.org/10.1186/s40479-021-00164-8.

Pazzagli, A., & Monti, M. R. (2000). Dysphoria and aloneness in borderline personality disorder. *Psychopathology*, *33*, 220–226.

Paris, J., & Lis, E. (2013). Can sociocultural and historical mechanisms influence the development of borderline personality disorder? *Transcultural Psychiatry*, *50*(1), 140–151. https://doi.org/10.1177/1363461512468105.

Pollack, G. H. (2001). Vulnerability to psychopathology: A biosocial model. *American Journal of Psychiatry*, *158*(7). https://doi.org/10.1176/appi.ajp.158.7.1172.

Potter, N. (2009). *Mapping the edges and the in-between: A critical analysis of borderline personality disorder*. Oxford University Press.

Potter, N. (2019). Listening well to psychiatric service-users: What does it mean to give uptake? *European Journal for Person Centered Healthcare*, *7*(3), 499–505.

Price, A., Mahler, H., & Hopwood, C. (2020). Construction and validation of a self-report subjective emptiness scale. *Assessment*, *29*(3), 397–409. https://doi.org/10.1177/1073191120968275.

Ratnayake, S., & Merry, D. (2018). Forgetting ourselves: Epistemic costs and ethical concerns in mindfulness exercises. *Journal of Medical Ethics*, *44*(8), 567–574.

Robins, C., Schmidt III, H., & Linehan, M. (2004). Dialectical behavior therapy: Synthesizing radical acceptance with skillful means. In: S. Hayes et al. (eds.), *Mindfulness and acceptance: Expanding the cognitive-behavioral tradition*. Guilford Publications. http://ebookcentral.proquest.com/lib/miami/detail.action?docID=330580.

Rodriguez-Seijas, C., Eaton, N., & Krueger, R. (2015). How transdiagnostic factors of personality and psychopathology can inform clinical assessment and intervention. *Journal of Personality Assessment*, *97*(5), 425–435.

Sani, F., & Herron, S. (2021). Many of us feel 'empty' – Understanding what it means is important for improving our mental health. *The Conversation*: *Neurosciencenews.com*. July 3, 2021. https://theconversation.com/many-of-us-feel-empty-understanding-what-it-means-is-important-for-improving-our-mental-health-163035

Scherpiet, S., Herwig, U., Opialla, S., Scheerer, H., Habermeyer, V., Jäncke, L., & Brühl, A. (2015). Reduced neural differentiation between self-referential cognitive and emotional processes in women with borderline personality disorder. *Psychiatry Research*, *233*(3), 314–323. https://doi.org/10.1016/j.pscychresns.2015.05.008.

Schmidt, C., Soler, J., Carmona i Farrés, C., Domínguez-Clavé, E., Vega, D., & Pascual, J. (2021). Mindfulness in borderline personality disorder: Decentering mediates the effectiveness. *Psicothema*, *33*(3), 407–414. https://doi.org/10.7334/psicothema2020.437.

Stanford encyclopedia of philosophy. Online encyclopedia. https://plato.stanford.edu/entries/hegel-dialectics/.

Stone, B. (2024). The pathogenesis of borderline personality disorder: Evolution of evidence and treatment implications for two prominent models. *Psychology Reports*, *127*, 2762–2783. https://doi.org/10.1177/00332941221127618.

Tao, Y., Chen, Y., Zhou, W., Lai, L., & Liu, T. (2022). The effectiveness of the moving to emptiness technique on clients who need help during the COVID-pandemic: A real-world study. *Frontiers in Public Health*, *10*, 1–9.

Treadway, M., & Lazar, S. (2009). The neurobiology of mindfulness. In F. Didonna (ed.), *Clinical handbook of mindfulness* (pp. 45–57). Springer.

Van Gelder, K. (2010). *The borderline and the Buddha: A memoir.* New Harbinger Publications.

Van Gordon, W., Sapthiang, S., Barrows, P., & Shonin, E. (2021). Understanding and practicing emptiness. *Mindfulness in Practice*, *12*, 1845–1848.

Williams, J., Gifford, W., Vanderspank-Wright, B., & Phillips, J. (2021). Violence and health promotion among First Nations, Métis, and Inuit women: A systematic review of qualitative research. *Trauma, Violence, and Abuse*, *22*(5), 996–1012.

Wilson, N., Robb, E., Gajwani, R., & Minnis, H. (2021). Nature and nurture? A review of the literature on childhood maltreatment and genetic factors in the pathogenesis of borderline personality disorder. *Journal of Psychiatry Research*, *137*, 131–146.

Winsper, C. (2018). The aetiology of borderline personality disorder (BPD): Contemporary theories and putative mechanisms. *Current Opinion in Psychiatry*, *21*, 105–110.

Zanarini, M. C. (2018). *In the fullness of time: Recovery from borderline personality disorder.* Oxford University Press.

Zanarini, M., & Frankenburg, F. (1994). Emotional hypochondriasis, hyperbole, and the borderline patient. *Journal of Psychotherapy Practice and Research*, *3*(1), 25–36.

20 Empathy Deficits in the Development and Maintenance of Narcissistic Personality Disorder

Thomas Schramme

In this chapter, I want to scrutinize an understanding of Narcissistic Personality Disorder (NPD) as involving different forms of empathy deficits. I will argue that because empathic processes function interactively and interpersonally, pertinent deficits are often not simply due to specific psychological traits of people affected by a disorder, but at least partly constituted in relation to other people. This potentially undermines the common diagnostic criterion of lack of empathy, because empathic deficits might be due to circumstantial impact. Empathy is foremost an epistemic mechanism, leading to different forms and levels of interpersonal understanding. I argue that interactive difficulties can result in profound interpersonal misunderstanding, which leaves some people in persistent doubt about other people's perspectives and also about their own social standing. Such status blindness, as I will call it, can explain some specific symptoms of NPD.

This chapter is written from the perspective of philosophy. More specifically, I make use of philosophical thinking about empathy. Philosophical reasoning is mainly theoretical and conceptual, although often empirically informed. My own argument bears some similarities with psychological theories, such as Heinz Kohut's account of NPD (Kohut, 1971), the interpersonal perspective on personality disorders (e.g., Hopwood et al., 2013; see also Wright, this edition), or relational psychoanalysis (e.g., Greenberg & Mitchell, 1983). I am not an expert in these theories and therefore, from a psychological point of view, some elements of my argument might seem naive and potentially ignorant. Nevertheless, I hope that my contribution will be interesting for any theorist interested in NPD, especially through the conceptual clarifications provided in relation to empathy.

I would like to contribute towards developing a more adequate clinical construction by discussing NPD as a pathology of empathy. Empathy impairments are commonly mentioned in relation to NPD, also in the DSM, as we will see shortly. However, it seems to me that the understanding of empathy in relevant clinical and psychological publications is insufficient. For instance, the DSM-5 describes "lack of empathy" in terms of being "unwilling to recognize or identify with the feelings and needs of others." This formulation throws together different elements, cognitive aspects of empathy ("recognizing"), affective aspects ("identifying with feelings"), and motivational aspects ("unwilling"). Given this confusing picture in the clinical and psychological discussion, my philosophical contribution accordingly lies in the conceptual clarification of a central diagnostic criterion of NPD. Such a need has been mentioned in the clinical and psychological literature as well (see, e.g., Cuff et al., 2016; Miller et al., 2021; Wright et al., 2021).

I will proceed by setting the context of my discussion in the first section. I will then introduce, in the second section, relevant conceptual distinctions regarding the notion of empathy. The analysis will help us to understand the complexity of the idea, especially the common confusion of epistemic and pro-social functions of empathy. In the third section I devise a complex map of empathy that describes four types and four features. I will apply the conceptual distinctions specifically to NPD in the fourth section. Here, I describe different ways in which NPD can be seen as involving empathy deficits. Finally, in the fifth section I zoom in on a specific impairment. Human beings are not just actively empathizing with other people, but they are also regularly the targets of the empathy of others. I argue that impartments in relation to this element of empathy are of particular interest when explaining NPD, because such issues lead to a form of ignorance about the esteem a person has in the eyes of others. I call the resultant psychological condition status blindness. The sixth section concludes.

20.1 The Context of Discussing Empathy Deficits in Relation to Narcissistic Personality Disorder

This chapter focuses on NPD, although my argument will hopefully also be useful when analyzing non-pathological versions of narcissism. Narcissistic Personality Disorder, the pathological version of narcissism, might be seen as an extreme version of narcissism or as a condition that has certain qualities that non-pathological versions of narcissism do not share. Many people would agree that personality characteristics fall on spectra of comparatively higher or lower degrees. A person might, for instance, show a much higher level of self-esteem than others, perhaps in combination with other altered levels of personality functioning. These alterations as such, however, do not give us sufficient reason to assume a personality disorder. We might accordingly settle on a certain threshold of excessively high self-esteem that is deemed grandiose, and grandiosity can then be used as a descriptor of NPD. In a word, even if we see a continuity between normal and pathological narcissism, for clinical purposes we will need to draw a line somewhere. This line-drawing problem constitutes the context of my contribution, although I will not be able to confidently draw the line myself. Rather, I see my contribution as making progress toward a better understanding of the issues in determining the boundaries of NPD in contrast to normal forms of narcissism.

The fifth edition of the *Diagnostic and statistical manual of mental disorder* (APA, 2013) describes the "essential feature" of NPD as "a pervasive pattern of grandiosity, need for admiration, and lack of empathy that begins by early adulthood and is present in a variety of contexts" (APA, 2013, 669f.). DSM-5 in addition lists nine diagnostic criteria, of which at least five need to be met for diagnostic purposes. In contrast, the "alternative model" in DSM-5 uses impairments in four different areas of personality functioning as diagnostic criteria of NPD. Elements of personality functioning are identity, self-direction, empathy, and intimacy (APA, 2013, p. 762). In terms of the area of identity, for instance, the relevant impairment is described as "excessive reference to others for self-definition" (APA, 2013, p. 767).

There is no need for us to go into the philosophical aspects and politics of different types of psychiatric classification (but see, e.g., Zachar, 2017; Miller et al., 2022). Some psychologists and psychiatrists adhere to a traditional categorical model, which supposedly carves out the specific conditions of pathological entities. Others support a more recent dimensional model, which sees pathology along scalar dimensions, albeit falling below a specific threshold of functioning. In the end, both models use very similar diagnostic criteria for NPD, despite the nosological disagreements. Dimensional and categorical models also agree on the general idea that specific psychological impairments underlie personality disorders. As mentioned before, dimensional models need to create diagnostic entities by drawing the line of functioning somewhere, so end up with psychiatric categories as well, not just spectra or scales.

Narcissism has been described by reference to psychological and behavioral features. An example of behavioral features is self-interested or even exploitative conduct towards others. In terms of psychological features, narcissism is often said to go along with high levels of self-esteem (Dawood et al., 2020, p. 280). It seems to me that we need to, right from the start, draw a clear distinction between psychological and behavioral features of narcissism. These are sometimes distinguished in terms of primary and secondary features. My point is also about the site of pathology, as it were. I understand the concept of mental disorder and accordingly of personality disorder to apply to psychological features. Certain behavior might be a sign or symptom of disorder but is not itself the site of disorder (Schramme, 2010). Accordingly, exploitative and other types of conduct that often go along with narcissistic traits are themselves not narcissistic; such conduct is the possible result of mental constellations of persons in interaction with others. Our conceptual focus, when discussing mental pathology, should therefore be on psychological traits and mechanisms. Resulting conduct can be important, of course, in terms of being symptomatic of psychological features of people, but I would argue that conduct is not the site of mental dysfunction. In other words, if apparent symptoms of NPD are maintained by circumstances or by other people, as opposed to being caused by psychological mechanisms internal to the affected person, then it is questionable whether the phenomena are actually pathological.

Commonly mentioned psychological characteristics of narcissism, such as grandiosity or self-centeredness, are intuitive; they seem to be in line with the folk concept of narcissism and with the experiences of experts (Ackerman et al., 2017). All of us know some people who show such traits and who we might have called narcissistic for these reasons. As long as the label is used for common purposes of succinct assessment and categorization of individuals, there does not seem to be much harm done. Admittedly, it might not be pleasurable to be deemed a narcissist by others, but neither do we like to be judged, say, a miser or a bore, and still not many really think that these labels are altogether harmful or never justified. Indeed, folk-psychological labels help us to get along in our lives, to quickly deal with people and our expectations toward them. Psychological labels also seem to be rather fleeting; someone who we judged to be narcissistic or boring might turn out to be quite moderate or interesting. However, the construct of narcissism is also used to introduce the clinical label of NPD. This changes the normative landscape and should make us specifically wary of the label of narcissism. After all, we do not assume, in analogy, the existence of a miserly personality disorder or a boring personality disorder.

Interestingly, the presence of relevant psychological traits in NPD is dependent on a person's relation to others. Grandiosity, for instance, is partly determined by other people's assessment. They deem a narcissistic person's psychological self-assessment as grandiose, that is, as potentially inadequate. Still, the narcissistic trait also seems to be internal to a person in that she deems herself better in a specific respect and in relation to others. Another commonly mentioned characteristic is entitlement (Krizan & Herlache, 2018), which refers to an attitude toward others. Again, it is not simply the internal, psychological condition of a person that supports the application of the NPD label in these cases. Rather, entitlement is a condition that is only explainable in relation to an attitude of a person toward others. In brief, it is a relational attitude. Entitlement is a psychological stance of assumed elevated status, often including assumptions about special claims in relation to others. Altogether it is a form of presumption or hubris. This attitude seems inadequate from the point of view of others. So, narcissism is at least partly constructed in reference to relational psychological traits and determined by assessment via social norms.

Of course, this value-laden aspect does not by itself make the construct inadequate or non-medical (Banicki, 2019; cf. Charland, 2006).

20.2 Empathy and Sympathy in Philosophy

As many know, the term *empathy* was only introduced at the beginning of the twentieth century. Before, the term *sympathy* had been used to pick out very similar phenomena. In consequence, some of the undertones that the concept of sympathy used to have are now merged with the concept of empathy. It is not possible to come up with authoritative definitions for either term, which would state necessary and sufficient conditions. Some level of stipulation is unavoidable. Still, it is important to keep different elements separate (Wispé, 1986), as the exact functions of empathy and sympathy have often been misunderstood.

Numerous authors have highlighted that empathy has a "sympathetic component" (Hoffman, 2011, 234f.) or that there are versions of a "proto-sympathetic empathy" (Darwall, 1998, 271f.). The psychologist Dan Batson refers to *empathic concern*, a notion that others might prefer to call *sympathy* (Batson, 2011, 11ff.; cf. Maibom, 2020, p. 61). In modern moral psychology – a branch of philosophy that is empirically informed – it is commonly stipulated that the concept of sympathy refers to the capacity (and the performance of this capacity – the psychological mechanism) of *feeling for* another being (Maibom, 2020, 60ff.). Sympathy is hence usually interpreted as a kind of moral or pro-social concern for others. This is a specific modern reading of the term (Mercer, 1972, p. 19). Historical authors, such as David Hume and Adam Smith, did not readily include moral elements in their theories of sympathy. Accordingly, their notion of sympathy is said to pick out the modern notion of empathy (see, e.g., Fleischacker, 2019, 3ff.). Empathy is not, as such, a moral concept. Rather, it is an epistemological notion, because it primarily addresses a mechanism of understanding mental phenomena experienced by another person.

The modern notion of empathy accordingly picks out mechanisms of interpersonal knowledge acquisition and understanding. There can be different relevant mechanisms. For instance, empathy is often understood in terms of *feeling as* another being. This can be a mirrored feeling or a vicarious feeling that we feel on behalf of someone else. Because this type of empathy implies some kind of feeling in the empathizing person, it is usually called affective empathy or emotional empathy (Maibom, 2014, 3f.). Yet the concept of empathy can additionally refer to an intellectual understanding or grasping of the mental state of another person, be it an emotional or cognitive state of the target. This is usually called perspective-taking, or cognitive empathy (Spaulding, 2017). The latter phenomenon clearly does not imply any concern for others and – in fact, in the case of con artists or sadists – can be effectively used for anti-social personal aims. Whether affective empathy involves concern is open for debate.

The epistemic stance of empathy does, however, promote some form of acknowledgment of others. *Acknowledgment* is not meant as a form of full-fledged recognition of the moral status of others, but rather as some kind of epistemic insight about the other. Once we do (and occasionally fail to) understand others, we cannot escape noticing their perspective. If we would not acknowledge others as centers of subjectivity at all, it would be difficult to account for our occasional – although of course not guaranteed – interest in their welfare. Indeed, without our ability to understand others we could not even care whether others sympathize with our point of view; we would be incapable of feeling the sting of their disagreement and the pleasure of their fellow feeling. In that case, the lack of understanding or disagreement of others would not represent another person's point of view, but would rather be like a material resistance that is either to be overcome or succumbed to. In other words, an epistemically purely self-oriented perspective cannot lead to sympathetic concern. In contrast, epistemic empathy – acknowledging others as subjects – seems to naturally lead to such concern. "It is our ability to enter into the interests and feelings of other people which provides the source of morality" (Wright, 2009, p. 288). So, moral concern might well be a developmental outcome of empathy and other contributory factors, but empathy itself is an epistemic instrument for interpersonal understanding.

In summary, empathy facilitates epistemic access to other minds – a form of understanding – and it enables alignment of mental states – a form of adjustment of perspectives. Empathy, if successful in the sense of resulting in shared mental states, is usually pleasurable to the empathizer and the target. It is both an unconscious and a conscious mechanism, sometimes working effortlessly, sometimes requiring effortful and deliberate feeling-into another person. Empathy can be honed and cultivated like other skills. It is accordingly not developed by purely affective processes, rather its cultivation "involves reflective judgement" (Taylor, 2015, pp. 194, 199). The latter implies cognitive mechanisms, for instance emotion regulation and control. Finally, and importantly, empathy is itself not a form of concern or moral sentiment, although it plays a role in enabling and determining moral capacities.

20.3 A Conceptual Map of Empathy

Empathy is not something that we simply have or show. Rather, it is a skillful process, a type of performance. It really is, as the German origin of the term (*Einfühlung*) suggests, a process of feeling into another person. As such, empathy needs to be developed, trained, and honed. It also requires adequate conditions. Fairly often, successful empathy relies on interaction with others.

Table 20.1 *A map of empathy*

Type \ Feature	Capacity	Process	Hindrance	Effect
Basic	Perceiving	Recognizing behavioral expressions	Insufficient experience; limited social cues	Acknowledging mindedness; minimal understanding
Affective	Feeling	Interactive aligning	Affective resistance; emotion dysregulation	Shared or vicarious emotion; affective understanding
Cognitive	Ascribing mental states	Perspective-taking	Cognitive resistance; poor imagination; restricted interactive engagement	Representation of other's condition; cognitive understanding;
Concern	Relating to others; valuing	Acknowledging well-being of others	External pressure; moral beliefs; distraction	Fellow-feeling

It then builds on a joint performance, which can obviously go wrong in many ways. Accordingly, empathy is often laborious, and its success depends on the quality of interpersonal relationship we have with others.

On a more theoretical level, I argue that in addition to distinguishing types of empathy, we need to delineate different aspects of empathy. In this section, I will accordingly suggest a complex map of the landscape of empathy (Table 20.1). I distinguish four types of empathy, adding to the complexity introduced in the previous section: (1) basic empathy, (2) affective empathy, (3) cognitive empathy, and (4) empathic concern. These types can be described by referring to different features, namely (i) capacities or (ii) processes, which can be (iii) affected by hindrances, and which will (iv) result in specific effects. Altogether, my map of empathy is hence a four-by-four matrix. I believe that such a complex picture will help us to improve hypotheses and eventually empirical research regarding the specific empathy deficits of people with NPD.

In the context of psychological research on NPD, we find relatively little detailed conceptual work on empathy (cf. Baskin-Sommers et al., 2014; Urbonaviciute et al., 2020). To be sure, the common distinction between cognitive and affective empathy is usually mentioned (Ritter et al., 2011; Blötner et al., 2021) and there are occasional nods toward acknowledging the differences between empathy and sympathy (see, e.g., Eisenberg, 2018). But there are also more indiscriminate claims about the alleged lack of empathy or empathy deficits in people with NPD (cf. Morey & Stagner, 2012, p. 912). These generalizations are due, it seems to me, to a too broadbrush approach to the nature of empathy (see also Hart et al., 2018). Distinctions are required not merely in terms of types of empathy, but also in terms of capacities involved, their performance, including possible hindrances, and as regards effects of empathy.

What is more, some of the alleged empathic deficits of patients with NPD might be due to a breakdown of interpersonal empathy in relation to them. We – relatives, friends, therapists, etc. of people with NPD – might be the ones who cannot fully empathize with these patients, because we fail to fully understand their attitudes and behavior. Empathy requires interaction between people (Vreekea & van der Mark, 2003; Betzler, 2019). If this interaction breaks down, it might not be due to specific personality traits of people, that is, their persistent psychological dispositions, but to circumstantial limitations in the interactive process of empathy, which undermine its functionality.

In view of that assumption, a person might be fully capable of feeling what another person feels, but they might struggle to perform the relevant psychological mechanisms, for instance due to so-called affective resistance. In cases of affective resistance, people struggle to understand another person's perspective due to normative disagreement, which results in problems to empathically align their own perspective with that of a target, that is, to feel into the other. We probably all have experienced such impaired performance of empathic mechanisms in our lives. Say, a colleague is very upset because they have failed at performing an insignificant task. We might struggle, in such a scenario, to really empathize with the colleague, because we feel that the colleague's emotion is way over the top, given the triviality of the performance within the grand scheme of work. In such a case, breakdown of empathy is probably due to the fact that we cannot easily align our own perspective to the colleague's and hence cannot share their feeling. This failure of empathy is not due to any lack of capacity but to the contextual circumstances. The example illustrates one of the numerous complexities of empathic processes, which overall put into doubt sweeping generalizations regarding lack of empathy (cf. Hart et al., 2018).

Empathy is usually not simply the result of a single interpersonal encounter. Rather, we often empathize with people we meet regularly. The level of personal relationship has impact on the context of the process of empathy. For instance, as regards the case mentioned in the previous paragraph, we might have previous knowledge about the colleague and their ambitions. Perhaps the task was something they set themselves as a challenge, or it was something their brother, who they shared a competitive relationship with for decades, was particularly good at. Knowledge of such facts can help us to empathize. More importantly, empathy can be developed in interaction or a series of encounters. The colleague might explain to us why they are so upset, and we might accordingly start affectively aligning with their feeling of failure. Empathic processes, in a word, are interactive and intertemporal phenomena. Only if these processes succeed will we reach adequate outcomes. This insight would need to be reflected when discussing empathic deficits in relation to NPD.

20.4 Empathic Impairments in Narcissistic Personality Disorder

In the following paragraphs, I will describe features of narcissism in relation to the map of empathy introduced in the previous section. My primary aim is not to identify specific traits that would qualify as diagnostic criteria of NPD. Rather, I want to show that empathy deficits in NPD can be due to multiple causes, including interactive failures and, importantly, deficits in other than narcissistic people. As I have said earlier, I would argue that pathological traits are forms of impaired psychological mechanisms, that is, mental dysfunctions. Therefore, I argue that some of the alleged symptoms of NPD to do with empathy failures are not actually due to pathological mechanisms.

(1) Basic empathy. A basic form of empathy is involved in the perception of other people's expressions. To be sure, basic empathy has not always been discussed under this label, other descriptors used are, for instance, "direct social cognition" (Walsh, 2014, p. 215) or "direct social perception" (Michael & de Bruin, 2015). However, it seems adequate to refer to empathy for describing the relevant processes (Zahavi, 2011) and in the history of philosophy the phenomena have indeed often been discussed under this rubric (see, e.g., Stein, 1964). We can occasionally "see" other people's anger or joy, especially in facial expressions. *Seeing* is here put in scare quotes, because there are more background capacities and knowledge involved than in simple perception when we realize the mental states of others in their expressions. Empathic perception has accordingly been called "smart" (Gallagher, 2008, p. 536). The relevant performance consists of the realization and interpretation of other person's expressions. Such a process can be disturbed by external and internal hindrances. For instance, in specific contexts our access to social cues is restricted. Seeing someone online can preclude knowledge of their body posture, which might deny us important information about their affective state. In terms of our own restrictions, we might have only limited experience with cultural impregnations of specific expressions and hence misread the mental states of others.

If everything goes right, we will achieve a minimal form of understanding of the perspective of another person via this process, especially about their currently experienced basic emotions, such as happiness or fear (Ekman, 1992). Importantly, empathizers will also normally acknowledge the other person, whose expressions they perceive, as a minded creature. Otherwise they would struggle to see the perceived behavior and movements of others as expressive. In other words, empathizers recognize that other persons' expressions stem from conscious experiences.

In general, basic empathy does not seem to be connected to specific symptoms of NPD. The effects of basic empathy are mainly due to internal capacities of empathizers, so in cases where persons consistently struggle to acknowledge the mindedness of others and fail to recognize their behavioral expressions, we can justifiably assume that this is due to a pathological psychological trait. But such pathologies do not seem to be specific to NPD.

(2) Affective empathy. Although there is no widely accepted definition of affective empathy, theorists and researchers usually agree that affective empathy involves a felt experience of the empathizer as a result of the experience of others (Maibom, 2017; Sodoma, 2022). For instance, an empathizer might feel sad due to the sadness of their friend. The fact that others' experiences are the target of affective empathy requires certain cognitive features, such as a conscious acknowledgment of the source of affect. In other words, there needs to be a clear self-other differentiation. Hence, affective empathy is not purely affective, and should in fact be distinguished from emotional contagion (Coplan, 2011, 15ff.). It is contested how much the change in affect needs to be in alignment with the target's affect. Some speak of a shared specific affect, which seems to imply a close association with the target, others only refer to the same valence (positive or negative) of the affect in empathizer and target (Hoffman, 2000, 29ff.; Schwan, 2019). There is also the problem that we seem to be able to affectively empathize with people who do not themselves experience relevant affects, for instance when a target of our vicariously felt anger is oblivious to a slight by another person. So, we can generate feelings on behalf of someone else or, to use a technical term, vicariously.

A required capacity for experiencing affective empathy is the capacity to experience affect and emotions in oneself. A person who struggles with feeling and identifying emotions in themselves will also have difficulties to feel and identify affect and emotions in others. This is one of the reasons as to why alexithymia, a form of emotional blindness where patients are less capable to identify and describe emotions, is researched in relation to empathy deficits (Adshead, 2014). However, possessing the capacity for affective empathy does not guarantee success. After all, the emotions of others need to be recognizable. If a target hides their affect or presents it in a misleading way, aligning one's own affect with theirs will become harder. As we have seen before, empathic processes are usually maintained in an interaction over time. This implies that sometimes the target of empathy can undermine the achievement of empathy's usual effects.

Aligning emotions with a target can also be hindered by affective resistance in empathizers. If they do not at least minimally endorse the adequacy of the target's affect, they will struggle, at least initially, to affectively empathize.

In this respect, sometimes lack of affective empathy can be due to other than impaired psychological mechanisms, more specifically to profound evaluative differences between empathizer and target.

Another problem, more to do with the required self–other distinction, is the potential misalignment of affective states between empathizer and target due to emotion dysregulation. If someone is overwhelmed by their own emotions, they will struggle to align them to others. For instance, if a person is fully immersed in their own grief, they will not easily feel empathic joy for someone else. Narcissists seem to be similarly restricted to their own experiences to a degree that makes it hard for them to connect with others. This struggle might not be due to incapacity for affective empathy but rather to a form of emotion dysregulation in the process of aligning one's own affect with targets.

If all goes well, however, the successful outcome is some level of affective alignment between empathizer and target. We can perhaps call this affective understanding, corresponding to the minimal understanding mentioned before. Affective empathy also seems to deepen the mainly epistemic recognition that goes along with basic empathy. It results in a form of nascent interpersonal relationship with the target person, not just an acknowledgment as a minded creature.

Affective empathy deficits seem particularly relevant for explaining behavioral symptoms of NPD, specifically anti-social conduct (Ritter et al., 2011, p. 245; but see Lishner et al., 2015). This is because aligning affect between persons is relevant for building rapport and eventually moral respect between persons. Affective states are especially significant for motivating behavior. For instance, realizing the pain of others that is caused by our conduct usually leads to changes in our attitude. If we, however, fail to align our own affect to the other person's affect, we might stay oblivious to their needs. It would be important to further clarify whether the mentioned behavioral effects of impairments in the process of affective empathy are due to primary, psychological traits of narcissism and therefore potentially pathological.

(3) Cognitive empathy. The most theorized and researched type of empathy is cognitive empathy. It is sometimes discussed under the rubrics of mind-reading or perspective-taking. Cognitive empathy has also been at the forefront of philosophical debate for some time, because the human capacity to gain knowledge about psychological processes of others is relevant in human agency. For instance, to predict the behavior of others and accordingly adapt to it, we require relatively detailed access to other people's minds, not simply via the relatively simple interpretations of perceivable expressions, as theorized earlier. However, how we access other minds is actually a major philosophical problem, given that the mind of others is not understandable by usual means of knowledge generation, such as observing or measuring. Cognitive empathy appears to be the solution to this problem. Indeed, in philosophy and cognitive

science we even find assumptions about a natural mental module, a genetic trait of a human Theory of Mind (cf. Gerrans, 2002).

One of the main capacities involved in cognitive empathy is therefore the ability to adequately ascribe mental states to others. These psychological conditions of others can themselves be affective or cognitive states, for instance that they are jealous or that they believe that there is beer in the fridge. Importantly, empathizers going through the relevant process do not themselves feel anything in relation to their target. Rather, they imaginatively take the point of view of other persons and consciously represent the others' perspectives in their own mind. This can be a laborious process, but it can also be fairly straightforward, especially if an empathizer is immersed in a situation or if they have had very similar experiences. The process again involves the target's input, for instance a form of communication and a general preparedness to being understood. The latter can occasionally require modifications of a target's expressions. If everything goes well, cognitive empathy will result in a sufficiently accurate representation of the perspective of another person. Again, in line with the previous terminology, we can call this a form of understanding, as it is first and foremost leading to knowledge about other minds.

Cognitive empathy can fail if empathizers have a very poor imagination. After all, they need to take the perspective of someone else, and the perspective might be hard for them to decipher. The empathic process can also end without success if there is no sufficient interaction between empathizer and target. It is easy to misread the mental states of others in cases where an empathizer has very little clues to work with. The process of cognitively empathizing can finally go awry if there is a form of cognitive resistance, similarly to the previous example if an empathizer does not agree with the assumed perspective of the target.

In general, narcissists do not seem to struggle to an unusual degree with cognitive empathy. They seem to be usually capable of forming adequate beliefs about others' perspectives and their mental states. Occasional difficulties seem to be due to environmental and interactive hindrances in achieving the relevant effect of gaining a sufficiently adequate representation of another person's perspective. This is a normal situation everyone is facing and does not point at specific pathological traits in NPD.

(4) Empathic concern. I will discuss empathic concern, that is, an acknowledgment of the significance of others, as a type of empathy, although this is contested, as we have seen before. Empathy and full-blown sympathy are different phenomena. However, some kind of concern for the other seems to be part and parcel of real-life empathic processes and it can therefore be characterized as an additional, theoretically distinguished, type of empathy (cf. Bailey, 2022). Empathic concern is targeted at others and their perspective. Another person can of course also be of concern to an agent in an instrumental

way, for instance when they are seen as competitors. However, empathic concern is based on the capacity to relate to others in some way, not simply to perceive them as relevant to one's own concern. The pertinent process consists of an acknowledgment of the normative significance of others and their perspectives. This acknowledgment as such does not guarantee pro-social behavior. Indeed, a lot can go wrong in the process of developing a pro-social disposition, which is the outcome of successfully relating to others. For instance, external pressure not to acknowledge others, maintained through social sanctions or cultural beliefs, but also one's own personal moral beliefs, can prevent the occurrence of empathic concern. Simple distraction has also been shown to undermine empathic concern, up to a point where philosophers started doubting the existence of any relevant persistent pro-social traits in humans (see, e.g., Doris, 2002).

In the context of NPD, it seems important to stress that it has occasionally been alleged that patients are unwilling to show empathic concern, as opposed to being unable to empathize (Hepper et al., 2014). As mentioned earlier, according to the current description in the DSM, a person suffering from NPD lacks empathy when they are "unwilling to recognize or identify with the feelings and needs of others" (APA, 2013, p. 670). But there is no information about the possible motivating reasons of such an alleged unwillingness. From a philosophical point of view, these reasons are most important, because they allow us to assess the relevant failure of showing empathic concern from a moral point of view. In a nutshell, the motivating reasons let us decide whether someone is evil or ill (Reznek, 1997). Again, the interactive nature of empathy is relevant here. It seems straightforward to assume that people usually show empathic concern toward people that have shown empathic concern towards them. In other words, empathic concern is often a reciprocal attitude. If someone with NPD is not empathized with by others or struggles to subjectively feel any empathic concern by others, then they will themselves be less motivated to show empathic concern. Indeed, this seems like a fully reasonable and normal reaction within a context of interactive empathic failures. The motivating reasons for such unwillingness are hence decisive for using empathic failures as a descriptor of pathology. To diagnose unwillingness to show empathic concern, as opposed to a lack of the capacity, is only the first step, but not itself sufficient, to adequately theorize the situation of people with NPD. This does not mean, of course, that the unwillingness to recognize or identify with the feelings and needs of others cannot be a sign of pathology, after all. But nevertheless, the fact of unsuccessful empathy as such does not qualify as a diagnostic criterion of NPD.

The experience that the other creature is a person, someone with a subjective point of view, usually involves a form of basic recognition. In the history of philosophy this has been described as a fellow-feeling; a recognition that the other is a fellow being (Smith, 2002, 12ff.). If someone does not develop this attitude of fellow-feeling toward others, anti-social behavior might be a pertinent outcome, because other human beings are then perceived like objects, as opposed to subjects who have normative significance in their own right.

In clinical psychological literature, the apparent anti-social traits of NPD are occasionally compared to anti-social personality disorder or psychopathy (cf. Zachar, 2014, 181ff.). Relatedly, narcissism is regarded as a one of the "dark triad" of personality types. It seems that specific deficits of NPD are explainable in terms of problems with empathic concern. Not to see another person as a minded creature but rather as a kind of object obviously will have an impact on social behavior. Apparently, NPD patients struggle to perceive the mindedness and significance of others. Partly, this impairment might be explainable through impairments of the other types of empathy. Indeed, there is some empirical evidence that narcissists are performing significantly worse in perceptual empathy tasks (Marissen et al., 2012). This underlines the fact that the types of empathy I have distinguished for systematic reasons will often be connected in reality. Empathic concern is indeed a complex phenomenon.

In this section I have laid out numerous distinctions as regard types of empathy, as well as their respective capacities, performances, possible hindrances, and effects. It has become clear that it is inadequate to generally refer to a lack of empathy in relation to NPD. We have seen that the different types of empathy require skillful performance. That is, they can be developed and honed. They also require the absence of certain hindrances to be successfully performed, that is, to fulfill their functions. Hindrances can be constituted by internal psychological deficits, which themselves have nothing directly to do with empathy, and external circumstances, including the conduct of other people. So, whether a person presents with empathy deficits is not necessarily due to psychopathological traits. Therefore, lack of empathy as such should not be used as a diagnostic criterion of NPD. Finally, it has been established that empathic processes are epistemic vehicles that help us to understand others and accordingly to adapt our behavior. This is, as such, not a moral or pro-social function of empathy. However, empathy usually comes with normative baggage, as it were. To empathize with others normally leads to a form of minimal recognition and pro-social dispositions, especially when they are reciprocated (cf. Jacobs, 2022). These attitudes do not build a full-blown moral stance, but they are developmental psychological foundations of human moral capacities (Schramme, 2017).

20.5 Being the Target of Empathy

In this final section, I want to look more closely at characteristics of being the target of others' empathy. In the literature on NPD, deficits of patients in their performance of empathy towards others are usually analyzed and researched, but not their problems in being the target of empathy. However, to develop one's own empathic skills seems to require that a person is at least occasionally the target of others' empathy. As social creatures we learn skills, at least partly, from others. For instance, the skill to read facial expressions correctly partly relies on our own expressions being successfully read by others. Otherwise, we would find it hard to personally experience the benefits of the mechanism as such and to develop the elaborate know-how required. To feel into another person and to align one's affect with them accordingly builds on personal experience of other people resonating with one's own feelings. What is more, to show concern for others requires confidence in others to show such concern toward oneself. In a word, being an empathic agent requires successful experience of being an empathic patient – where patiency is not a medical term, of course, but refers to being at the receiving end of others' agency (Reader, 2007).

If we now consider the situation of narcissists, we might wonder whether they can reliably experience such empathic patiency. After all, many features of their condition seem to undermine the maintenance of personal relationships and altogether make affected persons less likeable to others. When we describe NPD as a form of interactive empathy deficit – a kind of broken communication – we will notice the potential impact of others on the development of relevant symptoms. Similar ideas have been explored in relation to interactions between autistic and neurotypical people, and the relevant mechanism has interestingly been described as a "double empathy problem" (Milton, 2012; Mitchell et al., 2021).

Consider empathic failures due to affective or cognitive resistance. Say, if a narcissistic target of empathy seems to believe that they are well liked by others, but an empathizer has experienced numerous occasions of negative attitudes toward them, the empathizer might struggle to actually agree with the perspective of the target and therefore struggle to empathize with and eventually understand the attitude of the narcissist. This lack of understanding impacts on the targets of empathy, because they effectively do not receive sufficient signals by empathizers to understand their own social status.

Indeed, if we take a developmental point of view, we can also see how apparent psychological traits can be determined and maintained via recurrent interactive empathy failures. As we have seen, people with NPD often feel that they are more important than others, that they have earned constant admiration by others. They also seem to belittle the achievements of others in relation to their own successes. Occasionally, they even do all this contrary to facts, which are known to them, and despite explicit criticism by others. Once we deem narcissism an interactive condition, however, we can theorize that such apparent entitlement might be due to insufficient understanding of the real status of oneself and of others. As we have seen, empathic processes are epistemic vehicles to check the assessment of oneself by others and to align one's own assessment of others to theirs. In brief, empathic disruptions can lead to a kind of status blindness. People in such a condition will often fail to reliably know what level of respect they need to show others and what level of respect others owe to themselves, simply because they do not have sufficient understanding of others' perspectives. Accordingly, it seems inadequate to generally assume an exaggerated sense of superiority in NPD patients (cf. Zachar, 2006, p. 94). Rather, epistemic deficits in interpersonal interaction can lead to attitudes that are deemed inadequate and presumptuous by others.

Personal self-esteem is not simply a personal psychological trait. It is negotiated in relationships and joint interaction. This was already an insight of Hume (1978, 275ff.). Empathic processes play an important role in this negotiation, because they enable adequate understanding of other people's perspectives, including their relational value judgments. Such understanding is vital to build adequate self-esteem, that is, an estimate of one's social status relative to the assessment of others. A certain level of self-love and self-esteem is important to build relationships and to live a confident, self-determined life (cf. Frankfurt, 2000; Isserow, 2023). It should therefore be obvious that the epistemic roots of empathy have normative significance as well.

The fact that human beings rely on others' empathic responses additionally enables an important theoretical insight regarding the difference between vulnerable and grandiose versions of NPD, which is often highlighted in the psychological literature (Campbell & Miller, 2013; Pincus et al., 2015; Miller et al., 2017). A vulnerable version of NPD is often described as being based on low self-esteem, which is masked by specific symptoms. Alternatively, people with NPD might be deemed of the grandiose form, where patients have an unrealistically high level of self-esteem. However, given the analysis presented in this chapter, it seems more plausible to explain both types as being based on interactive empathy deficits and the subsequent status blindness. I would speculate that such status blindless, a persistent incapacity to successfully assess one's relation to others, is a relevant symptom of NPD that stems from defective psychological mechanisms.

Such deficits may lead to difficulties in developing positive self-esteem, due to the dearth of felt ego boosts by others, or, contrariwise, to the development of a kind of unfettered self-esteem, due to the scarcity of subjectively experienced threats to one's own ego. In both cases, patients experience a lack of orientation and subsequently an increased reliance on their own self-assessment, which lacks calibration with others. If a person with NPD does not gain the relevant information, support, and concern from others, then they end up in solipsistic extremes of very low or very high self-esteem. Their self appears inflated or deflated only relative to the assessment by others. Others' perspectives, however, are not sufficiently accessible to patients with NPD, and so they are in a “chronic state of self-under-construction” (Morf & Rhodewalt, 2001, p. 178), stuck in “primitive” self-regulatory mechanisms (Roche et al., 2013, 238ff.) and reliant on their “core beliefs” (Brummelman et al., 2018). Vulnerability, according to this perspective, is interpreted as a general feature of all human beings in relation to others’ empathic attitudes. It points toward the human relational need for recognition. Both grandiose and vulnerable NPD can be interpreted as versions of a status blindness that results from failures in interactive empathic processes due to mental incapacities.

20.6 Conclusion

I have argued that NPD can be explained as a pathology affecting empathic processes. Which psychological traits are relevant for the diagnosis of NPD is still an open question, and we should not loosely refer to any “lack of empathy,” because empathy failures are complex and can be due to many causes. I aimed to show that the relevant deficits result in impaired interpersonal understanding. Impaired understanding undermines interpersonal feedback mechanisms, and these issues eventually lead to insecurity regarding a person’s standing in the eyes of others – a situation I have called status blindness. Misunderstanding others can happen because of difficulties actively empathizing (not “getting” the other) or in being the target of empathy (missing out on feedback). In terms of behavioral consequences, these epistemic deficits can lead to difficulties in acknowledging the normative relevance of other people’s perspectives, including their interests and needs. From my point of view, impaired concern does not indicate moral failure but is evidence of difficulties in understanding others and being understood by others.

Acknowledgments: I would like to thank my Philosophy Master’s students at the University of Liverpool and the editors of this collection for helpful feedback. Work on this paper was supported by an AHRC-funded project on “How Does it Feel? Interpersonal Understanding and Affective Empathy” (AH/T012781/1).

References

Ackerman, R. A., Hands, A. J., Donnellan, M. B.t, Hopwood, C. J., & Witt, E. A. (2017). Experts’ views regarding the conceptualization of narcissism. *Journal of Personality Disorders*, *31*(3), 346–361.

Adshead, G. (2014). The words but not the music: Empathy, language deficits, and psychopathy. In T. Schramme (ed.), *Being amoral* (pp. 115–136). MIT Press.

American Psychiatric Association (APA). (2013). *Diagnostic and statistical manual of mental disorders* [DSM-5] (5th ed.). American Psychiatric Association.

Bailey, O. (2022). Empathy and the value of humane understanding. *Philosophy and Phenomenological Research, 104*(1), 50–65.

Banicki, K. (2019). From personality disorders to the fact-value distinction. *Philosophical Psychology, 32*(2), 274–298.

Baskin-Sommers, A., Ronningstam, E., & Krusemark, E. (2014). Empathy in narcissistic personality disorder: From clinical and empirical perspectives. *Personality Disorders, 5*(3), 323–333.

Batson, C. D. (2011). *Altruism in humans*. Oxford University Press.

Betzler, M. (2019). The relational value of empathy. *International Journal of Philosophical Studies, 27*(2), 136–161.

Blötner, C., Steinmayr, R., & Bergold, S. (2021). Malicious mind readers? A meta-analysis on Machiavellianism and cognitive and affective empathy. *Personality and Individual Differences, 181*, 111023.

Brummelman, E., Gürel, C., Thomaes, S., & Sedikides, C. (2018). What separates narcissism from self-esteem? A social-cognitive perspective. In: A. D. Hermann, A. B. Brunell, & J. D. Foster (eds.), *Handbook of trait narcissism: Key advances, research methods, and controversies* (pp. 47–55). Springer.

Campbell, W. K., & Miller, J. D. (2013). Narcissistic personality disorder and the five-factor model: Delineating narcissistic personality disorder, grandiose narcissism, and vulnerable narcissism. In T. A. Widiger & P. T. Costa, Jr. (eds.), *Personality disorders and the five-factor model of personality* (pp. 133–145). American Psychological Association.

Charland, L. C. (2006). Moral nature of the DSM-IV cluster B personality disorders. *Journal of Personality Disorders, 20*(2), 116–125.

Coplan, A. (2011). Understanding empathy: Its features and effects. In A. Coplan & P. Goldie (eds.), *Empathy: Philosophical and psychological perspectives* (pp. 3–18.) Oxford University Press.

Cuff, B. M. P., Brown, S. J., Taylor, L., & Howat, D. J. (2016). Empathy: A review of the concept. *Emotion Review, 8*(2), 144–153.

Darwall, S. (1998). Empathy, sympathy, care. *Philosophical Studies, 89*, 261–282.

Dawood, S., Wu, L., Bliton, C., & Pincus, A. (2020). Narcissistic and histrionic personality disorders. In C. Lejuez & K. Gratz (eds.), *The Cambridge handbook of personality disorders* (pp. 277–291). Cambridge University Press.

Doris, J. M. (2002). *Lack of character: Personality and moral behavior*. Cambridge University Press.

Eisenberg, N. (2018). Empathy-related responding and its relations to positive development. In N. Roughley & T. Schramme (eds.), *Forms of fellow feeling: Empathy, sympathy, concern and moral agency* (pp. 165–183). Cambridge University Press.

Ekman, P. (1992). An argument for basic emotions. *Cognition & Emotion*, 6(3–4), 169–200.

Fleischacker, S. (2019). *Being me being you: Adam Smith & empathy*. University of Chicago Press.

Frankfurt, H. (2000). The dear self. *Philosophers' Imprint, 1*, 1–14.

Gallagher, S. (2008). Direct perception in the intersubjective context. *Consciousness and Cognition, 17*, 535–543.

Gerrans, P. (2002). The theory of mind module in evolutionary psychology. *Biology & Philosophy, 17*, 305–321.

Greenberg, J., & Mitchell, S. (1983). *Object relations in psychoanalytic theory*. Harvard University Press.

Hart, C. M., Hepper, E. G., & Sedikides, C. (2018). Understanding and mitigating narcissists' low empathy. In: A. D. Hermann, A. B. Brunell, & J. D. Foster (eds.), *Handbook of trait narcissism: Key advances, research methods, and controversies* (pp. 335–343). Springer.

Hepper, E. G., Hart, C. M., & Sedikides, C. (2014). Moving Narcissus: Can narcissists be empathic? *Personality and Social Psychology Bulletin, 40*(9), 1079–1091.

Hoffman, M. L. (2000). *Empathy and moral development: Implications for caring and justice*. Cambridge University Press.

Hoffman, M. L. (2011). Empathy, justice, and the law. In. A. Coplan & P. Goldie (eds.), *Empathy: Philosophical and psychological perspectives* (pp. 230–254). Oxford University Press.

Hopwood, C. J., Wright, A. G. C., Ansell, E. B., & Pincus, A. L. (2013). The interpersonal core of personality pathology. *Journal of Personality Disorders, 27*(3), 270–295.

Hume, D. (1978, orig. 1739–40). *A treatise of human nature*, edited by L. A. Selby-Bigge. Clarendon Press.

Isserow, J. (2023). Self-esteem: On the form of self-worth worth having. *Pacific Philosophical Quarterly, 104*, 686–719.

Jacobs, K. A. (2022). The concept of Narcissistic Personality Disorder – Three levels of analysis for interdisciplinary integration. *Frontiers in Psychiatry, 13*, 989171.

Kohut, H. (1971). *The analysis of the self: A systematic approach to the psychoanalytic treatment of narcissistic personality disorder*. The University of Chicago Press.

Krizan, Z., & Herlache, A. D. (2018). The narcissism spectrum model: A synthetic view of narcissistic personality. *Personality and Social Psychology Review, 22*(1), 3–31.

Lishner, D. A., Hong, P. Y., Jiang, L., Vitacco, M. J., & Neumann, C. S. (2015). Psychopathy, narcissism, and borderline personality: A critical test of the affective empathy-impairment hypothesis. *Personality and Individual Differences, 86*, 257–265.

Maibom, H. L. (2014). Introduction: (Almost) everything you ever wanted to know about empathy (pp. 1–40). In: H. Maibom (ed.), *Empathy and morality*. Oxford University Press.

Maibom, H. L. (2017). Affective empathy. In H. Maibom (ed.), *The Routledge handbook of philosophy of empathy* (pp. 22–32). Routledge.

Maibom, H. L. (2020). *Empathy*. Routledge.

Marissen, M. A. E., Deen, M. L., & Franken, I. H. A. (2012). Disturbed emotion recognition in patients with narcissistic personality disorder. *Psychiatry Research, 198*(2), 269–273.

Mercer, P. (1972). *Sympathy and ethics: A study of the relationship between sympathy and morality with special reference to Hume's treatise*. Clarendon Press.

Michael, J., & De Bruin, L. (2015). How direct is social perception? *Consciousness and Cognition, 36*, 373–375.

Miller, J. D., Lynam, D. R., Hyatt, C. S., & Campbell, W. K. (2017). Controversies in narcissism. *Annual Review of Clinical Psychology, 13*(1), 291–315.

Miller, J. D., Back, M. D., Lynam, D. R., & Wright, A. G. C. (2021). Narcissism today: What we know and what we need to learn. *Current Directions in Psychological Science*, *30*(6), 519–525.

Miller, J. D., Crowe, M. L., & Sharpe, B.M. (2022). Narcissism and the DSM-5 alternative model of personality disorder. *Personality Disorders: Theory, Research, and Treatment*, *13*(4), 407–411.

Milton, D. E. (2012). On the ontological status of autism: The 'double empathy problem'. *Disability & Society*, *27*, 883–887.

Mitchell, P., Sheppard, E., & Cassidy, S. (2021). Autism and the double empathy problem: Implications for development and mental health. *British Journal of Developmental Psychology*, *39*, 1–18.

Morey, L. C., & Stagner, B. H. (2012). Narcissistic pathology as core personality dysfunction: Comparing the DSM-IV and the DSM-5 proposal for narcissistic personality disorder: Narcissistic pathology as core personality dysfunction. *Journal of Clinical Psychology*, *68*(8), 908–921.

Morf, C. C., & Rhodewalt, F. (2001). Unraveling the paradoxes of narcissism: A dynamic self-regulatory processing model. *Psychological Inquiry*, *12*(4), 177–196.

Pincus, A. L., Roche, M. J., & Good, E. W. (2015). Narcissistic personality disorder and pathological narcissism. In P. H. Blaney, R. F. Krueger, & T. Millon (eds.), *Oxford textbook of psychopathology* (pp. 791–813). Oxford University Press.

Reader, S. (2007). The other side of agency. *Philosophy*, *82*(4), 579–604.

Reznek, L. (1997). *Evil or ill? Justifying the insanity defence*. Routledge.

Ritter, K., Dziobek, I., Preißler, S., Rüter, A., Vater, A., Fydrich, T., Lammers, C-H., Heekeren, H. R., & Roepke, S. (2011). Lack of empathy in patients with narcissistic personality disorder. *Psychiatry Research*, *187*(1–2), 241–247.

Roche, M. J., Pincus, A. L., Lukowitsky, M. R., Ménard, K. S., & Conroy, D. E. (2013). An integrative approach to the assessment of narcissism. *Journal of Personality Assessment*, *95*(3), 237–248.

Schramme, T. (2010). Can we define mental disorder by using the criterion of mental dysfunction? *Theoretical Medicine and Bioethics*, *31*(1), 35–47.

Schramme, T. (2017). Empathy and altruism. In H. Maibom (ed.), *The Routledge handbook of philosophy of empathy* (pp. 203–214). Routledge.

Schwan, D. (2019). Does affective empathy require perspective-taking or affective matching? *American Philosophical Quarterly*, *56*(3), 277–288.

Smith, A. (2002; orig. 1759/1790). *The theory of moral sentiments*, edited by K. Haakonssen. Cambridge University Press.

Sodoma, K. A. (2022). Emotional gaslighting and affective empathy. *International Journal of Philosophical Studies*, *30*(3), 320–338.

Spaulding, S. (2017). Cognitive empathy. In H. Maibom (ed.), *The Routledge handbook of the philosophy of empathy* (pp. 13–21). Routledge.

Stein, E. (1964; orig. 1917). *On the problem of empathy*. Springer.

Taylor, J. A. (2015). Sympathy, self, and others. In D. Ainslie & A. Butler (eds.), *The Cambridge companion to Hume's treatise* (pp. 188–205). Cambridge University Press.

Urbonaviciute, G., & Hepper, E. G. (2020). When is narcissism associated with low empathy? A meta-analytic review. *Journal of Research in Personality*, *89*, 104036.

Vreekea, G. J., & van der Mark, I. L. (2003). Empathy, an integrative model. *New Ideas in Psychology, 21*, 177–207.

Walsh, P. J. (2014). Empathy, embodiment, and the unity of expression. *Topoi, 33*, 215–226.

Wispé, L. (1986). The distinction between sympathy and empathy: To call forth a concept, a word is needed. *Journal of Personality and Social Psychology, 50*(2), 314–321.

Wright, J. K. X., Grainger, S. A., Coundouris, S. P., & Henry, J. D. (2021). Affective empathy in neurodegenerative disorders: The importance of measurement type. *Neuroscience & Biobehavioral Reviews, 127*, 808–819.

Wright, J. P. (2009). *Hume's 'A treatise of human nature': An introduction*. Cambridge University Press.

Zachar, P. (2006). Pathological narcissism and its relationship to empathy and transcendence. *The Pluralist, 1*(3), 89–105.

Zachar, P. (2014). *A metaphysics of psychopathology*. MIT Press.

Zachar, P. (2017). Personality disorder: Philosophical problems. In T. Schramme & S. Edwards (eds.), *Handbook of the philosophy of medicine* (pp. 1005–1024). Springer.

Zahavi, D. (2011). Empathy and direct social perception: A phenomenological proposal. *Review of Philosophy and Psychology, 2*, 541–558.

21 Interaffectivity Disturbances in Narcissistic Personality Disorder

Susi Ferrarello

21.1 Introduction: Why Narcissists Are Who They Are

As embodied human beings we are charged with an affectivity that instinctively tunes us into the affectivity of others from birth and throughout life. As humans we are intrinsically relational beings because the affections that shape our being move us to connect with the world, by doing so generating emotions. By their nature, emotions (from Latin, *e-movere*) move us toward others while others affect us with their own emotions. By affection here I do not mean the feeling of tenderness or love we can have for someone but the etymological term *ad-facere*, which points to what impacts and influences us. A hug, the heat in a room, a stomach pain can be examples of affections from the environment and the people who populate it. Accordingly, interaffectivity is regarded as an intertwinement of two cycles of embodied affectivity in which a partner's affective affordances and bodily resonance continuously affects the other (Fuchs & Koch, 2014). Our body resonates with the body of others and vice versa through emotional interconnection (Zajonc, 1984; Hatfield et al., 1994). It is in this sense that we can refer to the experience of the other in terms of embodied perception. We do not need mental representations to feel what the other is going through because there is a bodily resonance in action that instinctively connects us to each other (Merleau-Ponty, 1964). People affected with narcissistic traits suffer from an interaffective disturbance because they might be able to understand what the other is feeling but they are not willing to connect with the level of affectivity that would allow them to feel in bodily resonance with others.

Although narcissistic behavior can be highly toxic, I believe it is important to maintain a position of compassionate understanding to be able to look at the reasons behind the development of narcissism and to recognize narcissistic traits in ourselves. Hence, this paper will focus on the types of affective intentionality that structure the major choices contributing to the constitution of narcissistic traits. I will briefly discuss narcissism through a myth and an anonymized case of a client from my philosophical counseling practice; then,

I will describe Husserl's notion of intentionality and articulate how a faulty interplay between passive, active and practical intentionality creates a lack of access to one's own affectivity. Then, I will expound upon the form of affective intentionality that animates the emotional choices that build the narcissistic persona and how that intentionality constitutes a disturbance within the interaffective community of persons suffering from narcissistic traits.

My thesis is that people suffering from narcissistic traits tend to experience "an intentionality" blockage that generates interaffective disturbances with the people in their lives. The lack of bodily resonance and embodied affectivity makes them unable to establish an intimate bond with themselves, and accordingly, to explore the intentional content of their lived experience. Hence, they are often left with a sense of emptiness and solitude. If given the tools for this exploration, they might regain a way to a more intimate and fulfilling life.

21.2 Narcissus and Other Stories

In my philosophical practice, I had encountered people that exhibit narcissistic traits, such as sense of grandiosity, problems with self-esteem, and difficulty establishing an intimate connection with a partner (which was often lamented as "my partner does not desire me" or "she does not initiate sex as often as I wish").

What brings them to my office is a slight sense of sadness and confusion about what to do next. I refrain from mentioning the concept of narcissism, but may cautiously introduce narcissism after our connection becomes a little more solid – primarily to assess their knowledge of the problem.

Because the phenomenological approach I use with philosophical counseling is goal oriented, my meetings with clients are often focused on the goal they wanted to pursue, which initially makes our encounters into a space to validate their behaviors and stories.

For instance, a client decided to meet with me because he had trouble sleeping at night. Through our conversations we realized that he was at a stage in his marital relationship where he was ready to move on. With his wife he experienced frustration and irritation and had already found another woman. His sense of grandiosity led him to despise his wife because she could not live up to his esthetic and social standards, or achieve the same goals as he did on a regular basis, such as reading the same amounts of books, practicing different languages, and keeping his body in flawless shape through exercise. Moreover, he was irritated by her tears and moments of desperation and often frustrated by what he perceived as the dismissive way she was connecting with his body. He demanded more sexual desire from her. With time, we understood that his self-esteem was low because of the way in which he felt his parents used to treat him, which often resembled the frustrations he felt toward his wife and his little son. Having interiorized a certain way of perceiving his parents' standards, he set for himself high goals that he pursued with harsh tenacity and very little space for any sense of embodied pleasure. He never gave himself the space to explore who he really was. Hence his sense of self was inflated, detached from feelings and incapable of establishing empathy toward those in his family. Although I do not believe that our consultations brought any radical change in his personality, it may have planted the seeds for a change in his intimate life that might sprout on the occasion of his crisis.

In his case, I used the points of irritation he would feel toward his wife as a bridge to connect with his intimate life. The feeling of irritation is one of the most powerful entrances to the space of intimate life as it represents an opportunity for awakening to a deeper self-awareness. During the hours spent together in my office we realized that a great part of his coldness, lack of compassion and being judgmental toward others in his life was, first of all, directed at himself because it was the ethical model he learned while growing up. In his view, the good person was the one pursuing excellence at everything; the good person was the one who gained the admiration of the people around him. Accordingly, his wife looked despicable in his eyes because she related to her sense of sadness and was almost paralyzed by it. He felt irritated at his wife's tears because when he was growing up crying was considered a weakness; he almost felt disgusted by her lack of interest in improving her appearance and her knowledge of foreign languages because those were considered strengths to cultivate in his original family. Looking at his upbringing it seemed that he kept within himself the wound of not having been fully accepted by his mother who felt trapped at home with children or by his father who was too busy and tired from work to have time to enjoy a relationship with him. Being able to touch that wound, even if for a very short time, allowed him to see how the need for external validation came from a lack of intimacy he had with himself. He was not allowed to tell himself that he was good enough because in his view his parents repeatedly showed him that he was not. He could not dedicate time to explore his real talents. What he learned was that self-validation was an ethically unacceptable act of weakness and vanity – it was wrong to feel good about oneself. Instead, he pushed himself to meet others' expectations (mostly his parents'), which in his view would give him the permission to feel good and (secretly) better than anyone else. Yet, that also came at a high price, that is, despising his true nature whenever certain expectations could not be met because of lack of energy, capabilities or skills. He was living each day in this dynamic, a Sisyphean search for peace and acceptance. For him only acceptance from external sources were valid – he did not know how to self-validate.

For this reason, we worked quite a bit on the notion of compassion, which originally sounded to him as a synonym for laziness. For him, being compassionate meant providing excuses for being weak and for not working on self-improvement. For example, when I asked him if he was feeling fulfilled in waking up at 4:30 a.m. to practice his French before his morning exercise, he replied that fulfilment was not what he was seeking, self-improvement was the goal. Although he felt burned out and demanded compassion from his wife, he, himself, could not have compassion toward himself because that would have felt lazy, at best. His sense of self-worth came strongly from the belief that the harsher he was toward himself the better results he could achieve in the eyes of others. His standards were high, rigid, and not based on any form of self-connection and self-exploration. He had no time for acceptance of his own objective limits or compassion for occasionally failing to meet his goals. In his world there was no space for contemplation of limits, the stakes of judgments were always quite high. The tears of his wife – often the recipient of this same treatment – were quite incomprehensible to him. Later, having gained insight into the old wound from which his self-serving behaviors originated allowed him to better understand, even if for a moment, himself and his close ones. He could enjoy moments of reconnection and true closeness with his wife, for example in holding hands while walking together in the city. Unfortunately, he discontinued our work before a new pattern of intentional affectivity could be consolidated. His need to move on with his relationship, I believe, reinforced the old intentional pattern.

21.3 The Myth of Cassius and Mariam

Similar to the myth of Narcissus there is a lesser-known myth that recounts the story of another "Narcissus" named Cassius, a young handsome man spoiled by a nymph who was desperately in love with him. Like Narcissus and Echo, these two did not make a good pair. A day arrived when she could no longer fulfill all his demands and he felt very lonely. As his nymph was not enough for him, Cassius started wandering around the forest in search of some company. There he saw her, Mariam, a young woman who was crossing the lake in a small boat. He greeted her and she greeted him back, from afar. When Cassius asked her where she was going, Mariam told him she was going back to her garden. "I want to come with you," he said. "But you don't know me," she replied. "We will get to know each other. For now, please, take me with you," he begged. Mariam accepted but with one condition: "It took me a long time to take care of my garden, growing my food, and creating a comfortable place for me and my people. I will take you with me if you respect my garden and give me a baby." "I will give you a baby," Cassius said without blinking. "This means that you will take care of everything when I am with the baby, and you will work to provide for us; you will play music to comfort me and the baby when we are in pain." "Yes, I will do all this," he said again without thinking twice. "Ok, then. Be aware that once this boat sails, you will not be able to come back to your life as it was. You will start your new life with me and the life as you lived it before will cease."

This last condition terrified Cassius. All the while the nymph had secretly observed Cassius' interactions with Mariam and feeling his hesitation, the nymph, still in love with him, took her chance and offered him even more gifts. She materialized in front of him, looking in every way so similar to Mariam that Cassius forgot about Mariam. He and the nymph spend one year together enjoying every kind of physical pleasure. One day, though, the memory of what he missed comes back to haunt him. He wanted to find Mariam and accept her offer. Yet, he was too late. The next time he meets Mariam she tells him that she found another man and they have a baby together. Cassius, desperate for this loss and the sense of loneliness, gives up on life and dies by suicide.

This story, similar to the myth of Narcissus, portrays an attractive young man who is missing something important in his life – the connection with himself. Cassius' world, similar to Narcissus', is populated by two-dimensional persons who exist only to serve his needs and whose lives are almost completely invisible to him. There is no interaffective connection with others. He cannot take pleasure from the affections of the people with whom he is in contact or with the beautiful natural landscape in which he lives. He cannot feel his affections. The people of his life are there only to mirror him. Although this is momentarily pleasing, it leaves him with a growing sense of desperation and emptiness that pushes him to try to connect to the real world. Yet, he is not willing to take the risk to change his world because he cannot give up on the image he has of himself; that image is all he has and giving that up would mean to die. Mariam's condition that he leave his old self behind is dreadful to him. Exploring a new real life would be a lethal threat to his very existence. Although dissolving the old patterns and enduring the transformation seems to be the only way to heal, taking that chance would mean to kill the image behind which his fragile ego hides and shields itself. According to this mythology, it seems that there is no escape from this existential situation. Narcissists are doomed to an excruciating loneliness unless they are willing to – metaphorically speaking – kill themselves, that is, to completely transform themselves and their lives.

Plato's *Symposium* offers a more optimistic solution to this problem. According to Symington (1993), Aristophanes' speech on the androgens is a way to resolve the narcissistic problem. In this dialogue Plato imagines Aristophanes telling the story of how human beings were originally self-fulfilled because they were androgens, that is both male and female. Then Zeus, envious of their completeness, split them into two parts, male and female. Since then, their sense of fulfilment would come through love, that is, by finding each other's perfect half. The split that takes place at the very origin of their creation is a metaphor for the traumatized event that splits the young life of people suffering from narcissistic traits. To heal this sense of incompleteness, the solution presented by Aristophanes is love. Finding your own other half can help incomplete persons to feel whole. Often, the problem is that people with narcissistic traits have great difficulties in experiencing real intimacy and love for others (Morf & Rhodewalt, 2001). For this reason, I propose a method that aims at developing intimacy with themselves through intentional reconnection and compassionate acceptance of their own limits. The goal is to put them in contact with their own affections.

21.4 Narcissism as an Interaffective Disorder

I propose that narcissism stems from a wounded interaffective system, which impacts self-esteem and the sense of connection that people should normally have with themselves and others. People with narcissistic traits cannot access their embodied affections and engage them with interest. This obstruction of intentionality also makes it difficult to develop resonance with other people's bodies or establish an interaffective connection with the world. Even though they might understand others, they do not tune to the affections coming from their interaffective network, probably because some affects are too painful to be felt. As a result, with artificial projections, such as externalized values and meanings, they obstruct the representational flow with which they could potentially make sense of their being-in-the-world. Accordingly, their ethical behavior might at times be questionable and not considerate of others.

Whenever life events threaten one of the bridges that connect individuals to their intimate cores (their job, their love life, their social status, etc.), then their sense of self (or at least the image with which they identify themselves) might feel threatened, potentially triggering the resurgence of a sort of narcissistic flu. In what follows I propose an intentionality-oriented maintenance treatment against the resurgence of this flu throughout life. The goal is to keep the individual open to and not scared of affections which would provide a foundation for self-acceptance, ego-integrity, and an unfolding of the feelings around the potential experiences that threaten the stable connection with their intimate core. Grounding the people affected from narcissistic traits to the affections of their own body as a part of a larger system of interaffection is a fruitful way to overcome painful blockages and recover intimacy.

According to phenomenological and enactive approaches, human sociality does not start from isolated individuals and their hidden inner states, but from interaffectivity (Husserl, 1973, 1981). We are embodied beings. We can survive in this world because we participate in an embodied interaffectivity (with others), which gives us a sense of vitality that allows us to engage our lives.

As a process of coordinated interaction, interaffectivity[1] allows bodily resonance, and mutual incorporation, to provide the basis for a primary empathetic understanding of oneself and others. A disturbance of interaffectivity might severely impair our ability to resonate with our body and the body of others and to feel empathy; hence a sense of emptiness and low vitality follows. Narcissistic traits might stem from a "detunement" (*Verstimmung*) of the resonant body that normally mediates our attunement and participation in the shared social space.

21.5 Active, Passive and Practical Intentionality

The etymology of the word intentionality refers to the connecting "tension" of "aiming at" something; this tension conjuncts our inner sense of reality to the outer world. Brentano (1874/2008) and later Husserl (2001) revived the studies around intentionality by emphasizing the reflective quality of the intentional arc. That is, intentionality is a reflective experience in which we become subjects of our lived experiences by reflecting on their content. To this extent the intentional content becomes the object of one's self-reflection and the means one uses to shape one's own reality by establishing meaningful bonds with the life-world. While we are living we are naive toward our experience, in the sense that we are one object among other objects and we do not interrogate how we relate to the world. When we reflect on the content of our lived experience, then we become subjects interested in the meaning that our lived experiences can offer.

The biologist Freeman (2000) writes, "All actions are emotional, and at the same time they have their reasons and explanations. This is the nature of intentional behavior" (p. 201). In particular, intentionality is a means to access these reasons without sticking to rigid pre-fixed emotional categories. As noted, intentionality expresses the continuous flow of our lived experiences.

In Husserl's phenomenology we find a multitude of ways of referring to intentionality. In my research (Ferrarello, 2016, 2018, 2019; Ferrarello & Zapien, 2018), I organize these forms of intentionality into three main groups: active, passive and practical intentionality. Active intentionality is the way in which we reflect on the content of our experience and assign a meaning to it (Husserl, 2001). For example, I realize that I skipped lunch today. I reflect on my action and explain that action by acknowledging the fact that I was not hungry then but I am hungry now. Using a more psychological example, I realize that I do not remember what my friend told me about his plans for

[1] "Interaffectivity includes body feedback (i.e., the impression function within self and other), which is necessary for interbodily resonance. Components of interbodily resonance are: mirroring or complementing movements, body awareness (via proprioceptive body feedback), and kinaesthetic empathy; they are psychotherapeutically important in phenomena such as somatic countertransference" (Pallaro, 2002, pp. 80–95).

the weekend. Upon reflection, I understand that while he was talking, I was getting worried about the late work piling up on my desk. In this latter example of active intentionality, subjectivity emerges from a state of passive listening that leads to take an interest in the affections that are presenting in the moment in order to form a meaning out of the feeling connected to that lived experience.

Any lived experience can be noticeable to the subject because of passive intentionality; without passive intentionality no event would potentially matter to us. This form of intentionality synthesized the embodied affections in a way that calls us to attend to them through feelings. Passive intentionality does not belong to me as a subject because it is the force of nature that makes my passive body, which is a thing among other things, into a subjective presence. Using the previous example, hunger alerts my body to a decision that I have to make. My stomach is telling me something. On this level passive intentionality is represented by the information that is offered to me as an emerging subject. Or, as my friend is talking about the weekend, a sense of anxiety is bothering me. I pay attention to this feeling and become aware of my presence. In passive intentionality the subject is a being to which a cluster of affections is presented; this emerging subject did not yet develop any interest toward its affections. The passive intentionality synthesized the affections together in a cluster of potential sense with which we can connect through feelings and emotions.

Practical intentionality is the crucial form of intentionality that bridges active to passive intentionality. It is in fact through this form of intentionality that the subject develops a form of interest that leads it to validate the cluster of affections that are passively presented to it and transform them in an active sense. Through practical intention the subject decides to feel the affections that are engaging with their body. In fact, coming back to the first example, while doing other things my body decides to stop and pay attention to the feeling of hunger and acknowledge its sense. Using the other example, my friend is talking about his plan, I want to be a good friend and keep listening to his plans, but more pressing affections are arising in that present moment. My practical intention takes an interest on it and validate those affections, which makes me aware of the fact that I am feeling anxious.

Practical intentionality is the connecting bridge between passive and active intentions. It expresses through an act of validation in which the volitional body (Husserl, 2012, p. 186) of the subject decides to pay attention to the affections and to transform them in sense through active intentionality. Thanks to practical intentionality the subject decides to be interested (Husserl, 2002, p. 81) in the affections, prompted by passive intentionality, that are poking its attention; then active intentionality will assign them meanings and values.

One's personality is built upon many of these moments that have the power to reduce or increase the distance with the people we love. Persons whose practical intentions repeatedly decide to cut themselves off from their affections and do not take an interest in what their affections are trying to communicate will as a result be distant and unauthentic because the sense and values that structure their actions is not rooted in their affections. Practical intention is that act through which subjects recognize the interconnection between passive syntheses and their own feelings. Ultimately, practical intentionality is what allows for bodily resonance and interaffectivity to function because it connects our passive synthesis (e.g., our organic nature) with our ability to feel it according to certain meanings and values. The bridge between active intention and passive synthesis is represented by the practical "*Ich will und ich tue*" (I want, I act), which operates through the means of the emotions that awaken the volitional body to a specific action. Being unaware of what is occurring during these moments results in a high level of emotional instability that significantly impacts our feelings of well-being.

The ego reacts to passive affections by deciding whether to accept and validate what awakes its interest. Some of the material contents provided to the ego will remain in the form of passive syntheses, others will be organized through values and meanings. Although the realm of passivity provides formless matter with a potentially graspable form, the realm of active intention is the constitutive pole through which a given number of affective layers are composed into a graspable meaning. Affective intentionality is one mode of practical intentions in which the affections call for a graspable determination of meaning (e.g., my stomach feels affected, I answer to these affections by acknowledging that I am hungry).

There is wide agreement among philosophers and psychologists that emotions are characterized by intentionality – they are about persons, objects, events and situations in the world (see, e.g., Solomon, 1976; Frijda, 1994; De Sousa, 2010). However, this intentionality is of a special kind: it is not neutral but concerns what is particularly valuable and relevant for the subject. In a sense, emotions are ways of perceiving, namely attending to salient features of a situation, giving them a significance and weight. Referring to Gibson's (1979) concept of affordances (that means, offerings in the environment that are available to animals, such as a tree being "climbable," water "drinkable," etc.), one could also speak of affective affordances: things appear to us as "important," "worthwhile," "attractive," "repulsive," "expressive," and so on. Without emotions, the world would be without meaning or significance; nothing would attract or repel us and motivate us to act (Fuchs & Koch, 2014).

21.6 The Intentional Answer

People affected with narcissistic traits use their active intentions to make meanings and values that are not based on their own passive intentions, that is, on what they affectively experience, but on an externalized sense of what they are expected to feel. In the case of my client, his parents educated him not to take an interest in his affections, as if these affections were almost despicable and reprehensible. Good behavior for his parents was all based on meanings and values construed from externalized affections. This leads to a general sense of coldness and meaninglessness as the self is not sustained by one's own embodied life. The first consistent step that leads to the constitution of narcissistic traits at a very young age is characterized by a disconnection from one's own feelings and the environment that elicits them (Lowen, 1983). Affections and the feelings stemming from the connection we make with those affections are the *via regia* to understanding our interaction with reality; shutting them out means living in an alternative uprooted reality. The reactiveness at small events displayed by people affected by narcissistic traits is one of the many outcomes of this affective uprootedness. Their rage tends to become very easily explosive because their emotions are not rooted in their affective life but are the artificial display of what is expected from them in the moment.

In the case of people affected with narcissistic traits, the interaffectivity disturbance is generated from a detachment between active and passive intentionality. The person does not exert their practical intentionality in a bridging way, that is, they do not connect with the affective awakenings that belong to their body or to the system of affectivity in which they are surrounded. They do not take an interest in their interaffective world, which, accordingly, remains for them inauthentic and poor in meaning. As we saw in the previous section, passive intentionality is what defines us as an object among other objects governed by biological and social norms; it does not require an ego to function –in fact, the subjectivity of the ego comes only at a very late stage of the process. Similar to Kohut's view of Narcissistic Personality Disorder (1971, 1977), we need to be part of an interaffective community, that is a social, geographical, emotional, physical, imaginative environment, in order to be and to become something (parents, friends, school, a home, etc.). The more qualities this environment shows us the richer our passive intentional life and accordingly our emotional world.

The role of the therapist is to help the client to reconnect with their own passive intentionality in order to heal the sense of primal exclusion from which the client is still suffering. This can be done by leveraging their practical intentionality, that is, on their volitional body that decides through an act of practical intentionality to make sense of what it is affectively experiencing in the moment. The new relationship with the therapist and exercises directed at making the client feel like a part of her social, geographical, emotional, physical, imaginative environmental support this reconnection. Through hypnotic, acceptance-based, mindful approaches, the intentional reconnection has the goal of recuperating the lower feelings and sensations that are still floating in the figurative rooms of the disconnection and give them space to become emotions.

The overall goal of therapy is to readjust the blocked interconnection of passive syntheses, practical intentionality, and active intentionality while tuning in body resonance to their interaffective community. Narcissists are not able to access the affections from the organic presence of their bodies. They have great difficulties in accepting any physical flaws or even their own age. What bodies are for them and what they do in their primal functioning (passive syntheses) feels almost shameful. This results in an inability to accept their own bodily functioning (practical intention) and assign them a meaning (active intention) that is commensurate with their possibility. Hence, the sense of grandiosity, the fixation on their image and the sense of disconnection from others' bodies. For this reason, the awakening, represented by practical intention, must be stimulated by bodily exercises until it reaches the real ground of the passive syntheses and not the empty one created from invalidating experiences. At that point, when that reconnection occurs, it is possible to revisit the old places where the invalidating experiences took place. If particularly difficult emotions arise and are not faced, they do not disappear in the linearity of time, but their affections persist in a timeless now. They must be lived in order to make space for new emotions to arise and fit the meanings to come. People affected by narcissistic traits feel emotional blockages and are often incapable of feeling pure joy or happiness because there is a long line of emotions waiting to be lived.

Hence, grounding the meanings (active intention) of their lives and their self-esteem on something unreal and untrustworthy (empty passive intentions) prevents any healing; only dealing with the still persistent and painful emotions would help a successful reconstruction of the interaffective community and positive reactivation of bodily resonance. In this step, the epoché – that is, a temporary moment of suspension of judgments and assumptions – should be used by therapist and client to suspend any temptation to make ethical judgments or assign quick meanings to the complexity of passive syntheses.

What often happens at this stage is that ethical judgment gets in the way of true healing. The temptation of invalidating certain affections with dismissive values and meanings can arise because it reinforces the need to run away from their intimate being. For my client, any self-exploration was dismissed as lazy and pointless. His life task was to inflate his self in the eyes of the others by showing his mastery of different languages, his muscular body, his expensive clothes. He did not take time to know what felt good for him, what made sense in his life.

For people suffering from narcissistic traits, it becomes easy to blame others for their misery, thus cutting off access to the constitution of new felt meanings in life. In their normal life, potentially neutral adjectives are transformed into ethically charged ones, thus creating a blockage to the constitution of new meanings: weak instead of sad, unappreciated instead of alone, failing instead of trying. Covering up real affections with ethical judgments is another way to block the interconnection between practical, passive and active intentions. The counselor's goal is to create an ethically neutral space of acceptance around the arousal of each sensation so that primal feelings and sensations can freely affect the subject and guide the therapist–client relationship toward a transformative healing process of sensations into affections, into emotions and then into meanings and values.

Once this acceptance is completed and habitualized, the client can proceed to the next step, which consists of the actual constitution of meanings based on their affective experiences. At that point, meanings would be formulated on a grounded, trustworthy and solidly based experienced reality as opposed to the grandiose empty reality created (or projected) as a shield to the distressed ego. From there the client can start rebuilding a personal value system that will be from the basis of their character and the way in which they want to embody their life in the real world. At that point, life will cease to be pointless, lonely, empty or without surprises.

Of course, this process is extremely difficult and painful because it implies an actual dissolution of old structures on multiple levels. Yet, if it occurs, the renewal will be complete. The person affected with narcissistic traits can transform themself into a more graceful and down-to-earth creature whose roots are safely protected by the "dirt" of the world, as the narcissus in Ovid's myth. The temptation to fall back into old habits would be continuously there as it is for the risk of any seasonal flu, but a way to recover from that sense of loneliness and desperation is possible.

21.7 Conclusions

In this chapter I have analyzed the main feature of narcissistic traits through mythology and an anonymized client's case. Then I discussed the intentional approach that I believe can help people with narcissistic traits to reconnect to their intimate environment as a first step to healing. Being able to resonate with their interaffective community and with their body is essential toward initiating a healing path. A reconnection to the passive intentions represented first by their present environment and then by their past experiences, especially the painful ones, is the best way to reconstruct the ground from which they can assign meanings and values to their present life (active intentions). Reconnection with their present and past environment helps people affected with narcissistic traits to fill the void left from the disruption of the intimate space caused by the eventual lack of parental (or primary caregivers') care. Giving them the tools to look at that space and find valuable essences there is, in my opinion, the first step to readjust the intentional arc.

References

Brentano, F. (1874/2008). Psychologie vom empirischen Standpunkt. In *Von der Klassifikation psychischer Phänomene*, edited by A. Chrudzimski. De Gruyter.

De Sousa R. (2010). Emotion. *Stanford encyclopedia of philosophy*. Available online at: http://plato.stanford.edu/archives/spr2010/entries/emotion

Ferrarello, S. (2016). *Husserl's ethics and practical intentionality*. Bloomsbury.

Ferrarello, S. (2018). Husserl's ethics and psychiatry. In M. Englander (ed.), *Phenomenology and the social context of psychiatry*. Bloomsbury.

Ferrarello, S. (2019). *Phenomenology of sex, love and intimate relationships*. Routledge.

Ferrarello, S., & Zapien, N. (2018). *Ethical experience: A phenomenology*. Bloomsbury.

Freeman, W. (2000). Emotion is essential to all intentional behaviors. In M. Lewis & I. Granic (eds.), *Emotion, development, and self-organization: Dynamic systems approaches to emotional development* (pp. 12–24). Cambridge University Press.

Frijda, N. H. (1994). Varieties of affect: emotions and episodes, moods, and sentiments. In P. Ekman, & R. J. Davidson (eds.), *The nature of emotion: fundamental questions* (pp. 59–67). Oxford University Press.

Fuchs, T., & Koch, S. C. (2014). Embodied affectivity: On moving and being moved. *Frontiers in Psychology*, *5*, 508.

Gibson, J. (1979). *The ecological approach to visual perception*. Houghton Mifflin.

Hatfield, E., Cacioppo, J. T., & Rapson, R. L. (1994). *Emotional contagion*. Cambridge University Press.

Husserl, E. (1973). *Zur Phänomenologie der Intersubjektivität. Texte aus dem Nachlass. Erster Teil. 1905–1920* [On the phenomenology of intersubjectivity. Texts from the estate. Part 1. 1905–1920], ed. I. Kern. Martinus Nijhoff.

Husserl, E. (1981). Phenomenology and anthropology. In P. McCormick & F. A. Elliston (eds.), *Husserl: Shorter Works* (pp. 315–323). University of Notre Dame.

Husserl, E. (2001). *Analyses concerning passive and active syntheses: Lectures on transcendental logic*, trans. A. J. Steinbock. Kluwer.

Husserl, E. (2002). *Natur und Geist. Vorlesungen Sommersemester 1919*, ed. M. Weiler. Kluwer Academic Publishers.

Husserl, E. (2012). *Einleitung in die Philosophie, Vorlesungen 1916–1919*, ed. H. Jacobs. Springer.

Kohut, H. (1971). *The analysis of the self: A systematic approach to the psychoanalytic treatment of narcissistic personality disorders*. International Universities Press.

Kohut, H. (1977). *The restoration of the self*. International Universities Press.

Lowen, A. (1983). *Narcissism. Denial of the true self*. Simon and Schuster.

Merleau-Ponty, M. (1964). *Phenomenology of perception*. Kluwer.

Morf, C. C., & Rhodewalt, F. (2001). Unraveling the paradoxes of narcissism: A dynamic self-regulatory processing model. *Psychological Inquiry*, *12*, 177–196.

Ovid. (2005). *The metamorphoses*. Barnes & Noble.

Pallaro, P. (2002). Somatic countertransference: The therapist in relationship. In P. Pallaro (ed.), *Authentic movement: Moving the body, moving the self, being moved* (pp. 176–193). Jessica Kingsley.

Symington, N. (1993). *Narcissism a new theory*. Karmac.

Solomon, R. (1976). *The passions*. Anchor/Doubleday.

Zajonc, R. B. (1984). On the primacy of affect. *American Psychologist*, *39*(2), 117–123.

22 Narrative Accounts of the Self

Differentiating Narcissistic from Non-Narcissistic Personalities

Louise Williams

22.1 Introduction

In its simplest form the narrative account of the self is the view that the self is a story. There are various debates around how to best understand this claim. Several philosophers have developed versions of the narrative account of the self, including Schechtman's Narrative Self Constitution View (2011), MacIntyre (1984), Taylor (1989), and DeGrazia (2005). What these views have in common is that they are trying to explain how the self is primarily a story.

In her articulation of the Narrative Self Constitution View, Schechtman claims that selves are constituted through "understanding our lives as narrative in form and living accordingly" (2011, p. 398). You can find similar statements in MacIntyre (1984, chapter 15), Taylor (1989, chapter 2), and DeGrazia (2005, chapter 3). This idea is central to some of the challenges with the way the narrative account of the self has been developed.

This version of the narrative account of the self has what I call the Epistemic Requirement.

> **Epistemic Requirement**: The organism understands its self as a narrative and uses that understanding in decision making.

Schechtman begins her description with the phrase "understanding" a term which is usually associated with epistemological concerns. How do we know what the self is? Well, we understand the self as a story.

One of the major objections to the narrative account of the self comes from philosopher Galen Strawson. Narrative accounts of the self which feature the Epistemic Requirement are most vulnerable to Strawson's objection. Strawson objects to narrativism by appealing to his own experience (2004). Although Strawson appears to have a self, he denies both (a) that he understands his self as a narrative and (b) that he uses this understanding in any way. Thus, Strawson does not identify with the same self for past, present, and future experiences.

Further, he does not make any choices with reference to such a narrative. Rather than understanding his self in terms of a single narrative, Strawson operates within short lived episodes. Although Strawson doesn't specify the length of a particular episode, his objection suggests that this kind of episodic living shows that the Epistemic Requirement doesn't track what is really needed in order for an organism to have a self. As the Epistemic Requirement is a key feature of most formulations of the narrative account of the self, Strawson claims that we should reject such accounts.

One way to formulate a version of the narrative account of the self that is resistant to Strawson's objection is to separate the metaphysical aspects of the account from the epistemological. In what follows, I will articulate what I call "Three-Tiered Narrativism," a framework for understanding the narrative account of the self that consistently separates the metaphysical aspects from the epistemological. This framework is not only useful in defending the narrative account of the self from Strawson-style objections, but it also provides a framework for differentiating folks with pathological narcissism and folks with healthy personalities.

According to my account, the claim that "The self is a story" is primarily a metaphysical claim. We can ask ourselves, "what is the self?" and the answer is: a story. This metaphysical claim is necessarily paired with an epistemological claim. Here the epistemological question is "how do we know what the self is?" and the answer is: "We understand our self as a story." As we will see, this distinction is quite important when it comes to unpacking the nuances of personality.

On the metaphysical level, we have a story that constitutes the self – let's call that M (short for metaphysical). On the epistemological level, we have a biological organism attempting to know that self and thus develop an understanding of M. Let's call that S for self-understanding.

Now, as social creatures, human beings do not exist in isolation. So in addition to Metaphysical (M) and Self-understanding (S), we also have to answer questions about how other humans come to know who we are. This is again a primarily epistemological consideration. There are two main ways that other humans come to know who we are. The first is through learning how the individual understands themselves. In other words, this other person comes to understand S. Next, the other person may observe this individual's behavior in real time. This is direct insight into the individual's story that constitutes who they are – M. Other people typically formulate their understanding of this individual through a combination of understanding S and experiencing M. Of these two sources of information, other folk's access to M is necessarily limited. Although an individual has access to lots of the information contained within M, other folks can only experience snippets of M. They do not have direct access to M prior to meeting this individual or to the majority of elements of the contemporary aspects of M. Instead, others can witness portions of M through the time they spend with the individual. Let's call "how others understand S and M" O for others.

That leaves us with the metaphysical reality of a story that constitutes who we are – M. Each individual's understanding of their own M, which we call S, and the way in which people outside of the given individual understand S and M, which we have labeled as O.

Others (O) – How others understand S and M
Self-Understanding (S) – Individual's understanding of M
Metaphysical (M) – Story that Constitutes the self

With this framework, we can explore how the narrative account of the self can help us identify people with Narcissistic Personality Disorder.

22.2 Three-Tiered Narrativism and Personality

22.2.1 Non-pathological Personalities

First, let's consider the relationship between M, S, and O for folks without any kind of personality disorder. Typically, these individuals try to ground their Self-Understanding (S) in the story that constitutes who they are (M). This means that their self-understanding is importantly connected with the actual story that makes them who they are. This has many practical implications. For example, someone who has no evidence of being a superhero in M will be unlikely to incorporate the narrative that they are in fact a superhero in S. The content of M acts as a guide for how S is developed for folks with non-pathological personalities.

Another important feature of individuals without pathological narcissism is that they typically have a significant degree of epistemic humility about S. This means that they are aware that their understanding of the story that constitutes who they are may be inaccurate at times. For example, someone may have the proposition "I was nice to Susan at the party" within the set of beliefs in S. But upon having a conversation with their other friend Julia, who was also at the party, they may learn new information about the interaction with Susan. Let's say that what was once understood as a nice gesture for Susan turned out to be something very upsetting to her because it reminded her of her recently deceased grandmother. Someone who does not have pathological narcissism would be willing to take this new information from Julia and revise their set of beliefs in S. Their new set of beliefs might look like "I tried to be nice to Susan at the party." In this case, Julia informed the individual that S did not accurately reflect the contents of M, and so a revision was made to S. This epistemic humility results in the individuals being able to acknowledge inaccuracies within S and, without too much dismay, revise S.

Finally, non-pathological personalities do not typically go to great lengths to enforce a particular version of others' understanding of S and M, which we refer to as O. All human beings care about O to some degree, and the extent to which we care can vary considerably over our lifetime. For example, teenagers typically care a great deal about the O of their peers. Someone working toward a raise or receiving some kind of career recognition may care a great deal about the O of their boss or colleagues. Non-pathological personalities may want to engage in particular behaviors in order to influence the shape of O, but most will not take it so far as to engage in enforcement tactics. Most people hope to positively influence O both through their actions (content of M) and the way they speak of themselves (S), but this hope to influence is not nearly as intense as the way someone with pathological narcissism relates to O. We might understand this as a healthy degree of narcissism rather than the more extreme end of pathological narcissism.

22.2.2 Pathological Narcissism

To begin, let's consider the first major way that folks with Narcissistic Personality Disorder (NPD) differ using Three-Tiered Narrativism. For someone with NPD, their Self-understanding (S) is not necessarily grounded in the story that constitutes who they are (M). Caligor and colleagues gesture at this deviation in individuals with narcissistic personality disorder: "Rather than the flexible and reality-based self-experience that characterizes healthy identity formation, the sense of self in narcissistic personality disorder is brittle and somewhat removed from reality" (Caligor et al., 2015). Instead, their self-understanding (S) is constructed with a specific goal in mind. S is designed to soothe the narcissistic insecurities. For whatever reason, there are some aspects of M which those with pathological narcissism have identified as deeply upsetting. This is where those insecurities are born. Once those have solidified, folks with pathological narcissism will then prioritize soothing those insecurities above all else.

One of the things most within their control is the set of beliefs in S. So rather than focus on having an S that attempts to reflect M, the way that most human beings are inclined to operate, someone with pathological narcissism will intentionally curate S independently of M. The main connection between the two is that the narcissistic insecurities usually stem from M.

We can start to see this coming out in Day, Townsend, and Grenyer's qualitative study (2020). Participants in this study were relatives of people high in narcissistic traits. Day et al. identified one of the ways participants described their relative is that they hide the self: "One way in which they described this was through the construction of a 'false self'. For instance 'He comes across very confident yet is very childish and insecure but covers his insecurities with bullish and intimidating behaviour'" (2020). Although the language of creating a false self doesn't exactly map onto Three-Tiered Narrativism, we can see how this statement is pointing to the authoring of an S that is not grounded in M. It is "false" in the sense that this S is not heavily tied to the real story of this person (M). Day et al. also specifically identify insecurity as one of the key ways the participants described their relative:

> Relatives were described as having an underlying sense of insecurity or vulnerability. For instance "He really is just a scared little kid inside of a big strong man's body. He got stuck when he was a child" (#1481); "At the core he feels unworthy, like a fake and so pretty much all introspection and self-growth is avoided at all costs" (#532) and "At night when the business clothes come off his fears eat him up and he would feel highly vulnerable and needs lots of reassurance" (#699). (2020)

From this we can see that insecurities and the lack of grounding S in M play a key role in folks with pathological narcissism.

Next, an individual with NPD aims to make others' understanding of them (O) identical with their own self-understanding (S). This means that O is often centered in the mind of those with pathological narcissism. The goal here is to get others to see them in exactly the same way the individual with pathological narcissism sees themselves independently of the content of M. Because the content of M is often in tension with, or even directly contradictory to, S, it is important to those with pathological narcissism that they control O. Otherwise they run the risk of O being too closely connected with M, which significantly increases the risk that the narcissistic insecurities will be triggered or more severely triggered than they usually are. The strength of commitment that individuals with pathological narcissism have to the project of making S and O identical can be seen in this quote from a participant in the Day et al. study: "'He is degrading to and about anyone who doesn't agree with him and he is very vengeful to those who refuse to conform to his desires' (#600)" (2020).

It is important here to point out that although folks with pathological narcissism center the project of enforcing S and O to be identical, the way this presents varies depending on the specific dynamics of the other person in question. For example, most individuals with pathological narcissism have a small in-group of people who are close to them. These in-group folks typically spend the most time with the individual with pathological narcissism and thus have access to a wide set of information regarding M. This means that they are naturally less able to accept the enforcement of S being identical with O. As a result, the person with pathological narcissism typically has to engage in much more severe enforcement tactics with this in-group. This explains why folks with pathological narcissism often treat the people close to them very differently from the people outside of their close circle. And this is somewhat captured by the DSM-5's identification of "Interpersonally exploitive behavior," which will be discussed in more detail in the next section.

Additionally, folks with pathological narcissism often have a tendency to discard people with some regularity. Even when a long-term relationship has been established, the individual with pathological narcissism may recognize that some individuals will never accept S being identical with O. Being around such people is so threatening to the narcissistic insecurities that at times the person with pathological narcissism will opt for discarding that relationship rather than continue the various enforcement tactics. However, these discard cycles are often not long-lived because the individual with pathological narcissism is often eager to come back around and see if the other person may be ready to accept S being identical with O. This is one of the ways that, "The specific pathology of identity formation that characterizes narcissistic personality disorder also lends itself to characteristic disruptions in interpersonal functioning" (Caligor et al., 2015).

22.2.3 Three-Tiered Narrativism and Narcissistic Personality Disorder According to the DSM-5

In this section, we'll take a look at how Three-Tiered Narrativism relates to the diagnostic criteria for NPD in the DSM-5. This is not necessarily to endorse the accuracy of these criteria, but simply to show the explanatory power of Three-Tiered Narrativism when it comes to the characteristics laid out here. Afterward, we will explore how Three-Tiered Narrativism relates to the dimensional model of personality, and what this might mean for the project of diagnosing folks with NPD.

According to the DSM-V, for an individual to be officially diagnosed with narcissistic personality disorder, they must present:

> A pervasive pattern of grandiosity (in fantasy or behavior), need for admiration, and lack of empathy, beginning by early adulthood and present in a variety of contexts, as indicated by five (or more) of the following:

1. Has a grandiose sense of self-importance (e.g., exaggerates achievements and talents, expects to be recognized as superior without commensurate achievements).
2. Is preoccupied with fantasies of unlimited success, power, brilliance, beauty, or ideal love.
3. Believes that he or she is "special" and unique and can only be understood by, or should associate with, other special or high-status people (or institutions).
4. Requires excessive admiration.

5. Has a sense of entitlement (i.e., unreasonable expectations of especially favorable treatment or automatic compliance with his or her expectations).
6. Is interpersonally exploitative (i.e., takes advantage of others to achieve his or her own ends).
7. Lacks empathy: is unwilling to recognize or identify with the feelings and needs of others.
8. Is often envious of others or believes that others are envious of him or her.
9. Shows arrogant, haughty behaviors or attitudes. (First, 2014)

In the rest of this section, I will go through each of these criteria and show how they relate to Three-Tiered Narrativism applied to NPD.

22.2.3.1 A Grandiose Sense of Self-Importance Having a grandiose sense of self-importance is a function of the connection between S and M. Because, in narcissism, S is not grounded in M, it is unproblematic for the individual with pathological narcissism to craft an S that makes them more important than the content of M would justify. A common insecurity many people, but especially folks with pathological narcissism, tend to have is that they are not very important in the world. Thus, constructing an S that overemphasizes just how important this person is works very nicely in the pathological narcissist's project of soothing their own insecurities.

22.2.3.2 A Preoccupation with Fantasies of Unlimited Success, Power, Brilliance, Beauty, or Ideal Love Although this reads to most people as a preoccupation, for folks with pathological narcissism, they are simply engaged in building their self-understanding (S) in the way that best suits their particular insecurities. Pathological narcissism leads to an understanding that it is perfectly possible for the individual to achieve unlimited success and so on because their self-understanding (S) is not primarily grounded in the actual metaphysical reality of who they are (M). By focusing their energy on these apparent fantasies, they are simply beefing up the S that they have chosen to make themselves feel more secure. Again, the reiteration of these fantasies to the people around them is a natural part of the pathological desire to make O identical with S. Somewhat operating on the principle that if you hear it enough times then it must be true, the person with NPD will consistently talk about these fantasies as if they were real in order to get as many people as possible to accept O being identical with S.

22.2.3.3 A Belief That He or She is Special and Unique and Can only be Understood by, or Should Associate with, other Special or High-Status People or Institutions A major goal of pathological narcissism is that the individual enforces O to be identical to S. As a way to disregard individuals who do not agree with the constructed narrative (S), the individual with pathological narcissism can throw away any criticisms or negative feedback by pointing out that they are just too special or unique to be understood by such simple people. This sort of mechanism is necessary in order for the individual with NPD to continue to hold onto an S that is disconnected from M. Otherwise, those with pathological narcissism may have to seriously consider feedback from outsiders when they point out that their S is flawed.

22.2.3.4 A Need for Excessive Admiration To outsiders this desire for admiration is excessive, but for the individual with NPD it's not excessive. The individual with pathological narcissism is aiming to enforce that O be identical with S. When someone expresses admiration it is taken as evidence that this other person does in fact understand this individual as the wonderful person they take themselves to be (S). It appears excessive to non-pathological personalities because most of us assume that other folks, like ourselves, desire to ground S in M. When we look at the metaphysical reality of who the individual with pathological narcissism is, we can see that the level of requested admiration is not in alignment with that content. But this isn't a problem for the person with pathological narcissism because they do not desire to have S be grounded in M. If admiration helps soothe their narcissistic insecurities and helps enforce O be identical with S, then the individual with pathological narcissism is going to seek admiration in excess.

22.2.3.5 A Sense of Entitlement The fact that an individual is not entitled to something is a fact about M. That is part of the metaphysical truth of who that person is. When dealing with individuals with pathological narcissism, they are uninterested in facts about M. Their focus is on an S that soothes their narcissistic insecurities. If any of those insecurities can be soothed by being entitled to something, there is no reason for the person with pathological narcissism not to act entitled. Pathological narcissism naturally lends itself to fostering this sense of entitlement, because by doing so this the individual has the opportunity to encourage others to ultimately accept that this individual is in fact entitled to whatever it is they desire. Again, this is a key aspect of the individual with pathological narcissism trying to actively enforce that O be identical with S.

22.2.3.6 Interpersonally Exploitive Behavior Individuals with pathological narcissism have an extremely robust commitment to enforcing O to be identical with S. It is seen as so essential to such individuals' well-being that they are often willing to engage in the exploitation of others. Consider the phrase "the ends justify the means." For folks with pathological narcissism, if exploitation will help, or at least appear to be helpful, then they will engage in that behavior. There is no reason for them not to; after all, such individuals are uninterested in

M and things like being exploitative can simply be edited out of S. In many situations, resorting to exploitation is necessary because it is very difficult to make O be identical with S. Most human beings ground S in M. To make someone believe that M is wholly unimportant is to go against many deeply ingrained norms. But for individuals with pathological narcissism, any evidence that M is important or should be a part of either S or O is a serious threat. So serious, in fact, that exploitation is permissible.

22.2.3.7 A Lack of Empathy Empathy does not function for individuals with pathological narcissism in the way most folks relate to empathy. Folks with pathological narcissism are capable of displaying empathy. For example, let's suppose someone with NPD sees that acting in an apparently empathetic manner might assist in the project of enforcing someone's O to be identical with their S. Because this act of empathy can further the goals of pathological narcissism, such an act is possible. However, we might think that this is insufficient to count as genuine empathy. Instead, this is a kind of masking that the individual with pathological narcissism engages in to serve their bigger insecurity-soothing goals. Authentic empathy, for most folks, involves things like active listening and responding in kind-hearted ways. But these are not things that the individual with pathological narcissism is centering in the moments they exhibit apparent empathy. Because the individual with pathological narcissism's self-understanding (S) is not grounded in the story that constitutes the self (M), the narcissistic individual doesn't need to engage in behaviors to support the beliefs in S. If beliefs related to empathy are soothing to the narcissistic insecurities, they can adopt those beliefs without having to exert the effort of genuine empathy. They simply assert or include the belief that "I am a good listener" or "I am kind-hearted" in their S and they do not actually need to engage in behaviors that are consistent with those beliefs. This generates conflict with other people because the majority of us ground S in M and find it frustrating when someone says things like "I am a good listener" and then fails to exhibit any of the behaviors that make someone a good listener.

22.2.3.8 Envy of Others or a Belief that Others are Envious of Them Why an individual with pathological narcissism might foster the belief that others are envious of them is somewhat obvious. If others are envious of the individual with pathological narcissism, then that person is validated in their construction of the amazing person they've built in S. This further soothes their insecurities because how could anything be wrong if other people wish to be as great as me? Individuals with pathological narcissism often have a lot of struggle in their lives because the way they relate to M and the force that they exert trying to control O is all-consuming. Such individuals may observe other people engaging in their lives with greater ease, or with a larger degree of success, and be envious of this. Although individuals with pathological narcissism do their best to disregard M and control O, they often struggle to accomplish this and that can foster envy of those who seem to avoid these struggles.

22.2.3.9 A Demonstration of Arrogant and Haughty Behaviors or Attitudes These behaviors and attitudes help demonstrate to other people that this individual is as great as their S reflects. This can contribute to the effort to enforce O to be identical with S. Additionally, the individual with pathological narcissism has no reason to hold back on such behaviors because their S is not grounded in M. These problematic behaviors cannot possibly undermine the set of beliefs within S because they can easily be edited out. This means that such individuals have little reason to refrain from such behaviors and good reason to engage.

As you can see, all the criteria laid out in the DSM-5 can be explained using Three-Tiered Narrativism. However, there is a lot of repetition in these explanations. This suggests that there may be a more direct way to evaluate whether someone has NPD. Let's look at an alternative model of personality and explore how it relates to Three-Tiered Narrativism.

22.3 Beyond the DSM

Three-Tiered Narrativism has significant explanatory power when it comes to narcissistic personality disorder. The core insight that this framework provides is that individuals with pathological narcissism relate to M, S, and O differently than non-pathological personalities. The key to identifying someone with NPD is to get clarity on how that individual is relating to these various aspects of the self, as well as seeking information on the degree to which the individual grounds S in M and enforces O to be identical with S.

This approach does present some challenges. For example, non-pathological personalities share some of the same dynamics as pathological narcissism. As you will recall from earlier, it is normal for human beings to care about O to different degrees depending on what stage of life they are in. However, the degree to which someone with pathological narcissism cares about O and the ways in which they will act to enforce a particular version of O is different from non-pathological personalities. This can in part explain why "as severity of narcissistic pathology increases . . . deficiencies in moral functioning become increasingly prominent" (Caligor et al., 2015).

We might also notice that within the group of healthy personalities, some people will care more about their self-understanding (S) being grounded in M than others. For example, some people will take it to be true that they are a nice person simply because their parents always called them nice, relying on a single piece of evidence from M, rather than evaluating whether the claim "I am a nice person" is true across multiple aspects of M. The more an individual cares to holistically evaluate statements in their S in relationship to the entirety of M, the more robustly this person seeks to ground S in M. However, although there is ordinary fluctuation in this aspect of people without NPD, the range of which such people fluctuate is going to cluster around the normal end of the spectrum. The degree to which an individual with pathological narcissism disregards M is such that it places the individual on the abnormal end of the spectrum.

We can also see this issue of degree when we consider the one thing that consistently connects individuals having pathological narcissism with M: their insecurities. Although all people have things that they are insecure about, it is the degree to which the individual with pathological narcissism centers these insecurities that differentiates them. Whereas most people acknowledge their insecurities and occasionally act out of character when those insecurities arise in various situations, folks with pathological narcissism construct their entire self-understanding (S) in order to create a specific dynamic between themselves and those insecurities. Such individuals put a lot of energy into making sure that their insecurities are never brought up or triggered, and this is significantly different from how individuals with non-pathological personalities behave.

This fact that folks with healthy personalities engage in the same kinds of behaviors as those with pathological narcissism but do so to a different degree naturally lends itself to the dimensional model of personality disorder. Here, individuals are evaluated in terms of the degree to which they express a particular set of characteristics. As Krueger and Hobbs describe the dimensional model "It essentially requires the diagnostician to make a dimensional (ordinal) determination of the degree of personality difficulty, in order to render any type of PD (personality disorder) diagnosis" (2020). Rather than the binary of either you have the symptom or not, the approach utilized by the DSM-5, the dimensional model allows for the possibility of considering the extent to which any individual expresses a characteristic. The dimensional model makes space for the fact that both folks with pathological narcissism and folks with non-pathological personalities sometimes fail to ground S in M and that at various points along the journey folks with non-pathological personalities may care a great deal about O while still acknowledging that the degree to which a pathological narcissist cares about O is distinct.

Three-Tiered Narrativism provides a framework for understanding the differences and commonalities with folks with pathological narcissism and folks with non-pathological personalities. In order to identify whether someone's behaviors are expressed to such a degree that an individual merits the label of "pathological narcissist," the diagnosing clinician needs to get a good understanding of how the individual relates to M, S, and O. From there, information needs to be gathered about the degree to which the individual grounds S in M and the lengths the individual is willing to go to in order to enforce O being identical with S.

Obviously, in order to see exactly how this works we would need to operationalize these criteria; however, doing that is beyond the scope of this chapter. But the general idea is that there are three key elements (M, S, and O) and two major relationships between them (S grounded in M and O being identical with S) for the clinician to investigate. This is a significantly shorter list of things to explore than what is required by the DSM-5 criteria.

One challenge with utilizing the Three-Tiered Narrativism framework in diagnosing individuals with NPD is that pathological narcissism often leads individuals to enforce that O be identical with S even when working with mental health professionals. This means that the patient may not provide accurate information, but instead provide information that they believe will most effectively get the professional to agree with the patient's S. These challenges of working with folks with pathological narcissism overall may help explain the "High dropout from treatment and challenges in building a therapeutic alliance with these patients" (Ronningstam, 2020).

Although this is a challenge for the Three-Tiered Narrativism framework, it is also a challenge for the DSM-5 criteria. The main advantage for the Three-Tiered framework is that the professional can more holistically explore the various reports of the individual and isn't necessarily looking at a narrow set of criteria that may or may not be relevant to the specific way this individual is developing and defending a particular S. This allows for more information to be considered and greater flexibility to account for the wide variety of behaviors of individuals with pathological narcissism. It has been pointed out by scholars such as Eve Caligor and Kenneth Levy that this wide range of behaviors make diagnosing someone with NPD quite challenging "it is far from self-evident what such individuals could have in common to justify a shared diagnosis" (Caligor et al., 2015). The Three-Tiered Narrativism framework offers enough commonality between individuals with pathological narcissism that it can account for the wide variety of subtypes of narcissistic personality disorder (Levy, 2012). Although it is beyond the scope of this chapter to explore in detail how Three-Tiered Narrativism can help clinicians navigate the sheer variety of ways pathological narcissism presents, we have seen the basic strategy of the framework. The focus is on unpacking the patient's relationship between M, S, and O and then examining whether S is grounded in M and to what lengths the individual is willing to go in enforcing that O is identical with S. Compared to the DSM-5's approach, there is much less emphasis on the specific content of M, S, and O, which allows more space for the greater variety of presentations of the disorder.

22.4 Conclusion

In this chapter I present Three-Tiered Narrativism, a framework based on the narrative account of the self. Although the focus of this chapter has been how Three-Tiered Narrativism relates to NPD and the dimensional model of personality, this framework may be useful in understanding the full range of cluster B personality disorders. Narcissistic Personality Disorder is defined by the individual's lack of grounding S in M and their enforcement of making O identical with S; other personality disorders may similarly be captured by the framework. I can only gesture at how these other disorders may relate because each deserves its own extensive study. Antisocial Personality Disorder may be the consequence of a complete disregard for O with permission to behave however the individual desires to support S; Borderline Personality Disorder may be focused on the consequences of someone experiencing a lot of instability of their S; and Histrionic Personality Disorder may be the consequence of needing to be at the center of O taking up as much space as possible in the minds and experiences of others. I would guess that a shared commonality with all the cluster B personality disorders is a lack of sufficiently grounding S in M. But as you can see, the thought here is that each disorder can be understood as focusing on different components of Three-Tiered Narrativism.

References

Caligor, E., Levy, K. N., & Yeomans, F. E. (2015). Narcissistic personality disorder: Diagnostic and clinical challenges. *The American Journal of Psychiatry*, *172*(5), 415–422. https://doi.org/10.1176/appi.ajp.2014.14060723

Day, N. J. S., Townsend, M. L., & Grenyer, B. F. S. (2020). Living with pathological narcissism: A qualitative study. *Borderline Personality Disorder and Emotion Dysregulation*, *7*(1), 19–19. https://doi.org/10.1186/s40479-020-00132-8

DeGrazia, D. (2005). *Human identity and bioethics*. Cambridge University Press.

First, M. B. (2014). *DSM-5® handbook of differential diagnosis* (1st ed.). American Psychiatric Publishing.

Krueger, R., & Hobbs, K. (2020). An overview of the DSM-5 alternative model of personality disorders. *Psychopathology*, *53*(3–4), 126–132. https://doi.org/10.1159/000508538

Levy, K. N. (2012). Subtypes, dimensions, levels, and mental states in narcissism and narcissistic personality disorder. *Journal of Clinical Psychology*, *68*(8), 886–897. https://doi.org/10.1002/jclp.21893

MacIntyre, A. C. (1984). *After virtue: A study in moral theory* (2nd ed.). University of Notre Dame Press.

Ronningstam, E. (2020). Internal processing in patients with pathological narcissism or narcissistic personality disorder: Implications for alliance building and therapeutic strategies. *Journal of Personality Disorders*, *34*(Suppl), 80–103. https://doi.org/10.1521/pedi.2020.34.supp.80

Schechtman, M. (2011). The narrative self. In *The Oxford handbook of the self*. Oxford University Press. https://doi.org/10.1093/oxfordhb/9780199548019.003.0018
Strawson, G. (2004). Against narrativity. *Ratio (Oxford)*, *17*(4), 428–452. https://doi.org/10.1111/j.1467-9329.2004.00264.x
Taylor, C. (1989). *Sources of the self: The making of the modern identity*. Harvard University Press.

Index

Printed by Integrated Books International,
United States of America